KV-632-891

DATE DUE

31/03/2014		
15/05/2014		
		PRINTED IN U.S.A.

Landmark Papers in Anaesthesia

Landmark Papers in . . . series

Titles in the series

Landmark Papers in Neurosurgery
Edited by Reuben D. Johnson and Alexander L. Green

Landmark Papers in Anaesthesia
Edited by Nigel R. Webster and Helen F. Galley

Landmark Papers in Cardiovascular Medicine
Edited by Aung Myat and Tony Gershlick

Landmark Papers in Nephrology
Edited by John Feehally, Christopher McIntyre, and J. Stewart Cameron

Landmark Papers in General Surgery
Edited by Graham J. MacKay, Richard G. Molloy, and Patrick J. O'Dwyer

Landmark Papers in Allergy
Edited by Aziz Sheikh, Tom Platts-Mills, and Allison Worth
Advisory editor Stephen Holgate

Landmark Papers in Anaesthesia

Edited by

Nigel R. Webster, BSc, MBChB, PhD, FRCA, FRCP Ed., FRCS Ed., FFICM

Professor of Anaesthesia and Intensive Care
School of Medicine and Dentistry
University of Aberdeen, UK
and Honorary Consultant in Anaesthesia and Intensive Care
Aberdeen Royal Infirmary, UK
and Chairman, *British Journal of Anaesthesia*

Helen F. Galley, PhD, FIBMS, FRCA

Professor of Anaesthesia and Intensive Care
School of Medicine and Dentistry
University of Aberdeen, UK
and Editor, *British Journal of Anaesthesia*

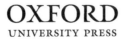

OXFORD
UNIVERSITY PRESS

OXFORD

UNIVERSITY PRESS

Great Clarendon Street, Oxford OX2 6DP,
United Kingdom

Oxford University Press is a department of the University of Oxford.
It furthers the University's objective of excellence in research, scholarship,
and education by publishing worldwide. Oxford is a registered trade mark of
Oxford University Press in the UK and in certain other countries

Published in the United States of America by Oxford University Press
198 Madison Avenue, New York, NY 10016, United States of America

British Library Cataloguing in Publication Data

Data available

Library of Congress Control Number: 2013938576

ISBN 978–0–19–958338–6

Printed and bound by CPI Group (UK) Ltd
Croydon, CR0 4YY

Dedication

We dedicate this book to anyone who is currently editing
a book—you have our sympathies!—but it turns out well in the end.

Preface

The first anaesthesia journal—*Anesthesia and Analgesia*—was founded in 1922, this was followed a year later by the *British Journal of Anaesthesia*. Since then, many national societies of anaesthesia/anesthesiology have followed suit in creating journals, so attesting to the underlying principle of anaesthesia having a strong foundation in research and evidence base. Many of the early papers were written in what would be considered a non-scientific style by today's standards. In fact many are gems of English literature and certainly warrant re-reading by today's generation of anaesthetists. Of course, it is recognized that anaesthetists also publish research articles in non-anaesthetic journals, making it sometimes difficult to keep up with the wide scope of the available anaesthetic-relevant literature.

The aim of *Landmark Papers in Anaesthesia* is to help classic papers resurface so that they can be read by the anaesthetists of today. We have rather arbitrarily divided the speciality of anaesthesia into sections and then invited experts in each of the specialist area to choose their own favourite papers. The concept is unique in that it aims to revisit seminal papers in the anaesthesia literature, based entirely on the personal opinion of an expert in the field. Each chapter starts with a short general introduction on the topic, followed by the author's choice of what they consider to be the ten most important papers in their field of expertise. The choice may be for positive or negative reasons and historical or more contemporary, but all are papers which have changed practice in some way. Most will contain lessons that are equally relevant today—both in terms of the actual content of the paper, but also in relation to the method of conducting the study or the serendipity of the findings and conclusions.

We have given the total number of citations for each article and these were obtained using Google Scholar in February 2012. Using other sources may give different results of course. Obviously this is only a surrogate, and a poor one at that, for the measure of the importance of a paper and is also subject to timeline bias. Coupled with this, at the end of the book is a table showing the 25 top cited articles from the journals *Anaesthesia, Anesthesia and Analgesia, Anesthesiology*, and the *British Journal of Anaesthesia*. We accept that this appendix in no way gives a flavour of the total output of anaesthetists but we saw no way of identifying the articles published by anaesthetists in non-specialist and basic science journals.

The choice of papers included in each chapter is clearly subjective. They are the personal choice of the chapter writers and so are subject to personal bias and likes and dislikes. This is what we feel is the strength of the book and actually what makes the chapters interesting to write and—we hope—read. Consider them in the same way as the choice of music to take to a desert island: 'Desert Island Discs', or the top ten motorcycles ever made. We hope you enjoy reading the book and perhaps it will make you think which papers you would have chosen . . .

Nigel Webster and Helen Galley

Acknowledgements

The editors wish to acknowledge and thank the contributors who rose to the challenge of selecting only ten papers, and who greeted our rather unusual book proposal with enthusiasm.

Contents

Contributors *xi*

Abbreviations *xiv*

1 Neuromuscular blockade *1*
  A Srivastava and JM Hunter

2 Anaesthetic equipment *33*
  NJ Allan and AT Cohen

3 Inhaled and intravenous anaesthetics *57*
  HC Hemmings Jr

4 Total intravenous anaesthesia *81*
  JK Oosterhuis and AR Absalom

5 Monitoring *103*
  PS Myles

6 Optimization *127*
  MPW Grocott and MG Mythen

7 Complications of anaesthesia *151*
  AM Møller

8 Mechanisms of anaesthesia *173*
  A Jenkins

9 Local anaesthesia *197*
  HBJ Fischer

10 Perioperative cardioprotection *221*
  ML Riess and JR Kersten

11 Neuroanaesthesia *245*
  K Ferguson and J Dinsmore

12 Thoracic anaesthesia *275*
  J Macdonald and A Macfie

13 Anaesthesia for vascular surgery *301*
  A Lumb and L Jobling

14 Anaesthesia for major abdominal surgery *327*
  MC Bellamy and S Flood

15 Liver transplantation anaesthesia *353*
  RM Planinsic, IA Hilmi, and T Sakai

16 Obstetric anaesthesia *375*
  G Lyons

17 Airway management *399*
CA Deegan and DJ Buggy

18 Paediatric anaesthesia *423*
P-A Lönnqvist

19 Malignant hyperthermia *445*
PM Hopkins and A Urwyler

Appendix *475*
Author Index *484*
Subject Index *489*

Contributors

AR Absalom
MB ChB, FRCA, MD
Professor of Anesthesia,
Anesthesiology Department,
University Medical Centre Groningen,
Groningen University,
The Netherlands

NJ Allan
MB ChB, FRCA, EDIC
Specialist Registrar in Anaesthesia and Critical Care,
Leeds General Infirmary,
Leeds, UK

MC Bellamy
MB BS, MA, FRCA, FFICM
Professor of Critical Care Anaesthesia,
and Consultant in Anaesthesia and Intensive Care,
St. James's University Hospital,
Leeds, UK

DJ Buggy
MB ChB, RCSI, MSc, MRCPI, MD
Professor of Anaesthesia,
School of Medicine and Medical Science,
University College Dublin,
and Consultant in Anaesthesia,
Mater Misericordiae University Hospital,
Dublin, Ireland

AT Cohen
MB ChB, DRCOG, FRCA, FFICM
Honorary Senior Clinical Lecturer,
University of Leeds and Consultant in Anaesthesia and Critical Care,
St James's University Hospital,
Leeds, UK

CA Deegan
MD, BMedSci, DIBICM, FCARCSI
Consultant in Anaesthesia and Intensive Care Medicine,
Mater Misericordiae University Hospital,
Dublin, Ireland

J Dinsmore
MB BS, FRCA
Consultant in Anaesthesia,
Department of Anaesthesia,
St Georges's University Hospital NHS Trust,
London, UK

K Ferguson
MB ChB, FRCA
Consultant Anaesthetist,
Department of Anaesthetics,
Aberdeen Royal Infirmary, UK

HBJ Fischer
MB ChB, FRCA
Consultant Anaesthetist,
The Alexandra Hospital,
Worcestershire Acute NHS Trust,
Redditch, UK

S Flood
BMedSci, BM BS, MRCP, FRCA
Specialty Registrar in Anaesthesia and Critical Care,
Leeds Teaching Hospitals NHS Trust,
Leeds, UK

MPW Grocott
BSc, MB BS, MD FRCA, FRCP, FFICM
Professor of Anaesthesia and Critical Care Medicine,
University of Southampton,
Director,
NIAA Health Services Research Centre,
Royal College of Anaesthetists,
and Consultant in Critical Care Medicine,
University Hospital Southampton NHS Trust,
UK

HC Hemmings Jr
MD, PhD
Professor of Anesthesiology and Pharmacology,
and Vice Chair of Research in Anesthesiology,
Department of Anesthesiology,
Weill Cornell Medical College,
New York, USA

IA Hilmi
MB ChB, FRCA
Associate Professor of Anesthesiology,
and Director of Quality Improvement/
Quality Assurance,
University of Pittsburgh Medical
Center, USA

PM Hopkins
MB BS, MD, FRCA
Professor of Anaesthesia, University of Leeds
and Consultant in Anaesthesia,
St James's Hospital,
Leeds, UK

JM Hunter
MB ChB, PhD, FRCA, FCARCSI
Emeritus Professor of Anaesthesia,
Department of Clinical Science,
University of Liverpool,
Liverpool, UK

A Jenkins
BSc, PhD
Assistant Professor of Anesthesiology and
Pharmacology,
Emory University School of Medicine,
Atlanta, USA

L Jobling
MB BS, BSc, MRCSEd, FRCA
Specialist Registrar,
Department of Anaesthetics,
St. James's University Hospital,
Leeds, UK

JR Kersten
MD
Professor and Senior Vice Chair,
Department of Anesthesiology,
Medical College of Wisconsin,
Milwaukee, USA

P-A Lönnqvist
MD, DEAA, FRCA, PhD
Professor of Paediatric Anaesthesia and
Intensive Care,
Karolinska Institute, Stockholm,
and Senior Consultant Anaesthetist,
Astrid Lindgrens Children's Hospital and
Karolinska University Hospital,
Stockholm, Sweden

A Lumb
MB BS, FRCA
Consultant in Anaesthesia,
Department of Anaesthetics,
St. James's University Hospital,
Leeds, UK

G Lyons
MB ChB, FRCA, MD
Consultant Anaesthetist,
St James's University Hospital,
Leeds, UK

J Macdonald
MB ChB, FRCA, FFICM
Consultant Anaesthetist and Lead Clinician
for Cardiac Anaesthesia,
Department of Anaesthetics
Aberdeen Royal Infirmary, UK

A Macfie
MB ChB, FRCA, FFICM
Consultant in Cardiothoracic Anaesthesia
and Critical Care,
Golden Jubilee National Hospital,
Clydebank, UK

AM Møller
MD, DrMS
Associate Professsor in Anaesthesia,
University of Copenhagen
and Consultant Anaesthetist,
Department of Anaesthesia,
Herlev University Hospital, Denmark

PS Myles
MB BS, MPH, MD, FCARCSI, FANZCA, FRCA
Professor and Director,
Department of Anaesthesia and
Perioperative Medicine,
Alfred Hospital and Monash University,
Victoria, Australia

MG Mythen
MB BS, MD, FRCA, FFICM
Smiths Medical Professor of Anaesthesia and
Critical Care,
University College London,
Director of Research at UCLH and National
Clinical Lead,
Department of Health Enhanced Recovery
Partnership Programme, UK

JK Oosterhuis
MD
Staff member,
Anesthesiology Department,
University Medical Centre Groningen,
Groningen University,
The Netherlands

RM Planinsic
MD
Professor of Anesthesiology, and
Director of Transplantation Anesthesiology,
University of Pittsburgh Medical Center,
USA

ML Riess
MD, PhD
Associate Professor of Anesthesiology and
Physiology,
Department of Anesthesiology,
Medical College of Wisconsin,
Milwaukee, USA

T Sakai
MD, PhD
Associate Professor of Anesthesiology,
Director of Resident Research Rotation,
University of Pittsburgh Medical Center, USA

A Srivastava
MB BS, MD, DNB, FRCA
Honorary Clinical Fellow,
Critical Care Research Unit,
Department of Clinical Science,
University of Liverpool,
Liverpool, UK

A Urwyler
MD
Professor of Anaesthesia and Intensive Care,
University of Basel,
and Co-Chairman Department of
Anaesthesia,
University Hospital Basel,
Switzerland

Abbreviations

AAA	abdominal aortic aneurysm *or* asleep–awake–asleep		DMV	difficult mask ventilation
			dtc	d-tubocurarine
ACT	activated clotting time		EC50	half maximal effective concentration
ACTA	Association of Cardiothoracic Anaesthetists		ECG	electrocardiogram
			ECMO	extracorporeal membrane oxygenation
ADH	antidiuretic hormone		EEG	electroencephalogram
ALI	acute lung injury		EIA	epidural infusion analgesia
APA	Association of Paediatric Anaesthetists		ET	endotracheal
aPTT	activated partial thromboplastin time		EVAR	endovascular aneurysm repair
ARDS	acute respiratory distress syndrome		FEV_1	forced expiratory volume in 1 second
ASA	American Society of Anesthesiologists *or* American Surgical Association		GA	general anaesthesia
			GCS	Glasgow Coma Scale
ATP	adenosine triphosphate		GDT	goal-directed therapy
AUC	area under curve		HMG-CoA	3-hydroxy-3-methyl-glutaryl-CoA
AVF	arteriovenous fistula		HPLC	high-performance liquid chromatography
BAL	bronchoalveolar lavage			
BBB	blood–brain barrier		HPS	hepatopulmonary syndrome
BP	blood pressure		ICI	Imperial Chemical Industries
BTS	British Thoracic Society		ICP	intracranial pressure
CABG	coronary artery bypass graft		iLA	interventional lung assist
CAD	coronary artery disease		ISAT	International subarachnoid aneurysm trial
CBP	citrated blood products			
CD	cyclodextrin		ITC	isothermal titration calorimetry
CEA	carotid endarterectomy		IVC	inferior vena cava
CI	confidence interval		IVCT	*in vitro* muscle contracture testing
CK	creatine kinase		JVP	jugular venous pressure
Cl	clearance		LA	local anaesthetic
CNB	central neuraxial block		LAD	left anterior descending [artery]
CNS	central nervous systems		LDL	low-density lipoprotein
CO_2	carbon dioxide		LED	light-emitting diode
CONC	concentration which causes unconsciousness		LMA	laryngeal mask airway
			LVP	left ventricular pressure
CPB	cardiopulmonary bypass		MAP	mean arterial blood pressure
CPP	cerebral perfusion pressure		MAC	minimum alveolar concentration
CPX	cardiopulmonary exercise		MELD	model for end-stage liver disease
CSF	cerebrospinal fluid		Mg^{2+}	magnesium
CVP	central venous pressure		MH	malignant hyperthermia
DBS	double burst stimulation		MHE	malignant hyperthermia equivocal
DLCO	carbon monoxide lung diffusion capacity		MHN	malignant hyperthermia normal

MHS	malignant hyperthermia-susceptible	portoPH	porto-pulmonary hypertension
MI	myocardial infarction	ppo	predicted postoperative
MV	mechanical ventilation	PRS	post-reperfusion syndrome
N$_2$O	nitrous oxide	PTFE	polytetrafluoroethylene
Na$^+$	sodium	PVB	paravertebral block
NCA	nurse-controlled analgesia	PVR	pulmonary vascular resistance
NHS	National Health Service	RCT	randomized controlled trial
NICE	National Institute for Health and Clinical Excellence	RVSP	right ventricular systolic pressure
NMBA	neuromuscular blocking agent	SAGM	saline–adenine–glucose–mannitol
NMDA	N-methyl-D-aspartate	SCI	serious clinical incident
NS	nerve stimulator	SpO$_2$	pulse oximeter oxygen saturation
NT-proBNP	lower N-terminal pro-brain natriuretic peptide	SRU	secondary recovery unit
		SvO$_2$	mixed venous oxygen saturation
O$_2$	oxygen	SWMA	segmental wall motion abnormality
OLT	orthotopic liver transplantation	TAP	transversus abdominis plane
OLV	one-lung ventilation	TBI	traumatic brain injury
OR	operating room *or* odds ratio	TCDB	Traumatic Coma Data Bank
PaCO$_2$	arterial partial pressure of carbon dioxide	TCI	target-controlled infusion
		TEA	thoracic epidural analgesia
PACU	postanaesthesia care unit	TIVA	total intravenous anaesthesia
PAP	pulmonary artery pressure	TMN	tuberomammillary nucleus
PAOP	pulmonary artery occlusion pressure	TOE	transoesophageal echocardiography
PCWP	pulmonary capillary wedge pressure	TOF	train-of-four
PEEP	positive end-expiratory pressure	TOFR	train-of-four ratio
PEFR	peak expiratory flow rate	TPG	transpulmonary gradient
PEG	percutaneous endoscopic gastrostomy	TRALI	transfusion-related acute lung injury
		TT	tracheal tube
PET	positron emission tomography	USGRA	ultrasound-guided regional anaesthesia
PMI	postoperative myocardial infarction	US	ultrasound
POISE	PeriOperative ISchemic Evaluation [trial]	VEGF	vascular endothelial growth factor
		Vmac	middle cerebral artery blood flow velocity
PONV	postoperative nausea and vomiting	Vt	tidal volume
POPC	postoperative pulmonary complications	WFNS	World Federation of Neurosurgeons

Chapter 1

Neuromuscular blockade

A Srivastava and JM Hunter

Introduction

Modern anaesthetic practice has only become established over the last 70 years because of the introduction of neuromuscular blocking drugs. Previously, deep anaesthesia was necessary using potent inhalational agents to produce sufficient (albeit often inadequate) neuromuscular block for abdominal and thoracic surgery. Recovery from anaesthesia was prolonged, with the potential risk of pulmonary aspiration of gastric contents. The seminal report of the use of d-tubocurarine (dtc) with light anaesthesia by Gray and Halton in 1946 allowed for the first time patients with a wide range of pathology across the age spectrum to be managed successfully. Although this approach became widely accepted, there were concerns expressed by anaesthetists that the side effects of dtc, and particularly its effect on blood pressure, limited its use. Hence the long drawn-out search for an ideal muscle relaxant began.

The first clinical report of a new aminosteroidal neuromuscular blocking agent, pancuronium, by Baird and Reid (1967) was also an important landmark, although this drug proved to be as dependant as dtc on renal clearance and to have different but significant effects on the cardiovascular system. Its variability of effect was also similar to dtc. Long-acting neuromuscular blocking drugs have since been shown to be associated with an increased risk of postoperative pulmonary complications (Berg et al., 1997). The advent of atracurium (Stenlake et al., 1983) and to a lesser extent vecuronium in the early 1980s, changed practice again. These shorter-acting agents, which were less dependent on renal elimination (Hunter et al., 1982), had fewer cardiovascular effects, and were more predictable in their effect, meant that the older agents fell into disuse. Soon the problem of prolonged block and recurarization was confined to history. But the search continued for the ideal non-depolarizing agent leading to the introduction of mivacurium, rocuronium, and cisatracurium. Indeed, this search still continues today.

To avoid inadequate or prolonged neuromuscular block it was soon realized that accurate clinical monitoring tools were required. The introduction of the train-of-four (TOF) twitch technique in 1970 by Ali, Utting, and Gray was another landmark in neuromuscular pharmacology: this technique is still practised throughout the world today, both as a research tool and also for routine clinical monitoring. It set landmarks for the required degree of recovery from block before extubation was permissible, and it was many years before the need for a TOF ratio (TOFR) >0.7 on recovery was disputed. Eriksson and colleagues in 1997 finally provided convincing evidence that a TOFR >0.9 was necessary in the adductor pollicis muscle to ensure adequate return of muscle power in the pharyngeal muscles. The problem was with accurate clinical detection of residual block in the later stages of recovery (TOFR >0.4), and the introduction of double burst stimulation (DBS) by the Copenhagen group was a major step forward in this respect (Engbæk et al., 1989). Viby-Mogensen's group demonstrated that in detection of the later stages of recovery, the use of DBS was more accurate than the use of the TOF in clinical practice.

Another major development in the last 30 years has been the ability to accurately measure plasma levels of neuromuscular blocking drugs. Since the first description in the 1970s of an assay to measure dtc (Matteo et al., 1974), the pharmacokinetics of all the neuromuscular blocking drugs in different disease states has been described, clarifying their disposition and guiding advice on drug dosage in different disease states. The original atracurium kinetic paper by Ward and Weatherley (1983) with an accompanying editorial by Hull, were the first to suggest that consideration should be given in a kinetic model to additional elimination of a muscle relaxant from a peripheral as well as the central compartment.

It was 10 years after the first description of the use of dtc by Gray and Halton before anticholinesterases became routinely used. Problems with residual block and pulmonary aspiration of gastric contents were threatening the continuation of the 'Liverpool technique' in the mid-1950s.

But anticholinesterases have side effects which, despite their regular use, are well recognized. The muscarinic effects of neostigmine including nausea and vomiting and its cardiovascular effects may prevent its use. In addition, it has always been recognized that recovery from block must be underway for neostigmine to be effective (Ali *et al.*, 1971) and in such circumstances the drug still takes at least 9 min to exert its full effect. Hence the introduction of the new reversal agent, sugammadex, is most exciting (Bom *et al.*, 2002). In suitable dosage, this γ-cyclodextrin can be used effectively immediately after administration of rocuronium, which could be useful in a 'cannot intubate, cannot ventilate' situation. No serious adverse effects have as yet been reported with its use. But sugammadex is expensive and it does not antagonize block produced by benzylisoquinolines. Its introduction may yet change anaesthetic practice.

What of the future? The ideal muscle relaxant with a speed of onset as rapid as suxamethonium, a short duration of action, predictability of effect, and fewer side effects still eludes neuromuscular pharmacologists.

Paper 1: A milestone in anaesthesia? (d-tubocurarine chloride)

Author details

TC Gray, J Halton

Reference

Proceedings of the Royal Society of Medicine 1946; **39**: 400–10.

Summary

This paper describes the voyage of Sir Walter Raleigh up the River Amazon in 1595 where he witnessed the use of arrow poisons by South American Indians to kill animals for food. The same techniques were described by Charles Waterton over 200 years later in 1812 when he detailed the effect of the poison on various animal species. Claude Bernard was to repeat these findings in the laboratory demonstrating, in 1840, that the poison acted at the neuromuscular junction. The substance being used was derived from the vine, Wourali. In 1943, Professor McIntyre (University of Nebraska) prepared a standardized extract of the alkaloids of this raw material which was first marketed by Squibb in the USA as 'Intocostrin'. Although it had been used clinically in the UK since 1934 for the treatment of tetanus, it was Griffith and Johnson in Montreal, Canada in 1942 who first reported the use of small doses of 'Intocostrin' in 25 spontaneously breathing patients as an aid to anaesthesia.

In November 1944 in Liverpool, England, John Halton used the purified extract, d-tubocurarine (dtc), for the first time during anaesthesia to overcome the limitations of using repeated boluses of barbiturate as the sole anaesthetic agent. He had found 'Intocostrin' to be of unreliable potency possibly due to its instability in solution. The crystalline extract, dtc, was prepared by Burroughs Wellcome & Co. and proved more reliable. The pharmacology of dtc is discussed in detail in this seminal paper. The crude extracts of Wourali were classified as 'Tube', 'Calabash', and 'Pot' curare and the alkaloids obtained from them are detailed. Gray and Halton presented the effects of dtc on various organs including the neuromuscular, central nervous (CNS), cardiovascular, respiratory, gastrointestinal, renal, and hepatic systems. Interestingly, Gray considered that dtc may have some action on the synapses of the CNS, as acetylcholine was the neurotransmitter in this system. Gray's theory was rebutted for decades but has recently undergone reconsideration.

Based on these observations, Gray and Halton defined three different techniques for the use of dtc:

1 *The single-dose method*: a small dose of dtc (15 mg) given on induction of anaesthesia with Pentothal, for short operations and upper and lower gastrointestinal endoscopies.

2 *For longer operations*: on induction of anaesthesia and with repeated increments of both the barbiturate and dtc (2–4 mg) throughout anaesthesia, without the use of an inhalational agent. Anaesthesia was maintained with cyclopropane or ether for operations requiring more than a total of Pentothal 1.5 g or Kemithal 3–4 g.

3 *As an adjuvant to inhalational anaesthesia*: in intermittent doses of dtc 15–30 mg.

For the first time in the scientific literature, the importance of using artificial ventilation of the lungs when a muscle relaxant is given was stressed.

As would be the case with the first report of the clinical use of a new muscle relaxant today, the paper describes the determination of its appropriate dose based on age, weight, and the type of operation. In this respect, this paper is similar to present-day scientific articles. It is noted that the effect of dtc is potentiated by concomitant use of intravenous barbiturates and potent inhala-tional agents such as cyclopropane and ether. It was appreciated that the conventional signs of determining depth of anaesthesia from the eyelash, corneal, and conjunctival reflexes were lost and respiratory signs modified when a small dose of muscle relaxant is used. Gray and Halton stated that the three aspects of clinical monitoring which are unchanged when using small doses of dtc are the 'pulse, respiratory rate and the anaesthetist's experience'. Monitoring the depth of neuromuscular block was crudely based on: (a) the paradoxical movement of the chest on the abdomen during respiration indicating intercostal paralysis and (b) the ease of manual ventilation with a rebreathing bag.

More than a thousand patients received dtc during various thoracic, abdominal, head and neck, and orthopaedic operations. Gray and Halton observed a significant decrease in postoperative respiratory morbidity after upper abdominal operations using their technique, compared with inhalational techniques (King, 1933; Campbell and Gordon, 1942). They considered the indica-tions for the use of dtc were limited to abdominal and thoracic operations, and in conditions such as peripheral circulatory failure and shock where deep anaesthesia is to be avoided due to its car-diovascular depressant effect. Their contraindications to the use of dtc were: the inexperience of the anaesthetist in taking care of apnoeic patients (which still holds true today); use with cyclo-propane for abdominal operations because of an increase in intestinal motility; and intestinal obstruction and distension because of the risk of aspiration (a point over which they were prob-ably not correct). It is also interesting that the authors commented that dtc should be avoided in the presence of renal failure: it was thought even at that time that dtc was excreted in the urine. Myasthenia gravis was also a contraindication. The paper concludes: 'The road lies open before us, and with a grave and insistent warning to the inexperienced that we are dealing with one of the most potent poisons known, we venture to say we have passed yet another milestone, and the distance to our goal is considerably shortened'. How true this statement was, and how little some aspects of our practice have changed in the interim.

Citation count

78.

Related references

1 King DS. Postoperative pulmonary complications. *Surg Gynec Obstet* 1933; **56**: 43–5.

2 Campbell SM, Gordon RA. Post-anaesthetic complications in a military hospital. *Can Med Assoc J* 1942; **46**: 347–51.

3 Griffith HR, Johnson GE. The use of curare in general anesthesia. *Anesthesiology* 1942; **3**: 418–20.

4 Beecher HK, Todd DP. A study of the deaths associated with anesthesia and surgery: based on a study of 599, 548 anesthesias in ten institutions 1948-1952, inclusive. *Ann Surg* 1954; **140**: 2–35.

Key message

For the first time it was possible using this technique to provide light anaesthesia in sick patients without a delayed recovery and the increased risk of pulmonary aspiration of gastric contents. This major change in technique led the way for the development of cardiac, neonatal, and neuro-surgery, and of intensive care. D-tubocurarine improved surgical operating conditions and decreased postoperative respiratory morbidity thus improving patient outcome. It had minimal cardiovascular effects with the small doses used at that time. Artificial ventilation of the lungs became established peroperatively. The 'Liverpool technique', consisting of sleep, analgesia, and muscle relaxation, had been born.

Strengths

This perfectly written but rather long paper was the first to systematically document the use of dtc in clinical anaesthesia in Europe. The study involved 1,049 patients. A detailed account of the history of dtc, its pharmacology, and the dose schedules are provided. Assessment of the degree of curarization and recovery from block are detailed. The observations extend into the postoperative period and a decrease in the incidence of respiratory morbidity was noted, although the duration of study was not clearly defined in this respect.

Weaknesses

In many ways, this paper is a huge case series, with no control group comparing the incidence of postoperative respiratory complications after an inhalational technique and no statistical analysis. Surprisingly, there is little mention of the use of an anticholinesterase to antagonize residual block: neostigmine or pyridostigmine were not used routinely at this time. Physostigmine was used in only two of the 1,049 patients and the authors state that it did not show 'impressive results'. It is uncertain what is meant by this statement. It would be another decade before the use of an anticholinesterase at the end of anaesthesia became established. Indeed, the omission of such drugs almost led to international rejection of the 'Liverpool technique' (Beecher and Todd, 1954).

Relevance

Presented at the Royal Society of Medicine in London in 1946, this paper heralded the advent of modern anaesthetic practice. By using light anaesthesia, it avoided the disadvantages of deep inhalational techniques, allowing sick patients to undergo prolonged and complex surgery for the first time.

Paper 2: The neuromuscular blocking properties of a new steroid compound, pancuronium bromide

Author details

WLM Baird, AM Reid

Reference

British Journal of Anaesthesia 1967; **39**: 775–80.

Abstract

The action of a new steroid compound, pancuronium bromide (NA97) on the myoneural junction in man has been studied. The drug was shown to produce myoneural blockade which was reversible with neostigmine. A 2-mg dose of pancuronium bromide produced a degree of blockade similar in intensity and duration to that of 10–15 mg of tubocurarine. Electromyography showed a rapid fall-off in tetanus followed by post-tetanic facilitation. These facts would point to the blockade being of the non-depolarizing or curariform type. On intravenous injection of the drug there were no changes in pulse rate or systolic blood pressure. Further investigation of the effects of pancuronium bromide in man would seem to be indicated.

Summary

In 1964, Hewett and Savege synthesized a new steroid compound, NA97, in an attempt to produce a muscle relaxant which was free of the cardiovascular side effects of tubocurarine (which were mainly due to histamine release in the clinical dose range). Animal studies by Buckett and Bonta, and Bonta *et al.* in 1966 had demonstrated that this new compound was 10 times as potent a neuromuscular blocking agent as tubocurarine in cats. In that animal species, the new relaxant also seemed to have fewer cardiovascular side effects due to its minimal vagolytic and ganglion-blocking properties.

Baird and Reid conducted this first pilot study on six healthy, female patients undergoing gynaecological procedures to determine the type and duration of block from pancuronium, and its ease of reversal with neostigmine. They also looked for cardiovascular side effects. The patients were premedicated and anaesthesia was induced with thiopentone and maintained with nitrous oxide, oxygen, and halothane (0.5%). Blood pressure and pulse rate was recorded at 1-min intervals. A Medelec electromyograph was used to record the twitch height using button-type EEG electrodes. Neuromuscular monitoring was carried out on the hypothenar eminence. Before administering pancuronium, the machine was calibrated with 1-mV twitches. The rate of ulnar nerve twitch stimulation at the elbow was once per second, of 0.1-ms duration and at 80mV (which is certainly supramaximal). The twitch response was monitored on one oscilloscope and a second one was used to photograph the recordings. The height of the twitch response was measured from the photograph using dividers.

After pancuronium has been given and when the twitch height had returned to one-third of baseline, a short burst of tetanic stimuli at 50 Hz was applied followed by single twitches to demonstrate post-tetanic potentiation, a sign of non-depolarizing block. When the twitch height had returned to baseline values, recovery was considered complete. Neuromuscular block was reversed with neostigmine and atropine in three of the six patients at a variable degree of recovery and in doses of neostigmine ranging from 1.25–3.75 mg. No change in heart rate or systolic blood pressure was found in any patient after pancuronium. The authors concluded that in humans, pancuronium is five times more potent than tubocurarine with a faster onset (20–50 s) but the same duration of effect. Considering the quicker onset of action of such a small dose of pancuronium (2–3 mg), Baird and Reid suggested that this new drug might replace suxamethonium.

Citation count

110.

Related references

1 Bonta IL, Buckett WR, Lewis JJ, *et al.* 2β, 16β-Dipiperidino-5α androstane-3α, 17β-diol diacetate dimethobromide, a potent neuromuscular blocking steroid. In *Proceedings of 2nd International Congress on Hormonal Steroids*, p.344. Amsterdam: Excerpta Medica, 1966.

2 Buckett WR, Bonta IL. Pharmacological studies with NA97 (2β, 16β-dipiperidino-5α androstane-3α, 17β-diol diacetate dimethobromide). *Fed Proc* 1966; **25**: 718.

3 Norman J, Katz RL, Seed RF. The neuromuscular blocking action of pancuronium in man during anaesthesia. *Br J Anaesth* 1970; **42**: 702–9.

4 Miller RD, Agoston S, Booij LHD, *et al.* The comparative potency and pharmacokinetics of pancuronium and its metabolites in anaesthetised man. *J Phamacol Exp Ther* 1978; **207**: 539–43.

Key message

This study suggested that a steroidal muscle relaxant may avoid the cardiovascular side effects of tubocurarine and produce profound neuromuscular block more rapidly. Pancuronium was shown at this early stage to be reversible with neostigmine and atropine once recovery from block had commenced.

Strengths

This was the first study of the use of small doses of pancuronium in humans. It suggested that in doses as small as 0.04 mg kg^{-1}, non-depolarizing neuromuscular block could be achieved in 180 s. The authors used stringent methodology for neuromuscular monitoring with fastidious positioning of the hand. They minimized skin impedance by cleansing with ether and used sophisticated electromyographic equipment including expensive electroencephalogram (EEG)-type electrodes to increase sensitivity. This approach is still essential to obtain accurate and reproducible neuromuscular research recordings. In this small study, no cardiovascular side effects were found following pancuronium.

Weaknesses

This study was carried out before the train-of-four (TOF) technique was described (1970), and used twitch stimuli, followed by tetanus and the post-tetanic count. So the data is not easily comparable with modern-day clinical research techniques where the monitoring methods would be more consistent, e.g. use of the TOF throughout the investigation. It would also have been more appropriate to standardize the dose of pancuronium and neostigmine. The time when the anticholinesterase was given should also have been related to twitch height. Their findings were somewhat surprising with durations of action of small doses of pancuronium as long as 77 min. The use of halothane would have potentiated neuromuscular block. Its end-tidal concentration should have been determined and standardized for each patient, but that would have been more difficult to achieve in 1967 than it is today. The variability of action of pancuronium (range 2–77 min) is no better than that of tubocurarine and is a weakness of all the older long-acting non-depolarizing neuromuscular blocking agents which are dependent on organ elimination.

Relevance

Following the successful clinical use of tubocurarine 20 years earlier, this was the first report of the use of a non-depolarizing muscle relaxant of a completely different chemical structure which was apparently devoid of cardiovascular side effects. Pancuronium, an aminosteroidal agent, was to be widely used throughout the world for the next 25 years. Despite these initial findings, it was found to have some vagolytic and sympathomimetic properties in humans in larger doses. These characteristics did have benefits in maintaining the blood pressure in hypovolaemic, hypotensive, or cardiovascularly unstable patients. But pancuronium proved ultimately to have as long an onset and as variable a duration of action as tubocurarine, as both drugs were dependant on renal elimination, as well as biliary excretion. However, newer aminosteroidal compounds with a more rapid onset (rocuronium), shorter duration of effect (vecuronium), and fewer side effects were subsequently synthesized from the original pancuronium molecule.

Paper 3: Quantitative assessment of residual antidepolarizing block (part II)

Author details

HH Ali, JE Utting, TC Gray

Reference

British Journal of Anaesthesia 1971; **43**: 478–85.

Abstract

An attempt to estimate residual neuromuscular blockade after the administration of antidepolarizing relaxants to anaesthetized patients is described. A train of four supramaximal nerve stimuli was applied to the ulnar nerve at the wrist and the twitch response (mechanical or electrical) was recorded. The frequency of the train used was 2–2.4 Hz with an interval of 10 seconds between the trains. Clinical recovery from the relaxant was assessed by the ability to lift the head. The ratio of the height of the fourth response of the train to that of the first, (ratio (c)), gave a good indication of the degree of residual neuromuscular block as indicated by this simple clinical test. As ratio (c) increased muscle power improved. Obvious muscle weakness was associated with values of ratio (c) of less than 0.6.

Summary

This paper is the third in a series of pioneering studies conducted in 1970–1971 in Liverpool by TC Gray and colleagues in an attempt to devise a reliable clinical method for assessment of residual neuromuscular block at the end of surgery. Clinicians had become aware by this time that more accurate tools were needed than simple clinical acumen to prevent residual neuromuscular block with all its complications postoperatively. In their first study, Ali, Utting, and Gray had selected a pattern of four twitch stimuli repeated at 10-s intervals. The second and the third papers discuss the use and limitations of this new monitoring technique. In their second study, Ali, Utting and Gray found a strong correlation between the relative decrease in height of the four twitch responses, which came to be known as 'fade' or 'decrement', and the degree of block. They referred to the ratio of the height of the fourth to the first twitch as 'ratio c', which was found to be a more sensitive index of the degree of curarization than the ratio of the height of the first and the control response (then called 'ratio a'), or the ratio of the second and the first response (then called 'ratio b') (Fig. 1.1). These abbreviations, which have been the cause of some confusion, have now changed. The four twitches are numbered 1, 2, 3, and 4. Ratio c, is now known as the 'train-of-four ratio' (TOFR) or T_4/T_1.

The introduction of this technique obviates the need to obtain a control twitch value before a muscle relaxant is given, which is of significant clinical relevance. In their third study, Ali, Utting, and Gray objectively correlated the clinical parameters used to assess recovery from non-depolarizing block, e.g. ability to lift the head for 5 s and to protrude the tongue, and the presence of tracheal tug, with the TOFR. They found that adequate clinical recovery as estimated using these variables is not complete until a TOFR >0.6 is attained. Nearly 40 years later this pattern, termed the 'train-of-four' (TOF) response, remains the gold standard for objective measurement of the depth of neuromuscular block.

Citation count

96.

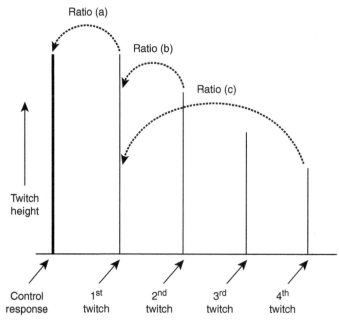

Ratio (a)

Ratio (b)

Ratio (c)

Twitch
height

Control   1st   2nd   3rd   4th
response   twitch   twitch   twitch   twitch

Fig. 1.1 The alphabetic labelling of the TOF as first described by Ali, Utting, and Gray (1970) is compared with the present numerical nomenclature.

Related references

1 Ali HH, Utting JE, Gray TC. Stimulus frequency in the detection of neuromuscular block in humans. *Br J Anaesth* 1970; **42**: 967–76.

2 Ali HH, Utting JE, Gray TC. Quantitative assessment of residual antidepolarizing block (part I). *Br J Anaesth* 1971; **43**: 473–7.

3 Ali HH, Savarese JJ. Monitoring of neuromuscular function. *Anesthesiology* 1976; **45**: 216–49.

4 Bevan DR, Donati F, Kopman AF. Residual neuromuscular blockade. *Anesthesiology* 1992; **77**: 785–805.

5 Kopman AF, Yee PS, Neuman GG. Relationship of the train-of-four fade ratio to clinical signs and symptoms of residual paralysis in awake volunteers. *Anesthesiology* 1997; **86**: 765–71.

Key message

This study described for the first time a unique clinical tool for defining adequate recovery from non-depolarizing neuromuscular block at the end of anaesthesia. The use of four twitch stimuli in close succession with the measurement of their fade was a new concept for anaesthetists at that time. The study demonstrated that a TOFR >0.6 correlated with adequate recovery from neuromuscular block as assessed clinically.

Strengths

This study demonstrated that the ratio of the fourth to the first twitch of the TOF response is a more important indicator of recovery than the ratio of the first to control or the second to the first twitch response. This landmark paper set the threshold for adequate clinical recovery from block at a TOFR >0.6: it remained at that level until the work of Kopman *et al.* (1997) increased it to 0.7, and later when Eriksson *et al.* (see paper 9) recommended it to be further raised to 0.9.

Weaknesses

For unknown reasons, in this small study, the authors used mechanomyography in ten patients and electromyography in another ten. Acceleromyography has since been shown to be a more sensitive tool for such clinical use than mechanomyography. Despite its findings, it is now known that full recovery from neuromuscular block is only achieved at a TOFR >0.9 at the adductor pollicis muscle. The clinical assessments made by Ali, Utting, and Gray are not able to accurately reflect the ability of pharyngeal muscle to protect the airway from aspiration of gastric contents.

Relevance

This was the first study to objectively correlate the TOF response with clinical signs of recovery from neuromuscular block. Previously, recovery was guided only by clinical criteria. Although the single twitch and tetanic responses were in use to assess neuromuscular weakness, they were research tools and not easy to apply in clinical practice. This study suggested that a TOFR >0.6 was an indication of adequate recovery from block: a recommendation that remained uncontested for over 25 years.

Paper 4: Atracurium: conception and inception

Author details

JB Stenlake, RD Waigh, J Urwin, JH Dewar, GG Coker

Reference

British Journal of Anaesthesia 1983; **55**: 3S–10S.

Summary

This review by the inventors of atracurium was part of a *British Journal of Anaesthesia* supplement based on an international symposium held at The Royal College of Surgeons of England in 1982. Atracurium was then a new non-depolarizing agent considered to have distinct advantages over established agents such as tubocurarine, pancuronium, alcuronium, and gallamine. This excellent paper discusses the limitations of older non-depolarizing agents including: the variable duration of action; cardiovascular side effects; and prolonged paralysis in patients with renal impairment. The new relaxant had been designed to undergo breakdown in the plasma by Hofmann elimination. This pathway for the spontaneous degradation of quaternary ammonium compounds was first identified for petaline, a constituent of the plant *Leontice leontopetalum*, which is similar in structure to tubocurarine. It broke down in mildly alkalotic conditions by spontaneous Hofmann degradation. Elimination of quaternary ammonium salts in this way was not thought to exist in mammalian metabolism. Hofmann (1851) had first described spontaneous breakdown at very high pH and temperature (100°C).

Stenlake and colleagues at Strathclyde University, Scotland, synthesized a series of bisquaternary compounds with selective neuromuscular blocking properties which incorporated a charged quaternary nitrogen from which an electron could be withdrawn to promote degradation to inactive components. These compounds were designed to break down *in vivo* at physiological pH (7.4) and temperature (37°C), but could be stored in solution at a lower pH (3.5) and temperature (2–8°C). Although the first two series of compounds were potentially degradable, they showed lack of potency, and unacceptable levels of vagal blockade. Most importantly, they proved unsuitable as they underwent reversible Hofmann equilibration to reform the original active quaternary ammonium compound. The third series still caused excessive vagal blockade. The fourth series of four compounds had a suitable combination of potency and biodegradability together with high specificity for the neuromuscular junction. Increasing the interonium distance not only increased the potency but also reduced the vagal blockade and hence any cardiovascular side effects.

Water solubility is a problem with iodide salts. The besylate salt of atracurium was chosen after testing mesylate, besylate, tosylate, and 1- and 2-naphthalenesulphonate salts because of its greater water solubility (60 mg ml^{-1} at 25°C). Thus, atracurium besylate was formulated as an aqueous injectable solution (10 mg ml^{-1}), and was claimed to be virtually free from cardiovascular side effects. Breakdown by Hofmann elimination produced laudanosine, which was thought to be devoid of neuromuscular or cardiovascular effects. In animals, this metabolite was subsequently demonstrated after pharmacological doses of atracurium to produce epileptiform activity. Later animal studies also showed that the breakdown of atracurium is independent of plasma cholinesterase or hepatic enzymatic activity as well as renal function.

Citation count

91.

Related references

1 Hofmann AW. Beiträge zur Kenntniss der fluchtigen organischen Basen. *Ann Chem* 1851; **78**: 253.

2 Stenlake JB, Urwin J, Waigh RD, *et al*. Biodegradable neuromuscular blocking agents 1. Quaternary esters. *Eur J Med Chem* 1979a; **14**: 77–84.

3 Stenlake JB, Urwin J, Waigh RD, *et al*. Biodegradable neuromuscular blocking agents 2. Quaternary ketones. *Eur J Med Chem* 1979b; **14**: 85–8.

4 Hughes R, Chapple DJ. The pharmacology of atracurium: a new competitive neuromuscular blocking agent. *Br J Anaesth* 1981; **53**: 31–44.

5 Payne JP, Hughes R. Evaluation of atracurium in anaesthetized man. *Br J Anaesth* 1981; **53**: 45–54.

Key message

Atracurium was the first custom designed intermediate-acting non-depolarizing neuromuscular blocking agent which underwent spontaneous degradation rapidly, primarily by Hofmann elimination at physiological pH and temperature and to a lesser extent by ester hydrolysis. Hence, it should not accumulate in the presence of organ dysfunction even when given in repeated doses or as an infusion. Prolonged neuromuscular block in acidotic patients should also be minimized with the use of atracurium.

Strengths

This project was a brilliant example of extensive structural modification of a molecule to produce an almost ideal neuromuscular blocking agent whose action was minimally affected by hepatic or renal dysfunction or by abnormalities of plasma cholinesterase. Atracurium had fewer side effects than its longer-acting predecessors.

Weaknesses

Storage is a problem with atracurium. Its stability in solution is dependent on temperature and pH, which if not strictly maintained leads to a decrease in potency. Although it was originally claimed to possess minimal cardiovascular activity, we now know that atracurium may cause hypotension, tachycardia, and bronchospasm, probably due to histamine release, and especially when used in high doses ($>0.6\,mg\,kg^{-1}$). In addition, there is a small risk that the metabolite of Hofmann degradation, laudanosine, may cause central nervous system irritation when atracurium is used for long periods by infusion in the critically ill, although this has never been demonstrated.

Relevance

Atracurium was the first of the new generation of non-depolarizing neuromuscular blocking agents which are less likely to cause prolonged block in the presence of renal or hepatic dysfunction. However, tachycardia, hypotension, and increased airway resistance due to histamine release has been an issue with its use in cardiovascular and respiratory patients. The later formulation of its 1R-*cis* 1′R-*cis* isomer, cisatracurium, has minimized these side effects, but with the effect of an increase in potency (which delays onset of block). Although there is the potential for the metabolite of atracurium, laudanosine, to induce seizures, it has been demonstrated in animals that this is very unlikely in the therapeutic dose range.

Paper 5: Use of atracurium in patients with no renal function

Author details

JM Hunter, RS Jones, JE Utting

Reference

British Journal of Anaesthesia 1982; **54**: 1251–8.

Abstract

Atracurium was given to 26 patients who had no renal function; in 21 of these neuromuscular block was monitored using the train-of-four stimuli. The results are compared with those obtained from normal patients presented for surgery. Unlike the non-depolarizing muscle relaxants currently in common use, it was possible to continue giving incremental doses of atracurium to the anephric patients without there being evidence of cumulation. Even when the total dose used (over a period of up to 2.5 h) was in the order of seven to eight times that previously described as the minimum required for endotracheal intubation (2.3 mg kg^{-1}) as opposed to (0.3 mg kg^{-1}) there was no evidence of residual curarization. This finding would seem to be compatible with what is known of the pharmacology of the drug. No adverse cardiovascular effects were demonstrated. It is concluded that atracurium may be especially valuable in patients with no renal function.

Hunter JM, Jones RS. Utting JE, 'Use of atracurium in patients with no renal function', *British Journal of Anaesthesia*, 1982, 54, 12, pp. 1251–1258, by permission of Oxford University Press and British Journal of Anaesthesia.

Summary

The older non-depolarizing relaxants such as tubocurarine, pancuronium, and gallamine are excreted in the urine to varying extents and hence can produce prolonged block in the presence of renal dysfunction. In these circumstances, accumulation of the relaxant or its metabolites (which can also have neuromuscular blocking properties) may occur. Atracurium is spontaneously broken down by Hofmann degradation and undergoes ester hydrolysis in the plasma. It is minimally excreted in the urine and less likely to accumulate in renal patients. This study was undertaken to determine the pharmacodynamics of atracurium in patients with no renal function compared to patients with normal renal function undergoing a range of surgical procedures. Twenty-six patients were recruited who were on regular haemodialysis. The anephric group consisted mainly of males (19/26) with a wide range of body weight (40–84 kg), age (21–61 yr), haemoglobin concentration (4.6–15.8 g dl^{-1}), metabolic acidosis, blood urea (6–48 mmol l^{-1}), and serum creatinine (358–1368 mmol l^{-1}).

All patients were premedicated and received fentanyl and droperidol: anaesthesia was induced with thiopentone 300 mg and maintained with nitrous oxide and oxygen using a face mask. Neuromuscular monitoring was established (21 of 26 patients) using a Grass nerve stimulator applied to the ulnar nerve at the wrist with needle electrodes and a control train-of-four (TOF) response was obtained from the adductor pollicis muscle. Atracurium 0.5 mg kg^{-1} was given and laryngoscopy attempted 90 s later. Neuromuscular monitoring was continued throughout the operation using the TOF response delivered at a frequency of 2 Hz and 0.3 s duration. The four responses were named in a similar way to the original Ali, Utting, and Gray report (1970): A, B, C, and D before atracurium was given and A′, B′, C′, D′ thereafter. The ratios A′/A and D′/A′ were measured to quantify the degree of block. Time to onset of action (the lag time, when the first depression of the TOF was noted), time to disappearance of the response, time to reappearance of A', time to 10% recovery A', time to the first increment of relaxant (given when A'/A was 20% in normal patients and 10% in anephric patients), and total number of increments were noted. Heart rate and systolic blood pressure were monitored at preset intervals and any change in haemodynamic parameters noted.

At the end of surgery, neuromuscular block was reversed in 16 renal patients with neostigmine 2.5 mg and 5 min later by a second dose of neostigmine 2.5 mg in a further five patients as A'/A was still <0.75. All the patients were able to lift their head off the pillow in the recovery room and did not suffer from diplopia the following day.

Citation count

49.

Related references

1 Fairley HB. Prolonged intercostal paralysis due to relaxant. *Br Med J* 1950; **2**: 986–8.

2 Hunter JM, Jones RS, Utting JE. Use of atracurium during general surgery monitored by train-of-four stimuli. *Br J Anaesth* 1982a; **54**: 1243–50.

3 Hunter JM, Jones RS, Utting JE. Comparison of vecuronium, atracurium and tubocurarine in normal patients and in patients with no renal function. *Br J Anaesth* 1984; **56**: 941–51.

4 Jones JE, Hunter JM, Utting JE. Use of neostigmine in the antagonism of residual neuromuscular blockade produced by vecuronium. *Br J Anaesth* 1987; **59**: 1454–8.

5 Jones JE, Parker CJ, Hunter JM. Antagonism of blockade produced by atracurium or vecuronium with low doses of neostigmine. *Br J Anaesth* 1988; **61**: 560–4.

6 Kirkegaard-Nielsen H, Helbo-Hansen HS, Lindholm P, *et al.* Time to peak effect of neostigmine at antagonism of atracurium- or vecuronium-induced neuromuscular block. *J Clin Anesth* 1995; **7**: 635–9.

Key message

This study confirmed that atracurium can be given in repeated doses to patients with no renal function without producing prolonged neuromuscular block. Incremental doses produced predictable effects with no signs of cumulation even after nine doses. The block was easily reversible with neostigmine 2.5 mg even after a total dose of atracurium 2.3 mg kg^{-1}. No pre-existing muscle relaxant could be given with such impunity to this patient population.

Strengths

This was the first report of the use of atracurium in renal patients. Since it is broken down spontaneously by Hofmann elimination at physiological pH and temperature, it does not accumulate in such patients. Atracurium would have similar advantages in patients with lesser degrees of renal impairment and patients whose renal function is transiently affected by, for instance, hypovolaemia. A change in those physiological parameters such as pH and $PaCO_2$ (arterial partial pressure of carbon dioxide) that could alter the metabolism of atracurium and hence its duration of action was prevented in this study and strict attention was paid to the details of neuromuscular monitoring.

Weaknesses

Although the paper investigates the dynamics of atracurium in anephric patients, the population studied was not homogeneous. They had various degrees of renal dysfunction and some were undergoing renal transplantation which could have affected the kinetics of atracurium intraoperatively. There is no mention of the use of core or peripheral temperature monitoring which is an important factor in the rate of breakdown of atracurium, especially during long operations when hypothermia is common. The older form of nomenclature (A, B, C, and D) was used in this study even though the numerical format was being used to label the TOF by 1982 (see Fig. 1.1).

A different degree of recovery of A'/A was fixed for the administration of incremental doses of atracurium between the healthy and anephric groups without a convincing explanation. Neostigmine was not administered at a fixed recovery of the TOF which would now be considered unacceptable. The second dose of neostigmine was given 5 min after the first dose if A'/A was <75%, even though it was known that the time to peak effect of neostigmine when given at the reappearance of T2 is about 9 min (Kirkegaard-Nielson *et al.*, 1995).

Relevance

Atracurium heralded the advent of a new era in neuromuscular pharmacology, ending the risk of prolonged block (or recurarization) as seen with the older neuromuscular blocking agents, especially in patients with renal dysfunction. This study showed that in conjunction with objective neuromuscular monitoring, atracurium can be used safely in repeated doses, even for prolonged surgery, and yet be reversed easily with neostigmine.

Paper 6: Pharmacokinetics of atracurium besylate in healthy patients (after a single i.v. bolus dose)

Author details

S Ward, EAM Neill, BC Weatherley, IM Corall

Reference

British Journal of Anaesthesia 1983; **55**: 113–17.

Abstract

The plasma decay of atracurium besylate was examined in two groups of six patients. Group I received atracurium 0.6 mg kg^{-1} and group II 0.3 mg kg^{-1} as a single bolus dose i.v. The plasma concentrations were measured by high performance liquid chromatography. An individual two-compartment pharmacokinetic model was used for interpretation. The results from the two groups were not significantly different, giving overall mean values of 2 min (±0.2 SEM) for the distribution half-life ($T_{1/2}\alpha$), 19.9 min (±0.6) for the elimination half-life ($T_{1/2}\beta$), 5.5 ml min^{-1} kg^{-1} (±0.2) for total clearance (Cl) and 157 ml kg^{-1} (±7) for total distribution volume (V_{area}).

Ward S, Neill EAM, Weatherley BC, Corall IM, 'Pharmacokinetics of atracurium besylate in healthy patients (after a single i.v. bolus dose)', *British Journal of Anaesthesia*, 1983, 55, 2, pp. 113–117 by permission of Oxford University Press and British Journal of Anaesthesia.

Summary

Ward and colleagues conducted this well-designed study on 12 healthy patients undergoing minor surgery to determine for the first time the pharmacokinetic parameters of atracurium in humans. They studied two groups of patients receiving either atracurium 0.3 mg kg^{-1} or 0.6 mg kg^{-1}. Patients were anaesthetized with thiopentone, nitrous oxide in oxygen, and halothane. Fourteen venous blood samples were taken at predetermined intervals until 120 min after administration of the drug. Plasma was separated within 30 s, and immediately transferred to glass vials and frozen. Neuromuscular block was reversed, if necessary, with neostigmine and atropine.

The plasma concentration of atracurium was measured in duplicate within 24 h of sampling by high-performance liquid chromatography (HPLC). The assay was accurate to 0.05 µg ml^{-1}. Each set of data was examined on a semilog plot and fitted to a standard two component exponential, $C = Ae^{-\alpha t} + Be^{-\beta t}$, to derive distribution and elimination half-lives and the volume of distribution of the central compartment.

The clearance was calculated from the graph by a traditional method:

$$\text{Clearance (Cl)} = \frac{\text{Total dose}}{\text{Area under curve (AUC)}}$$

There was no significant difference between the two groups. The overall mean (±standard deviation [SD]) elimination half-life was 19.9 (±0.6) min, total clearance 5.5 (±0.2) ml min^{-1} kg^{-1} and total volume of distribution 157 (±7) ml kg^{-1}.

In an excellent and frequently quoted editorial in the same issue of the *British Journal of Anaesthesia*, Hull (1983) used the data to analyse the pharmacokinetics of atracurium using two different models. The first, model A, was a conventional two-compartment model which he had previously described for pancuronium (Hull *et al.*, 1978) that assumes the elimination of atracurium occurs only from a central compartment (V_1). The second, model B, also took into account the additional elimination of atracurium directly from a second compartment (V_2) as the breakdown

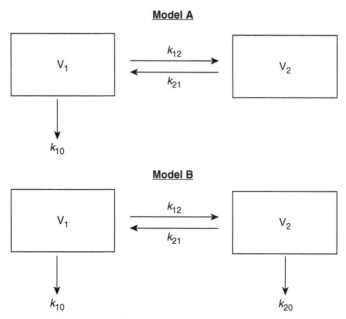

Fig. 1.2 The two models first described by Hull (1983) to determine the kinetics of atracurium. In model B, elimination is also considered from a second peripheral compartment (V_2). Reproduced from C. J. Hull, A Model for Atracurium?, *British Journal of Anaesthesia*, 1983, **55**(2), 95–96, Oxford University Press, by permission of British Journal of Anaesthesia. Data from S. Ward, E. A. M. Neill, B. C. Weatherley, and I. M. Corall, Pharmacokinetics of atracurium besylate in healthy patients (after a single i.v. bolus dose), *British Journal of Anaesthesia*, 1983, **55**(2), 113.

of atracurium is independent of any organ system (Fig. 1.2). In spite of its unique intuitive appeal, Hull showed that the more complicated model B offered no practical advantage over model A in determining the infusion regimes required to rapidly attain effective plateau plasma atracurium concentrations, although it helps in determining the kinetic microparameters, e.g. A, B, α, and β.

Citation count

65.

Related references

1 Matteo RS, Spector S, Horowitz PE. Relationship of serum *d*-tubocurarine concentration to neuromuscular blockade. *Anesthesiology* 1974; **41**: 440–3.

2 Hull CJ, Van Beem HBH, McLeod K, *et al.* A pharmacodynamic model for pancuronium. *Br J Anaesth* 1978; **50**: 1113–23.

3 Hull CJ. Editorial: A model for atracurium. *Br J Anaesth* 1983; **55**: 95–6.

4 Ward S, Weatherley BC. Pharmacokinetics of atracurium and its metabolites. *Br J Anaesth* 1986; **58**: 6S–10S.

5 Parker CJR, Hunter JM. Relationship between volume of distribution of atracurium and body weight. *Br J Anaesth* 1993; **70**: 443–5.

Key message

The distribution, elimination, and clearance of atracurium are independent of the dose administered as its breakdown is independent of organ function. The short elimination half-life of atracurium (19.9 min) was significantly lower than any other non-depolarizing muscle relaxant available at that time and the clearance (5.5 ml min^{-1} kg^{-1}) much higher.

Strengths

This study was meticulously designed to minimize the chemical breakdown of atracurium in the sample prior to HPLC analysis which is essential for accurate results. The plasma was separated in the operating theatre within 30 s of obtaining the blood sample and immediately frozen. The assay was accurate to very low concentrations and performed within 24 h of sampling. The kinetic data obtained for atracurium have since been verified repeatedly (Parker and Hunter, 1993). This was the first suggestion that elimination of a muscle relaxant from a second compartment (V_2) should be considered. This paper changed the approach to pharmacokinetic modelling of muscle relaxants from thereon.

Weaknesses

The number of patients studied in this investigation was small (12) and the kinetic data for the two different doses of atracurium were not provided separately. It has been shown that the disposition of atracurium in adults is independent of body weight (Parker and Hunter, 1993). It may have been more appropriate to give a fixed dose of drug to each patient. It proved impossible to determine the microkinetic parameters of the two-compartment model with a second rate of elimination using their methodology, so the area under the curve principle was used to drive A, α, B, and β.

Relevance

Atracurium was the first intermediate-acting non-depolarizing muscle relaxant which, due to its unique breakdown pathway, does not accumulate in the body. Its pharmacokinetics were shown in this study to be independent of the doses administered. There is evidence for giving a fixed dose of atracurium in adults rather than one related to body weight (Parker and Hunter, 1993).

Paper 7: Double burst stimulation (DBS): a new pattern of nerve stimulation to identify residual neuromuscular block

Author details

J Engbæk, D Østergaard, J Viby-Mogensen

Reference

British Journal of Anaesthesia 1989; **62**: 274–8.

Abstract

We present a new pattern of nerve stimulation–double burst stimulation (DBS)–to detect residual neuromuscular block manually. The DBS consists of two short lasting, 50-Hz tetanic stimuli or bursts separated by a 750-ms interval. The response to this pattern of stimulation is two single separated muscle contractions of which the second is less than the first during nondepolarizing neuromuscular blockade. The ability to identify fade manually at different train-of-four (TOF) ratios was compared in four DBS patterns in which different numbers of impulses in the individual bursts were combined. The DBS with three impulses in each burst ($DBS_{3,3}$) was considered to be the most sensitive and the least painful and thus most suitable for clinical use. The degree of fade in TOF and $DBS_{3,3}$ was almost identical at any level of blockade (correlation coefficient 0.96), and the major post- $DBS_{3,3}$ effect was a depression of the first twitch in TOF lasting less than 15 s. It is concluded that the DBS is more sensitive than the TOF in manual detection of residual block.

Engbæk J, Østergaard D, Viby-Mogensen J, 'Double burst stimulation (DBS): a new pattern of nerve stimulation to identify residual neuromuscular block', *British Journal of Anaesthesia*, 1989, 62, 3, pp. 274–278 by permission of Oxford University Press and British Journal of Anaesthesia.

Summary

The authors developed and evaluated a new pattern of nerve stimulation consisting of two tetanic bursts of 50 Hz separated by a short interval of 750 ms, which they named double burst stimulation (DBS). It was designed to improve the accuracy of assessing residual neuromuscular block manually. The TOF has recognized limitations in this respect, especially when the train-of-four ratio (TOFR) is >0.4. They first conducted a preliminary study on nine possible patterns of DBS based on three variables: the frequency of tetanic stimulation, the duration of tetanic stimulation, and the interval separating the two stimuli. Based on the ease of manual detection of fade, four patterns of stimulation consisting of a combination of two, three, or four stimuli in the first or second burst of the tetanus were selected for further study. The four patterns were represented as $DBS_{3,3}$ (two bursts each of three impulses), $DBS_{4,4}$ (four impulses in each of the two bursts), $DBS_{3,2}$ (three, then two impulses), and $DBS_{4,3}$ (four, then three impulses).

Forty-one patients were induced with thiopentone. Tracheal intubation was performed using suxamethonium and anaesthesia was maintained with halothane in a mixture of nitrous oxide and oxygen. Neuromuscular block was maintained with pancuronium 1–1.5 mg kg^{-1} and evaluated by stimulating the ulnar nerve at both wrists. One arm served as a control using the TOF pattern of stimulation and the other arm was used for assessing and recording various combinations of DBS patterns. Surface electrodes were used and the resultant thumb twitch measured by a force displacement transducer and recorded on a polygraph.

The study was divided into three parts. The first part was aimed at selecting the DBS pattern with the greatest sensitivity. Each of the four patterns was evaluated manually more than a hundred times and it was demonstrated that $DBS_{3,3}$ was the most useful pattern as it caused the least pain in conscious patients and was most closely correlated to the TOF response. The second part of the study was aimed at establishing the relationship between the TOF and DBS. Scattergram and regression analysis showed a close linear relation between the TOFR and DBS ratio represented by the equation:

$$\text{DBS ratio} = 1.07 \times \text{TOFR} - 0.032$$

The third part of the study assessed the possible decurarizing effect of $DBS_{3,3}$ from the mobilization of acetylcholine by the tetanic stimulus. The authors found that the TOF height was depressed significantly for only 3 s after $DBS_{3,3}$. No such depression was observed after 15 s and 27 s. The authors concluded that the DBS pattern demonstrated fade in almost all cases at a TOFR of <0.5, in about 50% of cases when the TOFR was between 0.5 and 0.7, but rarely demonstrated fade if the TOFR was 0.7 or greater. The study also showed that decreasing the number of impulses in the second burst rather than the first burst increases the ability to identify fade manually when the TOFR was >0.5, and this effect was increasingly exaggerated up to a TOFR >0.7.

Citation count
91.

Related references

1 Gissen AJ, Katz RL. Twitch, tetanus and posttetanic potentiation as indices of nerve muscle block in man. *Anesthesiology* 1969; **30**: 481–7.

2 Lee C, Katz RL. Fade of neurally evoked compound electromyogram during neuromuscular block by d-tubocurarine. *Anesth Analg* 1977; **56**: 271–5.

3 Viby-Mogensen J. Clinical assessment of neuromuscular transmission. *Br J Anaesth* 1982; **54**: 209–23.

4 Viby-Mogensen J, Jensen NH, Engbæk J, *et al.* Tactile and visual evaluation of the response to train-of-four nerve stimulation. *Anesthesiology* 1985; **63**: 440–3.

Key message

The aim of this study was to design a pattern of nerve stimulation which would be a more accurate clinical tool for tactile (or manual) detection of the later stages of recovery from neuromuscular block (when the TOFR is of limited use). $DBS_{3,3}$ was the most useful of all the patterns studied but even its sensitivity decreases when the TOFR reaches 0.7. The number of twitches in either burst can be increased or decreased, however, to obtain an optimal response depending on whether the TOFR is >0.5 or >0.7. Due to its subjective nature in the assessment of fade, the use of DBS is limited to clinical practice unlike the TOF which is quantifiable and reproducible and hence can be used a research tool.

Strengths

This study demonstrated that DBS circumvented the need to set up the complex equipment that was then required for quantitative measurement of the TOF to determine residual neuromuscular block during the later stages of recovery. DBS is a useful clinical tool especially in awake patients, as it is less painful than TOF stimulation.

Weaknesses

In spite of showing a close correlation with the TOFR, the $DBS_{3,3}$ ratio cannot quantitatively assess the degree of neuromuscular block. Only 50% of cases of fade as determined by a TOFR of

0.5–0.7 were judged to have residual block using DBS, implying that this new technique has a limited ability to detect residual block in the later stages of recovery. It is also more affected by the experience and tactile sensitivity of the observer than clinical estimation of TOF fade. Its benefits have been negated by more accurate clinical monitoring tools such as the TOF Watch SX which display and record the TOFR throughout recovery.

Relevance

This was the first study to demonstrate a pattern of stimulation, other than the TOF, which can be used to more accurately detect residual neuromuscular block manually during anaesthesia and into the recovery period. A close correlation between the TOFR and DBS makes it suitable for use in clinical practice, but not for research studies.

Paper 8: Residual neuromuscular block is a risk factor for postoperative pulmonary complications

Author details

H Berg, J Viby-Mogensen, J Roed, CR Mortensen, J Engbaek, LT Skovgaard, JJ Krintel

Reference

Acta Anaesthesiologica Scandinavica 1997; **41**: 1095–103.

Summary

In this large, prospective, randomized, and blinded study, Berg and colleagues first performed a power analysis based on a previous study by Pederson *et al.* (1992). They assumed a type I error with a probability of 5% and a type II error with a probability of 20%. This suggested that 549 patients were needed to find a significant difference between muscle relaxants in this study. Allowing for uncertainties and drop-outs they finally evaluated the effect of residual neuromuscular block on the incidence of POPC in 810 patients. The patients were divided into three groups, each of 270, receiving either pancuronium, vecuronium, or atracurium. Each group was further divided into three groups of 90 patients having either major surgery of the lower extremities, gynaecological and breast operations, or major abdominal surgery.

Patients were premedicated and anaesthesia was induced with thiopentone in the majority of cases. Various techniques were used to maintain sleep. Where epidural anaesthesia was used as an adjuvant to general anaesthesia, a morphine–bupivacaine mixture was given by bolus or infusion. Patients received either pancuronium or vecuronium 0.08–0.1 mg kg^{-1}, or atracurium 0.4–0.5 mg kg^{-1} for tracheal intubation. Maintenance doses of pancuronium or vecuronium 1–2 mg and atracurium 5–10 mg were given. Neuromuscular block was reversed with neostigmine 2.5 mg preceded by atropine or glycopyrrolate and incremental doses of neostigmine 1.25 mg were given if required, to a maximum of 5 mg.

All patients were monitored peroperatively for the depth of neuromuscular block using supramaximal TOF stimulation of the ulnar nerve, repeated every 12 s and evaluated manually. The depth of block was maintained at one to two twitches and reversal was only attempted when two twitches were detectable. The patient was extubated when all four twitches of the TOF were thought to be equal on palpation, and respiration considered adequate. Hand temperature was maintained above 32°C and core temperature above 36°C throughout the study. Neuromuscular monitoring was continued using mechanomyography into the postoperative period until the train-of-four ratio (TOFR) was ≥0.8. Patients were assessed clinically by a blinded anaesthetist in the recovery room, on their ability to lift their head for 5 s, to protrude the tongue, sustain eye opening, and lift the arm above and across the body. They were followed up on the second, fourth, and sixth postoperative day for symptoms of POPC: coughing, expectoration, or pain when breathing. Chest auscultation, oxygen saturation, and central temperature were recorded. If POPC was suspected, a chest X-ray and sputum culture were performed, and the presence of pulmonary infiltrates or atelectasis determined by a radiologist confirmed the diagnosis.

The study clearly demonstrated an increased incidence of residual block with a TOFR <0.7, and significantly increased incidence of POPC in the pancuronium group compared to the vecuronium and atracurium group (Table 1.1). Other factors that increased the incidence of POPC were abdominal surgery, increasing age, and anaesthesia lasting longer than 3 h.

Table 1.1 The incidence of postoperative pulmonary complications (POPC) in relation to the first postoperative TOF ratio recorded

	Pancuronium (n=226)		Atracurium or vecuronium (n=450)	
	No. of patients	POPC n (%)	No. of patients	POPC n (%)
TOFR ≥0.70	167	8 (4.8)	426	23 (5.4)
TOFR <0.70	59	10 (16.9*)	24	1 (4.2)

*P <0.02 compared to patients in the same group with TOF ratio ≥0.70.

From Berg H, Viby-Mogensen J, Roed J, *et al*. Residual neuromuscular block is a risk factor for postoperative pulmonary complications. *Acta Anaesthesiologica Scandinavica* 1997; **41**: 1095–103, 1997, with permission from John Wiley and Sons.

Citation count

352.

Related references

1 Bevan DR, Smith CE, Donati E. Postoperative neuromuscular blockade: a comparison between atracurium, vecuronium and pancuronium. *Anesthesiology* 1988; **69**: 272–6.

2 Pedersen T, Viby-Mogensen J, Ringsted C. Anaesthetic practice and postoperative pulmonary complications. *Acta Anaesthesiol Scand* 1992; **36**: 812–18.

3 Kopman AF, Ng J, Zank LM, *et al*. Residual postoperative paralysis. *Anesthesiology* 1996; **85**: 1253–9.

Key message

Residual neuromuscular block in the immediate postoperative period, especially following the use of long-acting neuromuscular blocking agents such as pancuronium, predisposes to POPC. Another important finding in this study was that increasing age, abdominal surgery and the duration of anaesthesia increased the incidence of POPC.

Strengths

This was the first attempt in a prospective, randomized study to compare the incidence of POPC following the use of the long-acting muscle relaxant, pancuronium, with the intermediate-acting agents, vecuronium and atracurium. The clinicians anaesthetizing the patients were allowed to administer the anaesthetic technique of their choice to mimic the diversity of clinical practice in anaesthesia. Strict adherence to the diagnostic criteria for determination of POPC with continued follow-up to the sixth postoperative day makes this a powerful study. It has been widely quoted in the literature in the last 12 years, mainly because the study has never been replicated. It would be apposite now to attempt to reproduce the results to reinforce the findings.

Weaknesses

Neuromuscular block was monitored using TOF stimulation, but assessed only by hand intraoperatively. It is well recognized that DBS is superior to the TOF for manual detection of fade in the later stages of recovery and it is surprising that, in the department where DBS was first described, this technique was not used. Supplemental doses of neostigmine were given to patients on recovery on the subjective decision of the anaesthetist, which may have confused the findings. It is not clear from the data how frequently epidural analgesia was used in the patients undergoing abdominal surgery which is significant, as this technique decreases the incidence of POPC.

Relevance

This study demonstrated for the first time that the use of pancuronium is a significant risk factor in the development of POPC, especially after abdominal surgery, long operations, and in old age. With the availability of newer, shorter-acting relaxants such as atracurium and vecuronium, which are associated with a significantly lower risk of POPC, the use of pancuronium should be abandoned.

Paper 9: Functional assessment of pharynx at rest and during swallowing in partially paralyzed humans: simultaneous videomanometry and mechanomyography of awake human volunteers

Author details

LI Eriksson, R Olsson, L Nilsson, H Witt, O Ekberg, R Kuylenstierna

Reference

Anesthesiology 1997; **87**: 1035–43.

Abstract

Background: Functional characteristics of the pharynx and upper esophagus, including aspiration episodes, were investigated in 14 awake volunteers during various levels of partial neuromuscular block. Pharyngeal function was evaluated using videoradiography and computerized pharyngeal manometry during contrast bolus swallowing.

Methods: Measurements of pharyngeal constrictor muscle function (contraction amplitude, duration, and slope), upper esophageal sphincter muscle resting tone, muscle coordination, bolus transit time, and aspiration under fluoroscopic control (laryngeal or tracheal penetration) were made before (control measurements) and during a vecuronium-induced partial neuromuscular paralysis, at fixed intervals of mechanical adductor pollicis muscle train-of-four (TOF) fade; that is, at TOF ratios of 0.60, 0.70, 0.80, and after recovery to a TOF ratio >0.90.

Results: Six volunteers aspirated (laryngeal penetration) at a TOF ratio <0.90. None of them aspirated at a TOF ratio >0.90 or during control recording. Pharyngeal constrictor muscle function was not affected at any level of paralysis. The upper esophageal sphincter resting tone was significantly reduced at TOF ratios of 0.60, 0.70, and 0.80 (P <0.05). This was associated with reduced muscle coordination and shortened bolus transit time at a TOF ratio of 0.60.

Conclusions: Vecuronium-induced partial paralysis cause pharyngeal dysfunction and increased risk for aspiration at mechanical adductor pollicis TOF ratios <0.90. Pharyngeal function is not normalized until an adductor pollicis TOF ratio of >0.90 is reached. The upper esophageal sphincter muscle is more sensitive to vecuronium than is the pharyngeal constrictor muscle.

Summary

Eriksson and colleagues recruited 14 volunteers to evaluate pharyngeal function and airway protection during various degrees of neuromuscular block in the awake state. Routine monitoring (electrocardiogram [ECG], saturation of peripheral oxygen [SpO_2], non-invasive blood pressure) was set up after intravenous cannulation. A catheter with four solid-state pressure transducers was placed under radiological control such that the most distal transducer lay within the upper oesophageal sphincter, the two intermediate sensors in the pharyngeal constrictor muscles, and the most proximal sensor at the base of the tongue. Once in position, the transducers were calibrated for pressure and temperature. Videoradiographic images of boluses of barium being swallowed were collated with the manometry recordings on a colour video screen for visual monitoring and recording.

Simultaneously, neuromuscular function was recorded using mechanomyography at the adductor pollicis muscle following supramaximal TOF stimulation to the ulnar nerve at the wrist and control values taken. Skin temperature above the adductor pollicis muscle was maintained over 32°C using warming blankets. Baseline manometry and radiographic variables were measured after giving five 10-ml iodine contrast barium swallows each separated by 10 s to the volunteers in the lateral position. Vecuronium 5 mg was then infused over 20–35 min to obtain train-of-four ratios TOFRs of firstly 0.6, then 0.7, then 0.8 and lastly >0.9, at which time the infusion was stopped and spontaneous recovery was allowed. The infusion rate was kept constant for 5–10 min at each level of neuromuscular block and a mean of five consecutive TOFRs were recorded. At each level of block, five barium contrast swallows were again given. Thus each volunteer received 250 ml of contrast material.

The authors recorded the following variables at control and for TOFRs of 0.6, 0.7, 0.8, and >0.9: (1) aspiration of dye into either the laryngeal vestibule or trachea; (2) peak amplitude, slope and duration of contraction of the pharyngeal constrictor muscle; (3) upper oesophageal resting tone; (4) coordination measured by the time from start of upper oesophageal sphincter relaxation until the start of pharyngeal constrictor contraction; and, (5) bolus transit time from the faucial isthmus to the upper oesophageal sphincter.

Laryngeal but not tracheal aspiration was evident at TOFRs of 0.6 (n=4), 0.7 (n=3), and 0.8 (n=1). No aspiration was observed at a TOFR >0.9. The authors noted only minor changes in the pharyngeal constrictor muscle contraction curve at each degree of block but marked reduction of the upper oesophageal sphincter tone at TOFRs ratios of 0.6, 0.7, and 0.8 which returned to near baseline values at a TOFR >0.9. The coordination of upper oesophageal sphincter relaxation with the start of pharyngeal constrictor muscle contraction and the transit time of the contrast bolus were impaired at a TOFR of 0.6. All volunteers reported diplopia, dysarthria, and subjective difficulty in swallowing at TOFRs of 0.6 and 0.7.

Citation count

191.

Related references

1 Pavlin EG, Holle Rh, Schoene RB. Recovery of airway protection compared with ventilation in humans after partial paralysis with curare. *Anesthesiology* 1989; **70**: 381–5.

2 Isono S, Ide T, Kochi T, *et al*. Effect of partial paralysis on swallowing reflex in conscious humans. *Anesthesiology* 1991; **75**: 980–4.

3 Manning B, Winter DC, McGreal G, *et al*. Nasogastric intubation causes gastroesophageal reflux in patients undergoing elective laparotomy. *Surgery* 2001; **130**: 788–91.

4 Sundman E, Witt H, Sandin R, *et al*. Pharyngeal function and airway protection during subhypnotic concentrations of propofol, isoflurane, and sevoflurane: volunteers examined by pharyngeal videoradiography and simultaneous manometry. *Anesthesiology* 2001; **95**: 1125–32.

Key message

This was the first evidence that recovery from neuromuscular block is not complete until the TOFR at the adductor pollicis muscle is >0.9. If the patient is extubated before this degree of recovery is achieved, pulmonary aspiration of gastric contents is still possible.

Strengths

This study was conducted on awake volunteers thus eliminating any influence of a potent inhalational anaesthetic agent on the muscles of the upper airway. Attempts to control the research conditions, e.g. by maintaining the temperature of the monitored hand using an active warming device, were made.

The authors measured objective functional variables in the upper airway and upper oesophageal sphincter such as: pressure measurements (amplitude, duration, and slope of pharyngeal constrictor muscle contraction), bolus transit time, laryngeal and tracheal penetration, and glottic closure. Synchronized measurement of the TOF response at the adductor pollicis muscle to these variables was used to correlate the routinely monitored skeletal muscle paralysis with impairment of the upper oesophageal sphincter and pharyngeal constrictor muscle. Thus this study recorded a range of variables which would not have been possible under clinical conditions. The study demonstrated that the upper oesophageal sphincter is more sensitive to neuromuscular blocking agents than the pharyngeal constrictor muscles even though both groups of muscles are striated.

Weaknesses

Reduction in upper oesophageal sphincter tone may occur in the presence of a foreign body such as a nasogastric tube in the upper airway (Manning *et al.*, 2001). The transducers used in this study were passed through the upper oesophageal sphincter which could have affected the control readings. The risk of aspiration may be higher even at a TOFR >0.9 in the anaesthetized or sedated patient. None of the volunteers were followed-up for any respiratory complications from silent aspiration, making the clinical implications of these findings uncertain.

Relevance

Since 1971, adequate recovery from neuromuscular block had been considered to be a TOFR >0.6 at the adductor pollicis muscle. This original paper demonstrated that the risk of pulmonary aspiration remains a possibility until the TOFR is >0.9 at that muscle. It raised, irrevocably, the threshold criteria for adequate recovery of neuromuscular function, and a TOFR >0.9 is still considered necessary for full recovery from block today.

Paper 10: A novel concept of reversing neuromuscular block: chemical encapsulation of rocuronium bromide by a cyclodextrin-based synthetic host

Author details

A Bom, M Bradley, K Cameron, JK Clark, J Van Egmond, H Feilden, EJ MacLean, AW Muir, R Palin, DC Rees, MQ Zhang

Reference

Angewandte Chemie International Edition 2002; **41**: 266–70.

Summary

This pioneering research aimed to develop an entirely new molecule to reverse the aminosteroidal neuromuscular blocking agent (NMBA), rocuronium, by encapsulation (chelation) rather than by its action as an anticholinesterase. The paper outlines the process of development of the molecule (Org 25969). Bom and colleagues measured the size of the cavity of a group of cyclic oligosaccharides, the α-, β-, and γ-cyclodextrins (CDs), which are known to encapsulate lipophilic molecules such as steroids. Gamma-cyclodextrins, consisting of a ring of eight glucopyranose units, were found to have the largest cavity (7.9 Å) and formed the most stable complex with rocuronium. The binding affinity of the cyclodextrin host to rocuronium was further enhanced by increasing the cavity depth using thioethers to link the glucopyranoside units. This also increased the hydrophobic interaction inside the cavity which improves its affinity for steroidal compounds. In contrast, introduction of anionic carboxyl groups on to the outer rim of the cavity maintained the water solubility of the host molecule. When tested *in vitro* in mouse hemidiaphragm, Org 25969 consistently formed a very tight binding complex with rocuronium. The association constant (K_a) as determined by isothermal titration calorimetry (ITC) is about $10^7 M^{-1}$, making it one of the most stable complexes between a cyclodextrin and an organic guest ever reported. It is comparable with the attraction of acetylcholine to the α-subunit of the postsynaptic nicotinic receptor. The complete and stable encapsulation of rocuronium by Org 25969 was confirmed by X-ray crystallography. When tested *in vivo* in guinea pigs, cats, and monkeys, Org 25969 demonstrated rapid, reproducible and complete recovery from rocuronium-induced neuromuscular block without significant adverse cardiovascular effects. Recovery from block was much faster than with the use of neostigmine and atropine.

Citation count

167.

Related references

1 Szente J, Szejtli J. Highly soluble cyclodextrin derivatives: chemistry, properties, and trends in development. *Adv Drug Deliv Rev* 1999; **36**: 17–28.

2 Epemolu O, Bom A, Hope F, *et al.* Reversal of neuromuscular blockade and simultaneous increase in plasma rocuronium concentration after the intravenous infusion of the novel reversal agent Org 25969. *Anesthesiology* 2003; **99**: 632–7.

3 Zhang M-Q. Drug-specific cyclodextrins: The future of rapid neuromuscular block reversal? *Drugs Future* 2003; **28**: 347–54.

4 Gijsenbergh F, Ramael S, Houwing N, *et al.* First human exposure of Org 25969. A novel agent to reverse the action of rocuronium bromide. *Anesthesiology* 2005; **103**: 695–703.

5 Duvaldestin P, Kuizenga K, Saldien V. A randomized, dose-response study of sugammadex given for the reversal of deep rocuronium- or vecuronium-induced neuromuscular blockade under sevoflurane anesthesia (Anesthetic Pharmacology: Brief Report). *Anesth Analg* 2010; **110**: 74–82.

Key message

This discovery heralds the advent of a completely different approach to reversal of steroidal NMBAs. The maximum effect of Org 25969 (now known as sugammadex) is significantly faster than with the use of anticholinesterases such as neostigmine (2 min versus 9 min respectively) or spontaneous recovery. Sugammadex does not, however, reverse the residual effects of benzylisoquinoline NMBAs.

Strengths

This is the first purpose-designed molecule to be developed for use in anaesthesia using the process of chemical encapsulation. A γ-cyclodextrin was systematically modified to enable it to completely encapsulate and form a highly stable host–guest assembly with rocuronium which is then excreted in the urine. In the correct dose, sugammadex reverses rocuronium-induced block at three times the rate of neostigmine with no significant side effects as yet reported. Sugammadex is unique in its ability to reverse profound block (post-tetanic count of 1–2) when used in the correct dose (4–8 mg kg^{-1}), which it is well accepted that neostigmine is unable to do. Sugammadex may be particularly useful in a 'cannot intubate, cannot ventilate' scenario when 8–16 mg kg^{-1} reverses block immediately after a high dose of rocuronium (1.2 mg kg^{-1}). Its use with rocuronium will also avoid the side effects of succinylcholine given during rapid sequence induction.

Weaknesses

Sugammadex only encapsulates the aminosteroidal NMBA, rocuronium, and to a slightly lesser extent, vecuronium. It has been reported anecdotally to reverse pancuronium, but its affinity for this older aminosteroid is much less than for rocuronium. It has no action on benzylisoquinoline NMBAs (although it is easy to imagine some anaesthetists trying to reverse these drugs with sugammadex).

The ability of sugammadex to encapsulate drugs of similar structure such as cortisone, atropine, hormonal contraceptives, remifentanil, fusidic acid, and flucloxacillin is 120–700 times less than that of rocuronium. Only after thousands of patient exposures will it be possible to determine whether such interactions have any clinical significance. Although it is considered to be biologically inert, there have reports in volunteer studies of allergic reactions to sugammadex, one of which has been substantiated by a positive skin test. It is therefore too soon in the clinical use of this drug to be certain of its side effects and their incidence. The excretion of the sugammadex–rocuronium complex almost entirely in the urine may alter its effect in patients with renal failure.

Relevance

It may be advantageous in certain patients to avoid the muscarinic effects of anticholinesterases. Previous attempts to develop reversal agents which act independently of the cholinergic system have been unsuccessful. Sugammadex will rapidly reverse profound neuromuscular block from rocuronium and vecuronium which neostigmine is unable to do. But neuromuscular monitoring is still advisable to determine the dose of sugammadex required for reversal. The much greater cost of sugammadex compared to neostigmine may well be a limiting factor to its routine use in anaesthetic practice.

Chapter 2

Anaesthetic equipment

NJ Allan and AT Cohen

Introduction

The design, manufacture, and evolution of specialist anaesthetic equipment is key to the development of the speciality of anaesthesia. Modern computer-driven technology continues this advance with particular emphasis on safety.

As with any evolutionary process, attempting to identify the key developments that have significantly led to a change in practice is difficult. We present a series of articles in chronological order identifying important papers from many aspects of anaesthetic practice. Papers identifying crucial advancement in the fields of airway devices, measurement, monitoring, and delivering of anaesthesia are discussed. Some of the earlier publications contain little information but were enough to change practice. We have selected one publication that is a modern review but makes remarkable reading.

Most hospital anaesthesia is delivered using a variant of Boyle's machine. Popularization of such machines allowed the practice of anaesthesia to become widespread. The original description (Paper 1) is remarkable in its brevity. Regional anaesthesia was hampered in popularity by the high incidence of post-dural puncture headache. Greene (Paper 2) suggested a solution to this problem by promoting atraumatic, small calibre spinal needles. Macintosh in Paper 3 describes the reasoning behind the creation of what is now one of the most widely used laryngoscopes worldwide. It seems unlikely that Seldinger, a radiologist, had any idea what the ramifications would be of a technique he described in Paper 4 to allow exchange of intravascular devices over a wire. The technique and equipment is widely used in many anaesthetic procedures, including vascular lines, emergency airways, and chest drains. Measurement of tissue and blood oxygen tension and saturation, as a consequence of Clark's electrode, Paper 5, and the pulse oximeter, Paper 7, are essential to safe anaesthetic practice. The Fluotec vaporizer (Paper 6) is the first in a series of temperature and flow compensated vaporizers allowing accurate administration of anaesthetic vapours. Painstaking work over many years resulted in the development of a new airway, Paper 8, that had many advantages over the tracheal tube, being easier to place without causing laryngeal irritation.

As computers became more commonplace and miniaturized, Kenny and White (Paper 9) showed that it was possible to use an electronic personal organizer to control a drug infusion using pharmacokinetic theory and data. We chose the last paper (Paper 10) as a description of the extraordinary risks to patients and staff of administering anaesthesia in the past.

Paper 1: New inventions: nitrous-oxide-oxygen-ether outfit

Author details

H Edmund and G Boyle

Reference

Lancet 1919; **1**: 226.

Summary

This is a short description of an early machine used to administer a combination of nitrous oxide, oxygen, and ether (see Fig. 2.1). The equipment included oxygen and nitrous oxide cylinders enclosed in a container. Each of the oxygen cylinders had a pressure gauge attached, with adjustable reducing valves. There is a small spirit lamp to warm the valves on the nitrous oxide cylinders to prevent obstruction from freezing of water vapour. An ether bottle is connected into the circuit, which is completed by a rebreathing bag, a three-way stopcock, and a face piece.

There are three different sizes of machine: a large size for work overseas; a medium size for work in domestic hospitals; and a small portable size version. The differences between these machines are their mobility and cylinder capacity.

Over 3,600 anaesthetics are described using this equipment, with no reported fatalities.

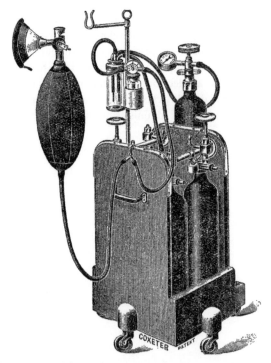

Fig. 2.1 Boyle's machine. Reprinted from *The Lancet*, **193**, 4980, H. Edmund and G. Boyle, New Inventions –Nitrous-Oxide-Oxygen-Ether Outfit, p. 226, 1919, with permission from Elsevier.

Citation count

Not available.

Related references

1 Gwathmey JT. Practical methods of anaesthesia. *Br Med J* 1917; **1**: 393–4.

2 Boyle HEG. The use of nitrous oxide and oxygen with rebreathing in military surgery. *Br Med J* 1917; **2**: 653–5.

3 Thompson PW, Wilkinson DJ. Development of anaesthetic machines. *Br J Anaesth* 1985; **57**: 640–8.

Key message

Boyle brought together all the components of a modern anaesthetic delivery system into a purpose built, portable machine allowing delivery of nitrous oxide, oxygen, and volatile agents.

Strengths

In this paper Boyle describes his invention, which was the forerunner of the modern anaesthetic machine. Many of the basic components remain.

Weaknesses

There is very little detail of the workings and structure of the machine. No description of the successful anaesthetics administered using the apparatus is presented.

Relevance

Henry Edmund Gaskin Boyle is a name that is synonymous with anaesthetic equipment history. His original Boyle's machine was produced by the instrument makers Coxeters and copied many of the features of the gas and oxygen machine produced by James Tayloe Gwathmey, an American anaesthetist. It contained cylinders, reducing valves, water-sight flowmeters, and a metal and glass ether vaporizer (a Boyle's bottle). One of the major differences was the connectivity of English oxygen cylinders. Cotton and Boothby designed the 'bubble bottle' flowmeters in 1912. The ability to control and measure, as well as humidify, gas flow was essential to this equipment.

The equipment gained popularity through its use with the British army treating wounded soldiers in France during World War I. Geoffrey Marshall used the machine on the front line, and suggested a number of modifications to the design such as the addition of a second vaporizing bottle. Further modifications have included exchanging the water-sight flowmeter with the more accurate variable area flowmeter and the introduction of a non-interchangeable pin index safety system.

Paper 2: Lumbar puncture and the prevention of postpuncture headache

Author details

HM Greene

Reference

Journal of the American Medical Association 1926; **86**: 391–2.

Summary

The paper describes methods to reduce the incidence of headache following lumbar puncture. Lumbar puncture is achieved using a four-step approach: the patient is kept still on a table; local anaesthetic is applied to the skin; a rounded tapering needle is inserted; and cerebrospinal fluid aspirated on visualization.

The size and the shape of the spinal needle are especially important. The needle tip is described as round, tapering, and sharp so that it may pass between the longitudinal fibres of the dura mater without cutting them. A small-gauge needle is preferable to both reduce the size of the hole made in the dura, and to allow the needle to bend rather than break.

Two hundred and fifteen lumbar punctures have been performed using the described technique with two headaches reported.

Citation count

67.

Related references

1 Hart JR, Whitacre RJ. Pencil-point needle in prevention of postspinal headache. *JAMA* 1951; **147**: 657–8.

2 Calthorpe N. The history of spinal needles: Getting to the point. *Anaesthesia* 2004; **59**: 1231–41.

Key message

The incidence of postpuncture headache can be reduced by using a finer, atraumatic needle.

Strengths

A clear description, with good illustrations, of a technique and equipment thought to be associated with less trauma to the dura supported by data showing a reduced incidence of headache.

Weaknesses

No true trial data is presented as evidence that this technique reduces postspinal headaches. The usual incidence of postdural puncture headache is not presented.

Relevance

Spinal anaesthesia, or the injection of analgesic and anaesthetic into the subarachnoid space, is a popular anaesthetic technique worldwide. It is commonly used for interventions below the umbilicus as a means to avoid the complications of general anaesthesia. It is frequently used for Caesarean sections, lower limb surgery, and urological surgery.

The idea of spinal regional anaesthesia was developed in the 1880s when J. Leonard Corning accidentally injected cocaine into the subarachnoid space of dogs, causing paralysis. Following this, Augustus Karl Gustav Bier (after practising on himself and his assistant), demonstrated spinal anaesthesia for surgical patients. The needles used tended to be large-calibre, cutting needles, causing damage to the dura resulting in cerebrospinal fluid (CSF) leakage. Postdural puncture headache was therefore a common occurrence. Needles of finer calibre with an introducer were designed to overcome the problem.

Despite the use of finer needles postdural puncture headache remained a significant problem, limiting the widespread use of spinal anaesthesia. This paper describes the first atraumatic spinal needle, which significantly reduced the incidence of headaches, and therefore made spinal anaesthesia a more attractive proposition. The Greene needle became extremely popular with manufacturing continuing until the 1980s.

The design of a completely non-cutting tip or pencil point needle was credited to Hart and Whitacre in 1951. This further reduced the incidence of postdural puncture headache.

Paper 3: A new laryngoscope

Author details

RR Macintosh

Reference

Lancet 1943; **1**: 205.

Summary

Macintosh's paper describes the first curve bladed laryngoscope. The short curved blade is inserted to the right of the tongue, pushing the tongue to the left. The blade is designed so that when in position its tip fits into the angle created by the epiglottis and base of tongue. The laryngoscope handle is lifted causing the base of the tongue to be pushed forwards and the epiglottis is drawn upwards revealing the larynx (Fig. 2.2).

It is postulated that as the blade does not come into contact with the back surface of the epiglottis, which is innervated by the superior laryngeal nerve, then the larynx can be exposed at a lighter plane of anaesthesia. The blade can be folded onto the handle when not in use, or removed for sterilization.

Citation count

64.

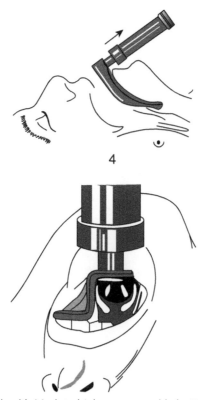

4

Fig. 2.2 View of the epiglottis with Macintosh's laryngoscope blade. Reprinted from *The Lancet*, **241**, 6233, R. R. Macintosh, A New Laryngoscope, p. 205, 1943, with permission from Elsevier.

Related references

1 Miller RA. A new laryngoscope. *Anesthesiology* 1941; **2**: 317–20.

2 Janeway HH. Intra-tracheal anesthesia from the standpoint of the nose, throat and oral surgeon with a description of a new instrument for catheterizing the trachea. *Laryngoscope* 1913; **23**: 1082–90.

3 Jepworth A. The Macintosh laryngoscope – A historical note on its clinical and commercial development. *Anaesthesia* 1984; **39**: 474–9.

Key message

Following his observation that a curved blade was associated with better visualization of the vocal cords and less airway stimulation Macintosh describes the first curved blade laryngoscope.

Strengths

The Macintosh blade has a number of successful design features. The strengths are compared to other blades currently available.

Weaknesses

There are no details of clinical trials or discussion of potential complications.

Relevance

The Macintosh blade is probably the most widely used laryngoscope in the UK and is extensively used throughout the world. This paper explains the reasons for the transition from the conventional straight blade, e.g. Miller's, to a curved blade. The straight blades are designed to pass beyond the epiglottis to evert it. This may lead to damage of the upper teeth or posterior pharyngeal wall. The Macintosh blade is inserted up to the vallecula and pulled forward to elevate the epiglottis. The blade was designed from a traditional Boyle–Davis gag, used for tonsillectomy, after it was recognized that visualization of the cords was better, at a lighter plane of anaesthesia, with an oversized Davis gag.

There are now several different Macintosh styles, depending upon their country of origin. The English (Classic), American (Standard), or German designs alter depending upon their flange shape and height, as well as their light position and type. Macintosh did not promote the need for different blade sizes depending on patient anatomy and size, although large adult, adult, child, and infant sizes are now widely available. There have been a number of developments of the Macintosh blade. A left-handed variety is available for when anatomical features of the airway require an endotracheal tube to be passed to the left side of the mouth. The McCoy blade is a more recent variation, which has an articulating distal tip connected to a lever on the laryngoscope handle. When activated the tissue at the base of the tongue is elevated, improving epiglottis lift and laryngeal exposure. Although it may make difficult laryngoscopy easier, it is also recognized to worsen laryngeal views in some patients.

Paper 4: Catheter replacement of the needle in percutaneous arteriography; a new technique

Author details

SI Seldinger

Reference

Acta Radiologica 1953; **39**: 368–76.

Abstract

The author describes a method by which it is possible, after percutaneous puncture, to insert a catheter of the same size as the needle used into an artery.

SI Seldinger, 'Catheter replacement of the needle in percutaneous arteriography; a new technique', *Acta Radiologica*, 1953, 39, pp. 368–376.

Summary

The paper describes current equipment and techniques used for inserting vascular catheters for angiography, highlighting the advantages of injecting contrast medium through an indwelling catheter as compared to a simple needle. One disadvantage of using a catheter is that it requires a larger puncture site than using a needle as the catheter is inserted through the lumen of a needle or trocar. This results in additional trauma to the artery as well as increasing the risk of haemorrhage.

Seldinger presents a technique used at Karolinska Sjukhuset, whereby a flexible leader (guide wire) is inserted into the needle used for puncture. A catheter, which is the same size as the original needle, is then fed over the guide wire (Fig. 2.3).

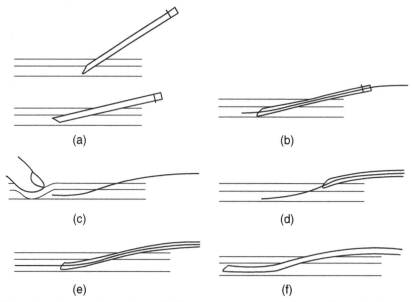

Fig. 2.3 Insertion of a vascular catheter. (a) The artery is punctured. The needle pushed upwards. (b) The leader inserted. (c) The needle withdrawn and the artery compressed. (d) The catheter threaded on to the leader. (e) The catheter inserted into the artery. (f) The leader withdrawn. Reproduced with permission from the Royal Society of Medicine Press Ltd. Seldinger SI. Catheter replacement of the needle in percutaneous arteriography; a new technique. *Acta Radiologica* 1953; **39**: 368–76.

The main advantage of this technique is that a smaller sized needle is needed for a given catheter, and so larger catheters can be used. The larger radius allows greater flow rates.

The paper presents a series of 40 catheterizations of both the femoral and brachial arteries. Complications such as failure to catheterize, resistance to threading the wire, damage to the arterial wall, and extravasations are reported.

Citation count

2,360.

Related references

1 Farinas PL. A new technique for the arteriographic examination of the abdominal aorta and its braches. *Am J Roentgenol* 1941; **46**: 641.

2 Higgs ZC, Macafee DA, Braithwaite BD, *et al*. The Seldinger technique: 50 years on. *Lancet* 2005; **366**: 1407–9.

Key message

A novel technique for minimizing traumatic complications when placing large-bore intraluminal lines is described.

Strengths

A very clear description of the equipment and technique required for the catheterization of the vascular tree. A case series is included.

Weaknesses

The case series is small with a high complication rate including extravascular injection of contrast and arterial damage. A larger case series is required to understand these complications.

Relevance

The equipment used and technique described by Seldinger in this paper have become important for many clinical procedures that could not have been envisaged by the author. The National Institute for Health and Clinical Excellence (NICE) recommends that all central venous access procedures should be performed using the Seldinger technique with ultrasound visualization. Arterial lines, tracheostomies, chest drains, pacemakers, percutaneous endoscopic gastrostomy (PEG) tubes, and many other invasive clinical procedures rely on the use of a catheter exchange method based on Seldinger's technique. Often dilators and stiffeners are also used to allow catheters larger than the initial needle to be inserted.

The Seldinger technique is an important part of interventional radiology, allowing diverse procedures such as balloon angiography and vascular and non-vascular stents to be inserted into various parts of the body. This has replaced some high-risk surgeries including coronary artery bypass and open abdominal aortic aneurysm grafting.

Paper 5: Continuous recording of blood oxygen tensions by polarography

Author details

LC Clark Jr, R Wolf, D Granger, Z Taylor

Reference

Journal of Applied Physiology 1953; **6**: 189–93.

Abstract

A shiny platinum cathode covered with a layer of cellophane has been found to be suitable for the direct measurement of oxygen tension in whole blood by polarographic procedures. The cellophane covering prevents the undesirable effects of the red cells which interfere with oxygen tension measurements using a bare platinum electrode, and in addition nearly abolishes the 'stirring effect.' A tiny cathode of this type (2 mm diameter and 8 mm long) mounted on a catheter can be passed into the major blood vessels and chambers of the heart, for continuous recording of oxygen tension. Such cathodes are easily calibrated and are stable, reproducible and sensitive.

LC Clark Jr, R Wolf, D Granger, and Z Taylor, 'Continuous recording of blood oxygen tensions by polarography', *Journal of Applied Physiology*, 1953, 6, pp. 189–193, by permission of the American Physiology Society.

Summary

This paper introduces a method of measuring oxygen content in electrolyte solutions and body tissues, describing problems encountered due to red cell interference. The circuit described uses a platinum cathode maintained at 0.6 volts with respect to a potassium chloride-calomel anode. The oxygen in solution is reduced causing current to flow, which is proportional to the oxygen content.

Clark *et al*. describe a solution to the problem of red cell interference by protecting the platinum cathode with a cellophane membrane (see Fig. 2.4).

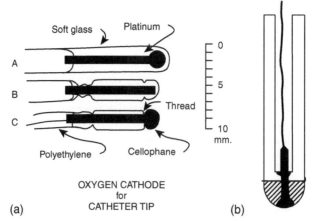

Fig. 2.4 Construction of cathodes. (a) The electrode constructed for measurement of oxygen tension *in vitro*—cathode is sealed in glass tubing A, moulded and ground to reduce diameter B, and surrounded by cellophane C. (b) A smaller electrode, sealed in capillary tubing, for measurement in the heart and vascular tree. With kind permission of the American Physiological Society. From Clark LC Jr, Wolf R, Granger D, Taylor Z. Continuous recording of blood oxygen tensions by polarography. *Journal of Applied Physiology* 1953; **6**: 189–93.

The paper describes the effects of the cellophane covering, commenting on the current flow, length of time required for equilibration, and temperature. Experimental evidence involving a cathode inserted into the aorta of a dog is presented.

Citation count

491.

Related references

1 Severinghaus JW, Austrup PB. History of blood gas analysis. IV. The Clark oxygen electrode. *J Clin Monit* 1986; **2**: 125–39.

Key message

Modification of polarographic electrode enables creation of a reliable method for measuring oxygen tension in blood and *in vivo* in tissue.

Strengths

A clear description of the development of the polarograph electrode is presented.

Weaknesses

Minimal trial data are available.

Relevance

Polarographic techniques had been previously investigated as a method of measuring oxygen tension in solutions and tissues, but had failed due to interference from red blood cells at the cathode. Clark's electrode overcame these problems by incorporating a cellophane covering allowing the accurate and calibrated measurement of the partial pressure of oxygen in blood.

With further development, including replacing the oxygen permeable cellophane membrane with PTFE (polytetrafluoroethylene), the Clark electrode has become a standard method for analysing oxygen *in vivo*. The electrode is incorporated into arterial blood gas analysers to give a reading of arterial oxygen tension as well as in intravenous catheters floated into the vasculature giving a continuous reading of oxygen tension. It is also used in transcutaneous monitoring of oxygen content in neonates. In addition to its use for measuring the tension of oxygen in blood samples, the electrode can also be used for measuring the oxygen in gas mixtures.

The electrode is used extensively in industry in several fields, including food manufacture, the aviation industry, and civil engineering.

Paper 6: Clinical evaluation of fluothane with special reference to a controlled percentage vaporizer

Author details

IM MacKay

Reference

Canadian Anaesthesia Society Journal 1957; **4**: 235–45.

Abstract

A series of 203 surgical and obstetrical patients anaesthetized with Fluothane at the Toronto General Hospital is presented. The methods and technique used and special apparatus available are discussed and clinical observations are given in detail.

With kind permission from Springer Science+Business Media: *Canadian Anaesthesia Society Journal*, 'Clinical evaluation of fluothane with special reference to a controlled percentage vaporizer', 4, 3, 1957, pp. 235–45, IM Mackay.

Summary

This paper primarily concentrates on a series of 203 cases of anaesthesia using a new anaesthetic vapour, 2 brom, 2 chlor, 1,1,1 fluoro-ethane, referred to as Fluothane (Halothane). Special reference is made of different methods and vaporizing chambers used to administer Fluothane. The new Fluotec (Cyprane) vaporizer is used in 144 of these cases.

The Fluotec Vaporizer is described as a temperature compensated, controlled percentage vaporizer manufactured in England. The concentration of Fluothane is most accurately controlled using a non-rebreathing technique with adequate gas flows, although it can also be used using a partial rebreathing technique using carbon dioxide absorption. It is calibrated to deliver 0.5–3.0% Fluothane within a gas flow of 4–16 l per minute at between 55–90°F, by means of a temperature compensated valve.

Fig. 2.5 demonstrate the mechanism of the vaporizer. Fig. 2.5a is in the 'off' position, with Fig. 2.5b in the open position.

In the off position, Fig. 2.5a, gas enters at A and passes through the bypass valve G to B and on to the patient. None of the vapour can mix into the gas flow. When the control, M, is rotated the spindle, F moves to the right, opening the vaporizing chamber, causing splitting of the gas flow (Fig. 2.5b). Some gas passes through port C into the vaporizing chamber, N. Here it picks up Fluothane. A bi-metallic strip, J, temperature regulates the outflow of the vaporizing chamber at H. From here the vapour rich gas flow mixes with the "clean" bypass gas at E to reach the patient. L is the filling funnel, and K is the level window.

The paper describes the most commonly encountered physiological effects of Fluothane, concluding that the most satisfactory and safest method at present available appears to be the non-rebreathing continuous flow circuit (nitrous oxide and oxygen) with the Fluotec temperature compensated vaporizer.

Citation count

35.

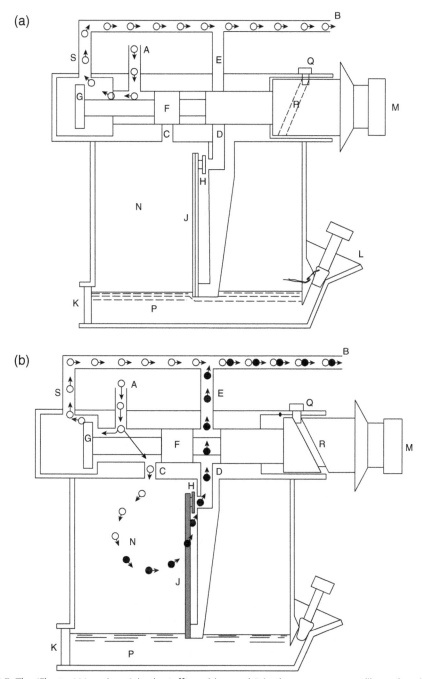

Fig. 2.5 The 'Fluotec' Vaporizer A in the 'off' position and B in the open or any calibrated position. With kind permission from Springer Science+Business Media: *Canadian Journal of Anaesthesia*, Clinical evaluation of fluothane with special reference to a controlled percentage vaporizer, **4**, 1957, pp. 235–245, I. M. Mackay.

Related references

1 Junker FE. A description of a new apparatus for administering narcotic vapours. *Med Times Gazette* 1867; 590.

2 Morris LE. A new vaporizer for liquid anesthetic agents. *Anesthesiology* 1952; **13**: 587.

Key message

Fluothane is a very potent anaesthetic agent in which minor variations in concentration can produce profound clinical effects. The Fluotec vaporizer is a safe and efficient vaporizer to provide control of the concentration of this uniquely potent agent.

Strengths

A new potent anaesthetic vapour is presented with potential pharmacological and physiological benefits and drawbacks. The temperature and flow compensated Fluotec vaporizer is a solution to some of these problems.

Weaknesses

The article seems to be two papers written as one. The presentation of a new potent anaesthetic vapour, Fluothane, and the presentation of a novel way of controlling the delivery of such a potent anaesthetic. It would have been better to separate these descriptions.

Relevance

The introduction of a temperature regulated, calibrated vaporizer was one of the key reasons for the success of the potent anaesthetic agent Halothane. Prior to Fluothane's introduction, two types of temperature compensated systems for the delivery of anaesthetic vapours had been developed. The first was Lucien Morris's Copper Kettle, developed in the USA, used for the administration of chloroform. The gas flow was percolated through the chloroform, causing it to become fully saturated. A thermometer was later added to indicate changes in temperature, which would allow, with some difficulty, calculation of the effect on vapour pressure. At the same time in Britain, an automated system, the TECOTA (Temperature Compensated Trichloroethylene Air) vaporizer, was being developed. This featured a bimetallic strip made of brass and nickel-steel. The technology from this vaporizer was incorporated in the 'Fluotec' vaporizer.

We believe this paper is the first article published with a full description of the Fluotec vaporizer. This vaporizer is the first in a series of 'Tec' vaporizers, manufactured by Cyprane, a British anaesthetic equipment manufacturer founded by William Edmondson and Wilfred Jones in Keighley, West Yorkshire. Tec vaporizers are now extensively used in anaesthesia throughout the world.

These vaporizers have evolved in a number of ways to minimize problems with use including positioning of the bimetallic strip, filling systems, and anti-spill mechanisms. The bimetallic strip is positioned inside the vaporization chamber in the Tec mark 2 whereas it has been moved outside in later models. Various safety features have been added to more recent vaporizers, including locking levers, preventing accidental switch on and interlocking extension rods preventing concurrent vaporizer use. Modern anaesthetic agents require differently calibrated Tec models, with the Tec mark 6 being exclusively used for Desflurane. This vaporizer has internal heating to compensate for Desflurane's unique physical properties.

Paper 7: Spectrophotometric monitoring of arterial oxygen saturation in the fingertip

Author details

I Yoshiya, Y Shimada, K Tanaka

Reference

Medical & Biological Engineering & Computing 1980; **18**: 27–32.

Summary

This paper describes the principle of operation, functional characteristics, and problems in clinical application of one of the first commercially available non-invasive pulse oximeters (Oximet Model MET-1471).

A halogen light source is transmitted via an optical transmitter to a finger probe. The light is then filtered to transmit only light of wavelengths 650 and 805 nm, the absorption coefficients of haemoglobin and oxyhaemoglobin. The attenuation produced by the tissues of the finger is subtracted out, leaving only that due to pulsatile blood. Using Beer's law, the percentage of oxyhaemoglobin to total haemoglobin can be calculated and displayed on a digital reading.

The accuracy of the instrument is assessed by comparing arterial oxygen saturations with blood-gas oxygen saturations in 15 intensive care patients, (Fig. 2.6). The oxygen saturation measured with the instrument is within ±5% of that obtained from the blood-gas method.

Reproducibility is assessed by measuring arterial oxygen saturation 60 times in a healthy volunteer breathing air.

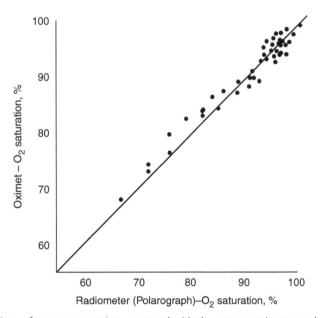

Fig. 2.6 Comparison of oxygen saturation measured with the present oximeter and the blood-gas method. With kind permission from Springer Science+Business Media: *Medical & Biological Engineering & Computing*, Spectrophotometric monitoring of arterial oxygen saturation in the fingertip, **18**, 1980, pp. 27–32, I. Yoshiya, Y. Shimada, K. Tanaka.

Problems relating to finger movement and blood pressure cuffs distorting readings are then explored.

Citation count

181.

Related references

1 Yelderman M, New W. Evaluation of pulse oximetry. *Anesthesiology* 1983; **59**: 349–52.

Key message

This is the first description we could find of a safe, non-invasive device that measures arterial oxygen saturation with compensation for variations in blood flow and haemoglobin.

Strengths

The authors describe the use of microprocessor and fibreoptic technology to allow arterial oxygen saturation to be estimated. The theoretical basis and electronics used in the equipment are detailed. The accuracy, reproducibility, and problems experienced are described.

Weaknesses

The clinical data supporting the claims for accuracy and reproducibility are limited. Calibration at low arterial oxygen levels in a healthy population is missing. There is no discussion of the effect of abnormal haemoglobin on the readings.

Relevance

The modern pulse oximeter is an essential piece of monitoring equipment in any hospital setting where a patient's oxygenation may be unstable. It is used extensively in operating theatres, recovery, intensive care, emergency departments, and wards. The monitor can quickly guide the effective use of supplemental oxygen therapy in critically ill patients. Prior to its development, measurement of arterial oxygenation was via intermittent sampling; transcutaneous oxygen tension measurement or 'arterialization' of the ear vasculature and measurement of light absorption. All of these methods were invasive, intermittent, or unreliable. The pulse oximeter indirectly measures the oxygen saturation of a patient's blood while compensating for changes in tissue blood volume, by subtracting the pulsatile component from the non-pulsatile flesh and bone.

This paper presents the theoretical and physical basis of a pulse oximeter, with a description of calibration and potential problems encountered. This is the forerunner of the modern light-emitting diode (LED), microprocessor-driven unit. Recent advances have reduced the size and incorporated batteries into monitors, making the equipment increasingly portable.

Paper 8: The laryngeal mask – a new concept in airway management

Author details

AIJ Brain

Reference

British Journal of Anaesthesia 1983; **55**: 801–5.

Abstract

A new type of airway is described, which may be used as an alternative to either the endotracheal tube or the face-mask with either spontaneous or positive pressure ventilation. The results of a pilot study involving 23 patients are presented and the possible merits and disadvantages of the device are discussed, bearing in mind that the study is of a preliminary nature.

Summary

This paper describes the concept, first clinical prototype and pilot trial of the laryngeal mask airway (LMA). The prototype was constructed of a Goldman paediatric dental mask stretched and fixed onto the diagonally cut end of a Portex 10-mm endotracheal tube. The device is easily inserted into the hypopharynx via the mouth, provided that it is inserted backwards and then rotated through 180 degrees as it is passed downwards into position behind the larynx.

A pilot trial using 23 patients is described, evaluating ease of use and feasibility in spontaneously breathing and ventilated patients.

Citation count

654.

Related references

1 Brain AIJ, McGhee TD, McAteer EJ, *et al*. The laryngeal mask airway – development and preliminary trials of a new type of airway. *Anaesthesia* 1985; **40**: 356–61.

Key message

The LMA may be a simple alternative to endotracheal intubation, avoiding complications arising from the requirement to visualize and penetrate the laryngeal opening.

Strengths

The paper describes in detail the concept and manufacture of the LMA prototype and presents a case series of patients in whom it is used. It is suggested that the important features were ease and simplicity of use and the fact that the device was well tolerated without serious side effects.

Weaknesses

This is a preliminary study. The case numbers are too small to reach firm conclusions about the LMA's likely success.

Relevance

Over time this has become a highly prophetic article. Laryngeal mask airways are now key equipment in both standard anaesthetic practice and in management of the difficult airway. This piece of equipment has popularized the use of supraglottic airway devices, where other equipment, such as the oesophageal obturator airway, failed. The LMA has allowed patients having short procedures to be cared for by an anaesthetist whose ability to respond to events is not restricted by holding onto a facemask. More complex cases are now preformed without the requirement for endotracheal intubation on both spontaneously breathing and mechanically ventilated patients. The LMA is also a key component of the difficult intubation drill. The device itself has evolved with paediatric, flexible, and disposable varieties now available. Newer designs have been produced to help with intubation for example with a silicon cuff and with suction and gastric tube insertion points.

Paper 9: A portable target controlled propofol infusion system

Author details

GNC Kenny and M White

Reference

International Journal of Clinical Monitoring and Computing 1992; **9**: 179–82.

Abstract

A portable target controlled infusion system for propofol has been developed based on a Psion hand-held microcomputer and the Ohmeda 9000 syringe pump. The system uses a pharmacokinetic model which describes the distribution and elimination of propofol to achieve and maintain any selected target blood concentration. Target blood concentrations of 1 μg/ml, 3 μg/ml and 5 μg/ml were selected in laboratory trials and the cumulative volumes delivered by the Psion system each minute were compared with the theoretical output calculated by the pharmacokinetic model. The results obtained showed that the computer system delivered volumes which were always within 2% of the theoretical values. This system offers a convenient and simple method of maintaining anaesthesia using propofol.

Summary

This paper describes a totally portable, battery-driven propofol infusion system using a simple handheld computer, a Psion organizer (an early personal digital assistant [PDA]), connected to a modified syringe pump (Ohmeda 9000). They are connected via a specially produced interface backbar by Ohmeda, which includes a rechargeable battery source. The control programme, written on the Psion organizer, requests details of the patient's age and body weight, and the initial target blood concentration of propofol. A bolus of propofol is then infused and the program predicts the blood concentration achieved every second. Once this is within 1% of the selected target, it is kept at this value by infusing propofol at the rate required to compensate for redistribution and elimination of the drug.

The device is calibrated against a previous designed, computer-based pharmacokinetic model, and has been shown to be accurate to within 2% of the theoretical values.

The paper comments on the successful trial of over 80 systems in 11 countries.

Citation count

34.

Related references

1 White M, Kenny GNC. Intravenous propofol anaesthesia using a computerised infusion system. *Anaesthesia* 1990; **45**; 204–9.

2 Glass PSA, Markham K, Ginsberg B, *et al*. Propofol concentrations required for surgery. *Anesthesiology* 1989; **71**(Suppl): A273.

Key message

This is the first description of a portable, battery-driven drug infusion system for use during routine anaesthesia. The system proves easy to use even when transporting patients.

Strengths

The paper summarizes previous attempts to produce a total intravenous anaesthesia (TIVA) delivery device. It describes a new system that obviates the need for an external mains powered computer. There is a description of the new equipment and its calibration.

Weaknesses

The author describes multiple trials of this equipment, but minimal data are presented.

Relevance

Interest in TIVA increased with the introduction of propofol during the 1980s, due to its desirable pharmacokinetic profile, its quality of recovery, and anti-emetic effects.

   The paper selected continues a series of papers describing the development of equipment required to produce safe, effective, and manageable TIVA. The mathematics of the pharmacokinetic model for target-controlled infusion (TCI) of propofol were derived and standardized several years prior to this publication, allowing the development of computer-driven systems. The first attempt was via a desktop computer (Atari 1040ST) connected to an Imed 929 volumetric pump via an RS-232 interface. Although the system worked, it was impractical due to its bulk. The key advantage of the system reported in this article is its portability and ease of use; however, safety features were not incorporated in this prototype. In 1996 the 'Diprifusor' system was introduced by Zeneca Pharmaceuticals. This system packaged the computer model and required safety features into one easy-to-use infusion pump. Since the development of accurate, usable target infusion pumps, TIVA has become increasingly popular.

Paper 10: A short history of fires and explosions caused by anaesthetic agents

Author details

AG MacDonald

Reference

British Journal of Anaesthesia 1994; **72**: 710–22.

Abstract

The first recorded fire resulting from the use of an anaesthetic agent occurred in 1850, when ether caught fire during a facial operation. Many subsequent fires and explosions have been reported, caused by ether, acetylene, ethylene and cyclopropane, and there has been one reported explosion involving halothane. Although some of the earlier incidents caused more consternation than injury, many of the later ones caused much death and destruction, particularly after the practice of administering oxygen, instead of air, became established. Many incidents have never been reported and many of those which have reached publication do not record essential details. The use of flammable agents has decreased significantly in recent years and although fires and explosions from non-anaesthetic causes, for example gastrointestinal gases, skin sterilizing agents and laser surgery, may continue to occur, those from gaseous and volatile anaesthetic agents may now be of historical interest only. This article reviews some of the more relevant and enlightening reports of the past 150 years.

Summary

The paper introduces the potential sources of fires and explosions in anaesthetic practice, giving a description of the criteria necessary for ignition to occur. Three ingredients are necessary: fuel, an oxidant, and a source of ignition. The fuel is most commonly an anaesthetic gas or vapour, particularly when mixed with oxygen; the oxidant is likely to be either oxygen or nitrous oxide; the source of ignition is traditionally an open fire or candle, a hot rod used for cautery, a defective electrical instrument, or static electricity. More recently laser surgery has evolved as a major cause of fires.

Chronological descriptions of fires and explosions in the medical literature are presented, highlighting the different agents used and the clinical consequences of each case. Incidents involving multiple agents are presented. Some of the reports are alarming. Some are barely believable such as the use of open flames in the operating room in the presence of inflammable anaesthetics to improve visibility or the following description:

> A sobering incident occurred during ophthalmic surgery in the early 1950s [J. I. Young, personal communication]. A junior nurse was told by the theatre sister to dispose of a half-full bottle of ether which had been on the anaesthetic machine. Not knowing quite what she should do with it, but aware that it was fairly dangerous, she decided to dispose of it in what she regarded as the safest possible way. She poured it down the lavatory, pulled the chain and went back to theatre. After completing the first cataract, the surgeon, a man who hated noise, went out for a quiet cigarette. Before going back into theatre, he went to the lavatory and, after sitting down, discarded his cigarette between his legs into the pan. There was a loud bang, followed by a sheet of flame upwards out of the pan. He had a very unpleasant fright but, although severely shaken, he was not badly burned, because ether burns with a cool flame.

An investigation into the hazards of fire and explosions by the American Society of Anesthesiologists was conducted in 1937. The subsequent report highlighted failings in knowledge of physics and chemistry, as well as poor safety measures. Recommendations as a consequence of this report included all anaesthetic equipment being made of conductive material; keeping humidification in theatres above 60%; using flooring in operating theatres of the appropriate resistance and con-ductivity; ensuring all personnel and equipment are in conductive contact with the floor; and removing all materials capable of generating static electricity from the operating room. Similar guidelines were introduced into UK practice.

The paper concludes that even though the risk of fire or explosion now seems remote, vigilance is still essential if future incidents are to be avoided.

Citation count

61.

Related references

1 Macdonald AG. A brief historical review of non-anaesthetic causes of fires and explosions in the operating room. *Br J Anaesth* 1994; **73**: 847–56.

Key message

The evolution of anaesthetic equipment safety is highlighted by case reports of fires and explosions whilst using anaesthetic agents.

Strengths

The paper provides a revealing series of case reports of fires and explosions from 1850, with an underlining serious safety message.

Weaknesses

The preventative message should be the key element of the paper.

Relevance

The approach to safety in the past as illustrated by some of the events described in this paper is remarkable. Safety is a key element of modern medicine. Medical equipment and hospitals are designed to operate efficiently and safely, exposing both patients and staff to minimal risk. Equipment undergoes regular strict safety tests to reduce the likelihood of fire, explosion, and electrical shock and is labelled to demonstrate these risks. Operators are required to have a thorough understanding of the potential hazards of using electrical equipment.

Operating theatres in the UK were previously designed to prevent the build-up of static electricity, which could provide the source of ignition for an explosion or fire. The floors were electrically conductive to allow the static to drain away, although a degree of resistance was required to prevent electrocution. All apparatus and trolleys had conducting wheels or supports to allow charges to conduct to the floor. The staff wore antistatic footwear.

Currently the operating theatre environment is controlled with a high relative humidity but many of the other antistatic precautions are no longer followed. Modern anaesthetic vapours are less flammable than those presented in this paper but nevertheless understanding and vigilance in relation to all aspects of safety remains essential.

Chapter 3

Inhaled and intravenous anaesthetics

HC Hemmings Jr

Introduction

Paracelsus (1493–1541), widely regarded as the father of toxicology and an early experimenter with ether, is famous for the following quotation that has been a guiding principle for anaesthesia since its beginnings:

> Alle Ding' sind Gift, und nichts ohn' Gift; allein die Dosis macht, daß ein Ding kein Gift ist.[1] [All things are poison and nothing is without poison, only the dose permits something not to be poisonous.]

The history of general anaesthesia is rich and storied. Even the concept of anaesthesia has roots in the parallel evolution of religious beliefs and medical science. While ether was known to Paracelsus in the 16th century (as sweet oil of vitriol), it took another three centuries for its use as an anaesthetic to be fully realized. Induction of general anaesthesia required inhalation of gases and vapours including nitrous oxide, ether, and chloroform, which often resulted in slow and occasionally dangerous inductions and emergence. The development of intravenous anaesthesia necessarily followed developments in chemistry and the introductions of hollow needles, syringes, and intravenous fluid therapy in the late 19th century. This paved the way for the introduction of rapidly acting intravenous anaesthetics for the induction of general anaesthesia.

This chapter highlights some of the landmark papers in the development and clinical pharmacology of inhaled and intravenous general anaesthetic drugs. There are three sections: inhaled anaesthetics, intravenous anaesthetics, and general anaesthesia. In some cases the choice of a single landmark paper is clear, but in others it was more difficult to select a single paper to recognize a major development; some of these are included as 'Related references'. Recognizing this element of subjectivity, I apologize in advance for any omissions or controversial choices. A number of important advances could not be highlighted in the limited space, and others will be found in other chapters of this book. The publications included were chosen for their impact on the development of the clinical pharmacology of general anaesthesia. The impact of these publications on the practice of anaesthesia is enduring.

---

[1] Gravenstein JS. Paracelsus and his contributions to anesthesia. *Anesthesiology.* 1965; **26**: 805–11.

Paper 1: Insensibility during surgical operations produced by inhalation

Author details

HJ Bigelow

Reference

Boston Medical and Surgical Journal 1846, **35**: 309–17.

Abstract

It has long been an important problem in medical science to devise some method of mitigating the pain of surgical operations. An efficient agent for this purpose has at length been discovered. A patient has been rendered completely insensible during amputation of the thigh, regaining consciousness after a short interval. Other severe operations have been performed without knowledge of the patients. So remarkable an occurrence will, it is believed, render the following details relating to the history and character of the process not uninteresting.

Summary

On 16 October, 1846, Dr John C. Warren performed the first public operation on a patient under ether anaesthesia administered by dentist William T.G. Morton at Massachusetts General Hospital. Dr Henry J. Bigelow was a witness and described the operation and others to the Boston Society for Medical Improvement on 9 November. His account, printed in *The Boston Medical and Surgical Journal* on 18 November, is the first medical publication on this groundbreaking achievement. The origins of anaesthesia are not without controversy however; other valid contenders include Crawford W. Long and Horace Wells (see Related references).

Citation count

110.

Related references

1 Long CW. An account of the first use of sulphuric ether by inhalation as an anaesthetic in surgical operations. *Southern Medical and Surgical Journal*, 1849; **5**: 705–713.
2 Wells H. *A History of the Discovery of the Application of Nitrous Oxide Gas, Ether, and Other Vapours, to Surgical Operations*. Hartford: Gaylord and Wells, 1847.

Key message

The inhalation of ether causes anaesthesia sufficient to permit a major operation.

Strengths

The report reviews the toxicity of ether including its troublesome excitatory effects, cardiopulmonary depression, and nausea and vomiting; describes the novel inhalation method of administration; and describes in detail a number of cases. The tremendous potential benefits as well as the serious problems that characterize general anaesthesia are all evident.

Weaknesses

No objective data are reported, as customary for the time. This is a narrative report of one of the greatest advances in human history.

Relevance

This is the first published account of the successful administration of ether as a general anaesthetic. This is the foundation upon which the modern specialties of anaesthesiology and surgery are built.

Paper 2: On chloroform and other anæsthetics: their action and administration

Author details

J Snow

Reference

On Chloroform and Other Anaesthetics: Their Action and Administration. London: Churchill, 1858.

Table of contents

Historical Introduction; General Remarks On Inhalation; Chloroform; Physiological Effects Of Chloroform; Circumstances Which Influence Or Modify The Effects Of Chloroform; Amount Of Vapour Of Chloroform Absorbed To Cause The Various Degrees Of Narcotism; Preparations For Inhaling Chloroform; Mode Of Administering Chloroform; Recovery From The Effects Of Chloroform; Occasional Sequelæ Of The Inhalation Of Chloroform; Cause And Prevention Of Death From Chloroform; Fatal Cases Of Inhalation Of Chloroform; Alleged Fatal Cases Of Inhalation Of Chloroform; Symptoms In Fatal Cases Of Inhalation Of Chloroform; Mode Of Death In The Accidents From Chloroform; The Two Kinds Of Syncope; Supposed Causes Of Death From Chloroform; State Of The Chief Organs After Death From Chloroform; Further Remarks On The Prevention Of Accidents From Chloroform; Treatment Of Suspended Animation From Chloroform; Effect Of Chloroform On The Results Of Operations; Administration Of Chloroform In The Different Kinds Of Operations; Chloroform In Parturition; The Inhalation Of Chloroform In Medical Cases; Sulphuric Ether, Or Ether; Amylene; The Monochlorurretted Chloride Of Ethyle.

Reproduced from 'On chloroform and other anæsthetics: their action and administration', Churchill Livingston, 1858.

Summary

In his magnum opus, Snow describes experiments conducted on the physical and pharmacological properties of chloroform and other inhaled anaesthetics; methods of administration; side effects and complications; and specific clinical applications. This monograph summarizes the development of anaesthesia and the state of knowledge at that time.

Citation count

Not available.

Related references

1 Snow J. On the Inhalation of the Vapour of Ether in Surgical Operations. *Lond Med Gaz.* 1847; **4**: 498–502. Reprinted in *Br J Anaesth* 1953; **25**: 53–67 [part 1], **25**: 162–9 [part 2], **25**: 253–67 [part 3], **25**: 349–82 [part 4].

2 Snow J. *On the Inhalation of the Vapour of Ether in Surgical Operations: Containing a Description of the Various Stages of Etherization, and a Statement of the Results of Nearly Eighty Operations in Which Ether Has Been Employed in St. George's and University College Hospitals.* London: Churchill, 1847.

3 Snow J. On the inhalation of chloroform and ether. With description of an apparatus. *Lancet* 1848; **1**: 177–80.

Key message

This was essentially a series of detailed case reports on the use of chloroform anaesthesia.

Strengths

This publication put anaesthesia on a firm scientific footing. Snow introduced inhalers to deliver a measured and accurate doses of anaesthetizing agent. As inscribed on his tombstone in Brompton Cemetery: 'he made the art of anaesthesia a science'.

Weaknesses

Like appropriate recognition for his contributions to medicine, his greatest work on anaesthesia was published posthumously, although it was largely complete at his death.

Relevance

Dr John Snow (1813–1858) was an epidemiologist and an anaesthesiologist, and one of the greatest physicians Britain, or the world, has known. In addition to establishing the field of epidemiology, Snow's contribution was to establish the scientific basis of anaesthesia by studying the human pharmacology of anaesthetic drugs. He introduced a chloroform inhaler and determined relationships between anaesthetic solubility, vapour pressure, and potency. His earlier work on ether first described five stages of etherization in response to increasing doses, presaging Guedel's description. This book on chloroform, published posthumously, describes the first dose–response relationship for an anaesthetic. Rightly considered by many the first anaesthetist, he elucidated many of the principles of anaesthesia that we take for granted today. Snow's iconic status is recognized by his depiction as one of the heraldic supporters of the Royal College of Anaesthetists.

Paper 3: Preliminary studies of the anesthetic activity of fluorinated hydrocarbons

Author details

BH Robbins

Reference

Journal of Pharmacology and Experimental Therapeutics 1946; **86**: 197–204.

Abstract

1 The anesthetic activity of forty-six hydrocarbons containing fluorine alone, or in addition to other halogens, has been determined in mice.

2 Eighteen of these forty-six compounds have been used on dogs to study their effect on blood pressure and changes in the cardiac rhythm as shown by electrocardioscopic examination.

   Data obtained with four of these compounds are such that further study of them as anesthetic agents is indicated.

Summary

Forty-six fluorinated hydrocarbons were tested for anaesthetic activity in mice, of which 18 were selected for further testing in dogs. Several had better therapeutic ratios than ether or chloroform with shorter induction and recovery times. Important structure–activity correlations noted included the marked increase in potency produce by a second halogen atom (bromine > chlorine). Dose-related reduction in blood pressure and cardiac dysrhythmias were identified as major complications with most of these agents.

Related references

1 Raventos J. The action of fluothane; a new volatile anaesthetic. *Br J Pharmacol Chemother* 1956; **11**: 394–410.

2 Johnstone M. The human cardiovascular response to fluothane anaesthesia. *Br J Anaesth* 1956; **28**: 392–410.

3 Bryce-Smith R, O'Brien HD. Fluothane: a non-explosive volatile anesthetic agent. *Br Med J* 1956; **2**: 969–72.

4 Suckling CW. Some chemical and physical factors in the development of fluothane. *Br J Anaesth* 1957; **29**: 466–72.

5 O'Brien HD. The introduction of halothane into clinical practice: the Oxford experience. *Anaesth Intensive Care* 2006; **34**: 27–32.

Citation count

80.

Key message

Fluorinated hydrocarbons have anaesthetic properties.

Strengths

A large series of compounds allowed useful structure–activity correlations. Characterization of pharmacokinetic properties and side effects provided a paradigm for selecting agents for further development. One of the first quantitative assessments of anaesthetic potency using multiple endpoints, a predecessor to the concept of minimum alveolar concentration.

Weaknesses

This was a single atom away from halothane!

Relevance

A major advance in anaesthesia was the introduction of safe and non-flammable inhaled anaesthetics in the mid 20th century. Although none of the compounds studied by Robbins were developed clinically, this landmark study demonstrated the potential of fluorinated hydrocarbons as non-flammable inhaled anaesthetics without convulsant activity. Based on Robbins's work, Suckling of Imperial Chemical Industries (ICI) developed halothane (Fluothane) as a non-flammable and non-explosive volatile anaesthetic that showed outstanding anaesthetic properties in animal testing (Raventos, 1956; Suckling, 1957). The clinical properties of halothane in humans were described by Johnstone in Manchester and by Bryce-Smith and O'Brien in Oxford, which marked the first major advance in anaesthetic pharmacology since ether. These newer agents replaced ether and cyclopropane, which were limited by their flammability and explosiveness, and chloroform, which was plagued by hepatic and cardiac toxicities. Although the introduction of halothane was a landmark in anaesthesia, it is difficult to pick a single paper that describes this, so I have selected this one as representative of the paradigm shift in anaesthetic chemistry that preceded development of all the modern agents.

Paper 4: General anesthetics. 1. Halogenated methyl ethyl ethers as anesthetic agents

Author details

RC Terrell, L Speers, AJ Szur, J Treadwell, TR Ucciardi

Reference

Journal of Medicinal Chemistry 1971; **14**: 517–19.

Abstract

Thirty-six halogenated Me Et ethers have been synthesized for evaluation as volatile general anesthetics. Eleven of the ethers were too unstable to test, and, of the remaining 25, 13 had promising anesthetic properties in mice and are suitable for study in larger species. Those ethers having one H with at least 2 halogens other than F or 2 or more H with at least one Br or one Cl were the best anesthetics.

Summary

A number of halogenated methyl ethyl ethers were synthesized and evaluated as anaesthetics in mice. Several structural features associated with desirable anaesthetic properties (volatility, stability, non-flammability, anaesthetic in mice) were demonstrated.

Related references

1 Vitcha JF. A history of Forane. *Anesthesiology* 1971; **35**: 4–7.

2 Terrell RC, Speers L, Szur AJ, *et al* General anesthetics. 3. Fluorinated methyl ethyl ethers as anesthetic agents. *J Med Chem* 1972; **15**: 604–6.

3 Terrell RC. The invention and development of enflurane, isoflurane, sevoflurane, and desflurane. *Anesthesiology* 2008; **108**: 531–3.

Citation count

38.

Key message

Certain structural features of halogenated compounds are associated with anaesthetic properties.

Strengths

This was a concise description of systematic synthesis and evaluation of a large number of related compounds allowed some correlations between properties and structure, facilitating clinical development of improved inhaled anaesthetics.

Weaknesses

The paper focussed on chemistry, with limited information on pharmacological testing.

Relevance

Progress in fluorine chemistry resulting from the US atomic weapons programme facilitated the synthesis of fluorinated anaesthetics, which exhibited greater stability and lower solubility than chlorinated or brominated analogues. In an effort to find a better anaesthetic than halothane, which had several problems including marked cardiovascular depression and arrhythmogenesis, and, rarely, fulminant hepatonecrosis, Terrell and colleagues at Ohio Medical Products synthesized and evaluated over 700 fluorinated compounds including enflurane, isoflurane, sevoflurane, and desflurane—mainstays of modern inhalational anaesthesia. The initial description in this paper led to testing in larger animals and eventually in humans.

Paper 5: The rate of uptake of nitrous oxide in man

Author details

JW Severinghaus

Reference

Journal of Clinical Investigation 1954; **33**: 1183–9.

Abstract

The volume rate of uptake of N_2O by the body was measured during surgical anesthesia. After 90 minutes of inhalation of an 80 per cent N_2O-20 per cent O_2 mixture, the body is still absorbing about 100 ml. of N_2O per minute from the gaseous phase in the lungs. Seven and one-half to 30 liters of N_2O are taken up in solution in the body during 1 to 2.5 hours of anesthesia.

The rate of uptake of N_2O during at least the first 2 hours of anesthesia is about 30 times the volume rate of elimination of nitrogen as reported by others (30 is the ratio of solubility of the two gases). This evidence supports the suggestion that the approximate uptake rate of other inert gases can be predicted from data on nitrogen elimination.

The average rate of uptake of N_2O in six subjects was described approximately by the equation: Rate $= 1,000\,t^{-0.5}$ ml. per min.

The experimental findings were discussed in relation to several clinical problems in anesthesia.

The method can be used to determine the oxygen consumption as an index of the metabolic rate during anesthesia with gases or vapors.

Summary

Severinghaus.determined the volume rate of uptake of nitrous oxide and oxygen in six surgical patients using spirometry and rotameters on a conventional anaesthesia machine. Oxygen and nitrous oxide flow rates were continuously adjusted to match their rates of uptake while maintaining the oxygen concentration at 20%.

Citation count

144.

Related references

1 Kety SS. The physiological and physical factors governing the uptake of anesthetic gases by the body. *Anesthesiology* 1950; **11**: 517–26.

2 Kety SS. The theory and applications of the exchange of inert gas at the lungs and tissues. *Pharmacol Rev* 1951; **3**: 1–41.

Key message

There is an inverse relationship between the solubility of an inhaled anaesthetic and its rate of uptake.

Strengths

Data obtained from human subjects were used to model uptake behaviour, which accurately predicted clinically observed phenomena.

Weaknesses

Manual adjustments of gas flow led to small changes in inspired concentration that required manual correction. Inspired gas concentrations were calculated rather than directly measured (which was not possible at the time). Gradual elimination of nitrogen from the tissues and diffusion of gases from the body to the atmosphere introduced small errors.

Relevance

This is the first study of the uptake of an inhaled anaesthetic in humans, which spawned the square root of time description of anaesthetic uptake. Work by Kety and others mathematically modelled the uptake and distribution of relatively insoluble inert gases in the body, but this was not applicable to whole body uptake of the more soluble anaesthetic gases and vapours. Using simple but precise spirometric methods, Severinghaus was able to show that previous assumptions that all body tissues were in near equilibrium with inspired anaesthetic gas after 20–30 min of anaesthesia did not hold for the soluble gas nitrous oxide, which continued to be taken up for several hours. This is shown to result from the large quantities of the soluble gas that are carried away from the lung in pulmonary venous blood, delaying the rise in alveolar gas tension. The data are used to predict the concentration effect during uptake and diffusion hypoxia during elimination. This study established the important inverse relationship between inhaled anaesthetic solubility and its rate of uptake, a fundamental concept in the kinetics of anaesthetic uptake and distribution.

Paper 6: A comparative study of halothane and halopropane anesthesia including method for determining equipotency

Author details

G Merkel, EI Eger II

Reference

Anesthesiology 1963; **24**: 346–57.

Abstract

Two fluorinated hydrocarbon anesthetics, halopropane and halothane, were compared in dogs during spontaneous and controlled respiration. Anesthetic equipotency was defined in terms of the minimal alveolar anesthetic concentration required to prevent muscular response to a painful stimulus. Halopropane was found a less potent anesthetic than halothane, with a narrower range between minimal anesthetic concentration and that required to produce respiratory or circulatory failure. Arterial pressure and cardiac output became depressed at relatively lower alveolar halopropane concentrations. Respiratory arrest also occurred at lower halopropane concentrations. With neither agent did the dogs demonstrate a significant tendency to compensate for increasing anesthetic depression.

Summary

A technique is described for determining the minimum alveolar (end-tidal) concentration (MAC) of anaesthetic required to prevent gross muscular movement in response to a painful stimulus in dogs. This approach was devised so that the physiological effects of different anaesthetics, halothane and halopropane in this case, could be compared at equivalent depths of anaesthesia. This index of potency was used to compare the effects of these two anaesthetics on arterial pressure, venous pressure, cardiac output, respiratory rate and volume, arterial blood gases, electrocardiogram, and electroencephalogram at multiples of MAC during spontaneous and controlled ventilation. MAC did not vary significantly with the degree of the painful stimulus, and was thus a reproducible measure of potency. The advantage of alveolar (exhaled) over inspired anaesthetic concentration is noted. Cardiovascular effects were proportional to anaesthetic depth, but were greater with halopropane at equivalent MAC. Both agents depressed respiration similarly, with respiratory arrest occurring at lower concentrations than circulatory arrest.

Citation count

142.

Related references

1 Eger EI II, Saidman LJ, Brandstater B. Minimum alveolar anesthetic concentration: a standard of anesthetic potency. *Anesthesiology* 1965; **26**: 756–63.

2 Saidman LJ, Eger EI II. Effect of nitrous oxide and of narcotic premedication on the alveolar concentration of halothane required for anesthesia. *Anesthesiology* 1964; **25**: 302–6.

3 Quasha AL, Eger EI II, Tinker JH. Determination and applications of MAC. *Anesthesiology* 1980; **53**: 315–34.

Key message

It is possible to compare the potency of different anaesthetic agents using a standardized measure.

Strengths

Detailed comparison of two drugs at multiple concentrations using multiple physiological assays.

Weaknesses

Data for different painful stimuli are not explicitly identified.

Relevance

Progress in the scientific study of inhaled anaesthetics required a standard measure of potency comparable to the effective dose for 50% of subjects (ED_{50}). This is the first description of MAC, a concept that continues to enable the study of inhaled anaesthetics at equipotent doses. This concept was extended from animals to humans by Saidman and Eger in 1964, and subsequently to many other species, which revealed a remarkable consistency in anaesthetic potency between organisms (<twofold variation). Although the quantal nature of MAC does not permit comparisons at multiples or fractions of the experimentally determined value, the practical validity of this approach has been demonstrated in many cases. The relative ease of MAC determinations, its consistency between species, and its direct relation to the partial pressure of anaesthetic at the site of action have made MAC the major index of anaesthetic potency for over 50 years. The concept has been extended to other end-points of anaesthetic action beyond the abolition of movement in response to pain (immobilization), the essence of general anaesthesia, including loss of consciousness and autonomic depression.

Paper 7: Intravenous anesthesia: preliminary report of the use of two new thiobarbiturates

Author details

JS Lundy

Reference

Proceedings of the Mayo Clinic 1935; **10**: 536–43.

Abstract

Increase in use of intravenous anesthesia has been delayed because of lack of a suitable agent, but at times when a general anesthetic is needed the intravenous method is the best; for example, if the cautery or diathermy is to be used, and thus an inflammable agent would be dangerous, or if portability is of importance. For intravenous anesthesia the barbiturates, particularly, have been employed. The ideal agent for routine intravenous anesthesia has not been found as yet but the available agents have been found to be satisfactory in certain types of cases.

Summary

This short report describes briefly the historical development of anaesthetic barbiturates focusing on effort to speed onset and recovery, introducing two new thiobarbiturates including thiopentone (barbiturate A). Methods of administration and its clinical effects are described in narrative form based on its use in 700 cases. Important features such as respiratory depression and obstruction, cumulative effects, tissue irritation, anticonvulsant effect, lack of analgesic effect, and use for induction of anaesthesia and for short ambulatory procedures are covered.

Citation count

46.

Related references

1 Tabern DL, Volwiler EH. Sulfur-containing barbiturate hypnotics. *J Am Chem Soc* 1935; **57**: 1961.

2 Pratt TW, Tatum AL, Hathaway HR, *et al.* Sodium ethyl(1-mentylbutyl)thiobarbiturate: preliminary experimental and clinical study. *Am J Surg* 1936; **31**: 464–6.

3 Dundee JW. Fifty years of thiopentone. *Br J Anaesth* 1984; **56**: 211–13.

Key message

Thiobarbiturates can be effectively used as anaesthetic agents.

Strengths

This paper was both highly practical and clinically orientated, highlighting both the advantages and disadvantages of this new drug.

Weaknesses

The report is narrative and anecdotal, not uncommon for clinical communications of this era. A more scientific description came from Waters' group in Wisconsin, who was probably the first to administer thiopentone to a human in 1934.

Relevance

In 1935, Lundy introduced thiopentone at the Mayo Clinic in Minnesota, a drug discovered by Tabern and Volwiler at Abbott laboratories earlier that year. Lundy also introduced the concept of 'balanced anaesthesia' in 1926, which he used to describe a combination of premedication, local anaesthesia, and general anaesthesia to reduce the dose of each individual agent and thereby improve safety by minimizing toxicity. This concept has evolved to include combinations of intravenous sedatives, hypnotics, analgesics, and muscle relaxants, often supplemented with inhaled anaesthetics. Lundy also recognized the undesirable properties of intravenous barbiturates, which led to continuing efforts to find other induction agents with reduced non-hypnotic side effects such as cardiovascular depression. Thiopentone became widely accepted, largely because of its lack of excitatory myoclonic movements, and is still in use 75 years later (although recent production issues have threatened its availability).

Paper 8: A dynamic concept of the distribution of thiopental in the human body

Author details

HL Price

Reference

Anesthesiology 1960; **21**: 40–5.

Abstract

A mathematical analysis of the kinetics of thiopental redistribution in the human body has been presented. This method has been validated by direct measurement of thiopental concentration in human tissue.

Summary

A mathematical model devised to describe the changes in tissue thiopentone concentration following a bolus intravenous injection or infusion was applied to published data on the perfusion, mass, and tissue:blood partition coefficients of various compartments of the human body. The assumption that metabolism and excretion are unimportant in the early phases of drug kinetics results in a model that accurately describes the central nervous system response to thiopental injection. Within a minute following a single dose of thiopental, 90% of the dose has left the central blood pool to enter the rapidly perfused viscera (heart, kidney, splanchnic area, central nervous system) to produce a rapid effect onset. Over the next 30 minutes, these tissues are depleted of drug as a result of redistribution of 80% of the dose to lean tissues (muscle), with the remainder entering fat. The rate of fall in the central nervous system drug concentration thus depends on the rate the lean tissues take it up, which is in turn dependent on their blood flow. After infusions of thiopental for over an hour, lean tissues are saturated and cannot participate in redistribution, which then requires the slower contribution of uptake into fat. Thus rapid emergence is unlikely after long infusion, and recovery becomes dependent on the duration of infusion and other causes besides fat uptake (metabolism).

Citation count

113.

Related references

1 Brodie BB, Mark LC, Papper EM, *et al.* The fate of thiopental in man and a method for its estimation in biological material. *J Pharmacol Exp Ther* 1950; **98**: 85–96.

Key message

This is a first step in describing the pharmacokinetics of thiopentone.

Strengths

The paper applies a simple pharmacokinetic model with few assumptions to make a number critical observations and novel interpretations about the pharmacokinetic behaviour of an intravenous anaesthetic.

Weaknesses

The model is not validated by direct measurements of plasma and tissue thiopentone concentrations, but did explain the limited available published data.

Relevance

This represents a landmark for the study of the pharmacokinetic behaviour of intravenous drugs in humans by applying a simple pharmacokinetic model to describe the disposition of thiopentone. The concept of redistribution with minimal contribution from metabolism is introduced to explain the ultra-short onset and short duration following intravenous injection and the prolonged recovery following infusion. Price's model focused attention on multiple sequential drug redistribution between compartments. The earlier hypothesis of Brodie *et al.* to suggest the importance of distribution to fat as the predominant mechanism for the effect offset is refuted by the model. A number of important observations are made including the rapid distribution of thiopentone from the central compartment to richly perfused tissues, the minimal role of metabolism in the early phases of drug administration, and the importance of saturation of the redistribution mechanisms to explain slow recovery following large doses or prolonged infusion. The concept of context-sensitive half time is even suggested by modelling infusions of increasing duration. These are many of the fundamental pharmacokinetic concepts crucial to intravenous anaesthesia, and they also influenced Eger's models of inhaled anaesthetic uptake.

Paper 9: Animal studies of the anaesthetic activity of ICI 35 868

Author details

JB Glen

Reference

British Journal of Anaesthesia 1980; **52**: 731–42.

Abstract

The activity of a new i.v. anesthetic agent ICI 35 868, a compound unrelated to currently used barbiturate, eugenol or steroid agents, has been examined in a range of animal species. Some of the properties of ICI 35 868 resemble those of thiopentone in that it is a rapidly acting agent which produces anaesthesia of short duration and without excitatory side-effects. Both agents have a similar therapeutic index and produce equivalent cardiovascular and respiratory effects. In the mouse ICI 35 868 is 1.8 times more potent than thiopentone as a hypnotic. However, the anaesthetic profile of ICI 35 868 differs from that of thiopentone in that recovery is rapid following repeated administration, no tissue damage is produced by perivascular or intra-arterial injection and greater reflex depression and more profound e.e.g. changes are produced at equipotent doses. This new agent has been shown to be compatible with a wide range of drugs used for preanaesthetic medication, inhalation anaesthetics, and neuromuscular blocking drugs.

Summary

A novel intravenous anaesthetic agent was evaluated in a number of species in comparison to thiopentone. The anaesthetic properties of ICI 35 868 (propofol) formulated in Cremophore were similar to those of thiopentone in its rapid onset with cardiovascular and respiratory depression, but differed in a significant way: repeated doses and continuous infusions could be administered without markedly prolonging recovery. There were no significant interactions with common anaesthetic drugs, but the need for an alternative vehicle is raised.

Citation count

162.

Related references

1 James R, Glen JB. Synthesis, biological evaluation, and preliminary structure-activity considerations of a series of alkylphenols as intravenous anesthetic agents. *J Med Chem* 1980; **23**: 1350–7.

2 Glen JB, Hunter SC. Pharmacology of an emulsion formulation of ICI 35 868. *Br J Anaesth* 1984; **56**: 617–26.

Key message

Propofol is an effective anaesthetic in animals.

Strengths

The study directly compared propofol to other current intravenous anaesthetics in multiple species using multiple indices of therapeutic and toxic effects, an impressive preclinical study of a novel anaesthetic.

Weaknesses

Pharmacokinetic analysis would have been useful in interpreting the cumulative effects.

Relevance

Thiopentone revolutionized anaesthesia by providing a rapid means for intravenous induction, but continuous intravenous anaesthesia was limited by its accumulation and slow recovery upon repeated or prolonged infusion. Working at Imperial Chemical Industries (ICI), James and Glen synthesized and evaluated a series of unique hindered phenolic compounds for their anaesthetic activity in animals. The most promising of these was ICI 35 868 (2,6 di-isopropylphenol), a chemical entity unrelated to any prior anaesthetic, which was selected for further development. This animal study showing reduced accumulation (prolonged recovery) following repeated administration provided the impetus for further development. Problems with formulating such a highly lipophilic and water-insoluble compound were a major stumbling block in commercialization. The initial vehicle Cremophor was dropped due to excessive anaphylactoid reactions in favour of a lipid emulsion, although initial clinical studies were done with the Cremophor vehicle. Problems with formulation still exist, but the successful introduction of propofol was revolutionary in allowing the development of total intravenous anaesthesia and ambulatory anaesthesia.

Paper 10: A study of the deaths associated with anesthesia and surgery: based on a study of 599, 548 anesthesias in ten institutions 1948–1952

Author details

HK Beecher, DP Todd

Reference

Annals of Surgery 1954; **140**: 2–35.

Summary

All deaths associated with surgery and anaesthesia in ten geographically separated US university hospitals occurring over 5 years (representing about 600,000 procedures) were recorded prospectively and analysed by cause and associated factors. These factors included: anaesthetic agents and techniques; provider; and patient physical status, diagnosis, and surgical procedure. Inhalation anaesthesia, mainly with ether, was the most common technique used, but use of intravenous anaesthesia doubled over the study. Spinal anaesthesia used mainly tetracaine, and local anaesthesia used mainly procaine. Endotracheal intubation was used mainly for inhalation anaesthesia, but use with intravenous anaesthesia increased probably due to combination with muscle relaxants. The overall death rate for hospitalized surgical patients was 1:75, and the primary anaesthesia death rate was 1:2680. This was disproportionately higher in men, and at the extremes of age. Since most anaesthetics employed various combinations of specific drugs, it was impossible to establish a specific death rate for individual agents. The important observation emerged that anaesthetics involving the use of muscle relaxants were associated with an increase in death rate of sixfold ('curare deaths') regardless of anaesthetist background or experience, patient risk, or procedure. These deaths implicated an inherent toxicity associated with muscle relaxant use involving both respiratory and circulatory failure. The authors conclude that muscle relaxants should be used with caution, and not for 'trivial purposes' or to supplement inadequate anaesthesia.

Citation count

461.

Related references

1 Abajian J, Arrowood JG, Barrett RH, *et al.* Critique of "A Study of the Deaths Associated with Anesthesia and Surgery". *Ann Surg* 1955; **142**: 138–41.

2 Beecher HK, Todd DP. Comment on the Critique. *Ann Surg* 1955; **142**: 142–4.

3 Bunker JP. The contribution of anesthesia to surgical mortality. *Int Anesthesiol Clin* 2007; **45**: 7–12.

Key message

Anaesthesia has an inherent risk of mortality.

Strengths

The first serious study to determine the incidence of mortality attributable to anaesthesia, this was a true landmark in the development of efforts to improve the safety of anaesthesia.

Weaknesses

Residual neuromuscular blockade (categorized as 'Respiratory failure (hypoxia)' as a cause of death) probably contributed to the many of the curare deaths, though its significance was overlooked by Beecher and Todd. This issue is still a concern today.

Relevance

This represents one of the first large prospective outcome studies. It was remarkable in that data was collected for all anaesthetics in ten hospitals (representing about 2.5% of all anaesthetics in US non-profit hospitals) and submitted to a central office. This was a milestone in clinical data information systems, and was done by hand on paper without the aid of computers. The resulting data reveal aspects of anaesthesia that are still relevant to practice today including the increased mortality associated with very young or old age. Anaesthesiologists were outraged that this was published in the surgical rather than the anaesthesia literature (Abajian *et al.*, 1955), and pointed out that overall mortality should have been examined to determine the extent to which surgical mortality might depend on the anaesthetic technique and agents. As a toxicological study, it was important that no specific anaesthetic agent was associated with poor outcome. This focused attention on clinical practice rather than pharmacology in patient safety.

Acknowledgements

Illuminating discussions with E.I. Eger II are gratefully acknowledged.

Chapter 4

Total intravenous anaesthesia

JK Oosterhuis and AR Absalom

Introduction

In the context of the history of medicine, anaesthesia is a relatively new development. This is especially true for intravenous anaesthesia, which only become commonplace in the 1990s. Intravenous *induction* of anaesthesia became widespread in the 1930s after the introduction of thiopentone, but in the absence of an intravenous agent with suitable pharmacokinetics for use by repeated boluses or infusion, maintenance of anaesthesia remained almost exclusively inhalational for several more decades.

During the 1970s, two drugs with pharmacokinetics suitable for use by infusion were introduced, but both provided a false dawn for total intravenous anaesthesia (TIVA), i.e. induction and maintenance of anaesthesia by the intravenous route. Etomidate infusions were found to be associated with impaired adrenocortical function, while althesin was withdrawn from human clinical practice after it was found to be associated with a high incidence of anaphylactoid reactions. Ironically, these reactions were probably the result of the vehicle, Cremophor EL, not the agent.

The modern popularity of TIVA began with the introduction of propofol, an agent with pharmacokinetic characteristics eminently suitable for use by infusion. After it was discovered by the team lead by Dr Iain Glen, propofol was initially solubilized in Cremophor, but owing to the experiences with althesin, it was unlikely to become a clinical success if supplied in this formulation. Thus, the first Landmark Paper is the report of a study showing that propofol in a lipid emulsion provided equivalent anaesthesia and improved safety in animals, compared with the Cremophor formulation. The 10% Intralipid vehicle may ironically be the cause of the metabolic derangements associated with the propofol infusion syndrome, a rare but serious complication of prolonged, high-dose propofol administration, and the topic of the second Landmark Paper.

In the past three decades our understanding of pharmacokinetics has expanded immensely, and no one has made a greater contribution than Professor Steven Shafer, the first author of the third Landmark Paper, in which the complexities of pharmacokinetics of drug infusions were clearly illustrated, along with the benefits of the use of computer simulations in rational choice of opioids for infusions. The best agent for infusion depends in part on how the decrement time changes as the duration of infusion increases, and this concept was further developed in the Landmark Paper by Hughes on the context-sensitive half-time.

The current popularity of intravenous anaesthesia was been promoted further by the discovery of a very short-acting opioid, remifentanil. Paper 5 is one of three publications in November 1993, when the pharmacokinetics and dynamics of this agent in humans were first described. Another major factor boosting the popularity of intravenous anaesthesia has been the development of target-controlled infusion (TCI) technology. The first commercially available TCI system was developed by a team in Glasgow lead by Professor Gavin Kenny. Their system used the 'Marsh' pharmacokinetic model for propofol. This model, intended for use in adults, was an adaptation of the model developed by Dr Elizabeth Gepts. It is a simple model, in which the parameters depend only on patient weight. The sixth Landmark Paper is by the Kenny group, in which the 'Marsh' pharmacokinetic parameters were first published. Ironically, and somewhat confusingly, this manuscript was not about the use of propofol in adults, but concerned the poor performance of the model in children, and the development of a more appropriate model for children.

In current practice, two main pharmacokinetic models are used for propofol TCI—the Marsh and the Schnider models. Schnider, while working with the Shafer group in California, investigated the pharmacokinetics *and* dynamics of propofol in a single group of volunteers, thereby producing a model able to predict both plasma and effect-site propofol concentrations. This work was described in two companion papers, the second of which concentrated on the important matter of the influence of age of propofol's kinetics and dynamics; and hence it was chosen as Paper 7.

Most TIVA practitioners use a combination of propofol and an opiate. Thus, the issue of pharmacokinetic and dynamic interactions is very important, leading to the inclusion of the very important paper by Dr Jaap Vuyk, on pharmacodynamic interactions, Paper 8. Although most anaesthetists will agree that propofol-based anaesthesia has very many benefits, there are rather few papers providing objective scientific evidence of improved outcomes. Two particularly important advantages of propofol are the beneficial effects on cerebral haemodynamics and the 8 low incidence of postoperative nausea and vomiting, and thus we end our chapter with two landmark papers on these subjects.

Paper 1: Pharmacology of an emulsion formulation of ICI 35 868

Author details

JB Glen, SC Hunter

Reference

British Journal of Anaesthesia 1984; **56**: 617–26.

Abstract

Studies with an emulsion formulation of ICI 35 868 (2,6-diisopropylphenol) indicate that this new formulation has anaesthetic properties in rats and mice, and haemodynamic effects in the mini-pig which are similar to those of the previously available Cremophor formulation. Administration of the emulsion formulation to dogs produced no untoward effect, whereas the Cremophor formulation produced a marked increase in plasma histamine concentration. In the mini-pig, no adverse response was produced by the repeated administration of the emulsion formulation of ICI 35 868, whereas the Cremophor formulation produced anaphylactoid responses when a second injection was given 1 week after an uneventful first exposure to this formulation. Behavioural responses in the rat suggest that the emulsion formulation may produce less discomfort in i.v. injection.

Glen JB, Hunter SC, 'Pharmacology of an emulsion formulation of ICI-35868', *British Journal of Anaesthesia*, 1984, 56, 6, pp. 617–626, by permission of Oxford University Press.

Summary

In a variety of animals, the lipid emulsion formulation of propofol was shown to provide equivalent anaesthesia but without the adverse (anaphylactoid) effects seen with a Cremophor emulsion.

Citation count

170.

Related references

1   Glen JB. The animal pharmacology of ICI 35 868: A new I.V. anaesthetic agent. *Br J Anaesth* 1980; **52**: 230P.

Key message

In a variety of animals, a lipid formulation of propofol provided safe, effective anaesthesia.

Strengths

Several animal species were studied and repeated doses used. Numerous clinically relevant end-points were studied (including anaesthetic activity, pain on injection, hypotension, tachycardia, lethal dosage).

Weaknesses

There were only small numbers of animals from each species.

Relevance

Propofol had earlier been discovered by Dr Iain Glen, working for Imperial Chemical Industries (ICI). It is insoluble in aqueous solutions, but was unlikely to be a commercial and clinical success if formulated in Cremophor. A previously discovered agent, althesin, had been withdrawn from clinical use, because of a high incidence of anaphylactoid reactions. Naturally, this had severe commercial implications for the manufacturer. It was also regrettable to the clinical community, since the drug (actually a combination of alphaxolone and alphadolone) had several highly desirable pharmacokinetic and pharmacodynamic properties. Later it became apparent that the anaphylactoid reactions associated with althesin were probably caused by Cremophor.

Thus, the demonstration, that a lipid formulation provided safe, effective anaesthesia, helped provide the evidence that prompted further studies in humans, and was thus crucial to the eventual success of propofol, the mainstay of modern total intravenous anaesthesia practice.

Paper 2: Metabolic acidosis and fatal myocardial failure after propofol infusion in children: five case reports

Author details

TJ Parke, JE Stevens, AS Rice, CL Greenaway, RJ Bray, PJ Smith, CS Waldmann, C Verghese

Reference

British Medical Journal 1992; **305**: 613–16.

Abstract

Objective: To examine the possible contribution of sedation with propofol in the deaths of children who were intubated and required intensive care.

Design: Case note review.

Setting: Three intensive care units.

Subjects: Five children with upper respiratory tract infections aged between 4 weeks and 6 years.

Results: Four patients had laryngotracheo-bronchitis and one had bronchiolitis. All were sedated with propofol. The clinical course in all five cases was remarkably similar: an increasing metabolic acidosis was associated with brady-arrhythmia and progressive myocardial failure, which did not respond to resuscitative measures. All children developed lipaemic serum after starting propofol. These features are not usually associated with respiratory tract infections. No evidence was found of viral myocarditis, which was considered as a possible cause of death.

Conclusion: Although the exact cause of death in these children could not be defined, propofol may have been a contributing factor.

Summary

Prolonged sedation with propofol for critically ill children may be associated with a syndrome involving lipaemia, metabolic acidosis, brady-arrhythmia, and progressive fatal myocardial failure.

Citation count

391.

Related references

1 Bray RJ. Propofol infusion syndrome in children. *Paed Anaesth* 1998; **8**: 491–9.

2 Cremer OL, Moons KGM, Bouman EAC, *et al.* Long-term propofol infusion and cardiac failure in adult head-injured patients. *Lancet* 2001; **357**: 117–18.

3 Kam PCA, Cardone D. Propofol infusion syndrome. *Anaesthesia* 2007; **62**: 690–701.

Key message

Propofol infusions for sedation of critically ill paediatric patients may be unsafe, and should not be used until further evidence of safe dosing limits are available.

Strengths

Clear, detailed descriptions of the clinical histories of the children involved are provided.

Weaknesses

This was a retrospective review of only five cases. In addition there was no proven causality—the authors simply showed an association between the syndrome and the introduction of a new agent for sedation.

Relevance

This landmark paper was among the first of several papers showing that prolonged higher dose propofol infusions for paediatric intensive care sedation may result in a potentially fatal syndrome of metabolic acidosis and progressive myocardial failure. Eventually, the health authorities of several countries issued safety alerts, resulting in an almost universal cessation of the use of propofol for intensive care sedation in children. Since then, this syndrome, which became known as the 'propofol infusion syndrome', has also been described in a handful of children undergoing shorter duration sedation or anaesthesia, and in some adults. Not all reported cases have been fatal. Several reports have shown that a fatal outcome can be prevented by propofol cessation and appropriate supportive and resuscitative procedures as soon as the syndrome is detected. The aetiology of the syndrome appears to be a defect of mitochondrial metabolism; but whether this is the result of propofol, or the lipid carrier, or both, remains subject to debate.

Paper 3: Pharmacokinetics, pharmacodynamics, and rational opioid selection

Author details

SL Shafer, JR Varvel

Reference

Anesthesiology 1991; **74**: 53–63.

Summary

In this study computer simulations were used to estimate the time it took for a 20%, 50%, and 80% decline in plasma and effect-site concentrations after bolus doses, and short and long infusions of alfentanil, fentanyl, and sufentanil. Published pharmacokinetic *and* pharmacodynamic (k_{eo}) parameters were used. When a rapid onset and offset of drug effect are required, then alfentanil is more appropriate than fentanyl or sufentanil. For infusions longer than 6–8 h, recovery from alfentanil is more rapid than from sufentanil and fentanyl. Surprisingly, for infusions shorter than 6–8 h, the authors estimated that a 50% decline in concentrations occurs more quickly for sufentanil than for alfentanil, because there is a faster initial decline in plasma concentrations with sufentanil. At 6 h, equilibration between plasma and redistribution compartments is complete with alfentanil, whereas for sufentanil, the concentration in the slow redistribution compartment is lower than in the plasma concentration, so that ongoing redistribution contributes to the initial decline when the infusion stops.

Citation count

422.

Related references

1 Stanski DR, Hug CC, Jr. Alfentanil: a kinetically predictable narcotic analgesic. *Anesthesiology* 1982; **57**: 435–8.

2 Maitre PO, Vozeh S, Heykants J, *et al*. Population pharmacokinetics of alfentanil: the average dose- plasma concentration relationship and interindividual variability in patients. *Anesthesiology* 1987; **66**: 3–12.

3 Scott JC, Stanski DR. Decreased fentanyl and alfentanil dose requirements with age. A simultaneous pharmacokinetic and pharmacodynamic evaluation. *J Pharmacol Exp Ther* 1987; **240**: 159–66.

4 Hudson RJ, Bergstrom RG, Thomson IR, *et al*. Pharmacokinetics of sufentanil in patients undergoing abdominal aortic surgery. *Anesthesiology* 1989; **70**: 426–31.

5 Shafer SL, Varvel JR, Aziz N, *et al*. Pharmacokinetics of fentanyl administered by computer-controlled infusion pump. *Anesthesiology* 1990; **73**: 1091–102.

6 Gepts E, Shafer SL, Camu F, *et al*. Linearity of pharmacokinetics and model estimation of sufentanil. *Anesthesiology* 1995; **83**: 1194–204.

Key message

Use the opioid which suits the expected duration of the surgical procedure, and the desired rate of recovery.

Strengths

The article applies knowledge of pharmacokinetics and pharmacodynamics, to provide a deeper understanding of the complexities of drug behaviour in the clinical setting. It demonstrates the sometimes surprising results that can arise when computer technology is used to understand complex polyexponential processes.

Weaknesses

The work is entirely theoretical (computer simulations). The accuracy of the results depends on the accuracy of the pharmacokinetic models and k_{eo} values used. The pharmacokinetic models used in the study are of questionable validity—Scott (fentanyl), Stanski (alfentanil), and Hudson (sufentanil)—and are no longer commonly used in present day practice. The models in current common use are Schafer (fentanyl), Maitre (alfentanil), and Gepts (sufentanil). The k_{eo} values are also of questionable validity. They came from studies of the electroencephalogram (EEG) effects of the agents. There are two problems with this. Firstly, these studies involved huge doses of opioids (since the EEG changes only occur with large doses), and secondly, there are likely to be marked differences in the time course of EEG changes and other more relevant clinical effects such as analgesia, respiratory depression, or sedation. Although the work gives an estimate of the time for a specified proportional decline in effect-site concentration, work is based on models.

Relevance

The direct current clinical relevance of the study is limited by the weaknesses of the pharmacokinetic models and k_{eo} values, and the fact that it did not include remifentanil. However, the longer-lasting relevance and value of the study is that it helped to establish and reinforce some very important concepts and principles:

- It reinforced the general concept of decrement time as a parameter for understanding pharmacokinetics.
- It demonstrated that time course of plasma and effect-site concentrations after an infusion are almost impossible to predict from the pharmacokinetics of a drug without computer simulations.
- It reinforced the principle that time course of clinical effect depends on effect-site concentration.
- It reinforced the principle that duration of effect after an infusion, has a complex relationship with the duration of administration.

Paper 4: Context-sensitive half-time in multicompartment pharmacokinetic models for intravenous anesthetic drugs

Author details

MA Hughes, PSA Glass, JR Jacobs

Reference

Anesthesiology 1992; **76**: 334–41.

Summary

This highly cited article introduced and promoted the concept of 'context-sensitive half-time' which is a specific instance of the decrement time (the time taken for plasma concentration of a drug to decrease by a specified proportion after administration ceases). Using computer simulations, Hughes was able to demonstrate, for six commonly used anaesthetic agents, the simplicity and utility of the concept. These simulations demonstrated very elegantly the influence of infusion duration on the context-sensitive half-time (and thus on the initial rate of decline in plasma concentration after an infusion) for the individual drugs. It highlighted the fact that the recovery profiles of the drugs were very different, and that duration of infusion affected context-sensitive half-time differently for each agent.

Citation count

512.

Key message

The rate of decline in plasma concentrations after an infusion depends on several interacting exponential processes, and is difficult to predict from the pharmacokinetics of the drug. The context sensitive half time gives a clinically useful summary of the recovery profile of a drug after an infusion of a specified duration.

Strengths

It used simulations of the behaviour of commonly used drugs. It is of clear clinical relevance. Finally, it is the development of a concept that is easy to understand.

Weaknesses

Context-sensitive half-time only describes the pharmacokinetics of a drug, and thus only gives a rough estimate of pharmacodynamics. After an infusion of a drug, the duration of *clinical* effect depends on the initial plasma concentration at the end of the infusion, *and* on pharmacodynamic factors such as the individual sensitivity of the patient to the infused drug (such as age, sex, pharmacodynamic interactions with other drugs, critical illness).

Relevance

This concept was very quickly accepted and used by the anaesthetic pharmacology community. For most anaesthetic agents, the pharmacokinetics can be described by a three compartment model. Consequently, the time-course of changes in plasma concentration after an infusion depend not only on the individual pharmacokinetic characteristics of the drug (metabolism/

elimination clearance, and fast and slow re-distribution clearance) but also on the duration of infusion. The individual pharmacokinetic parameters, such as elimination half-life, are difficult concepts for clinicians. But even for the mathematically gifted, the influence of infusion duration on poly-exponential drug behaviour after infusion is very difficult to predict from the pharmacokinetics of a drug. Thus, most anaesthetists are now also familiar with the concept, and those practising intravenous anaesthesia will routinely use the context-sensitive half-time concept in their clinical decision making process.

Paper 5: Preliminary pharmacokinetics and pharmacodynamics of an ultra-short-acting opioid: remifentanil (GI87084B)

Author details

PSA Glass, D Hardman, Y Kamiyama, TJ Quill, G Marton, KH Donn, CM Grosse

Reference

Anesthesia and Analgesia 1993; **77**: 1031–40.

Summary

In this study the kinetics of remifentanil were consistent with a two compartment mamillary model. The compartment volumes were small, while clearances were large, resulting from very rapid elimination and re-distribution. Furthermore, the main metabolite is essentially inactive. In addition to it being a very potent analgesic and respiratory depressant, remifentanil crosses the blood–brain barrier very rapidly.

Citation count

475.

Related references

1 Egan TD, Lemmens HJ, Fiset P. The pharmacokinetics of the new short-acting opioid remifentanil (GI87084B) in healthy adult male volunteers. *Anesthesiology* 1993; **79**: 881–92.
2 Westmoreland CL, Hoke JF, Sebel PS, *et al*. Pharmacokinetics of remifentanil (GI87084B) and its major metabolite (GI90291) in patients undergoing elective inpatient surgery. *Anesthesiology* 1993; **79**: 893–903.

Key message

Remifentanil is a very potent, very short-acting drug likely to have a useful role in clinical practice.

Strengths

The authors compared remifentanil with alfentanil. Numerous blood samples were taken, including several early and late samples. The study was pure in that volunteers received no other agents. In addition a wide range of doses (0.0625–2 µg kg⁻¹) were studied.

Weaknesses

Only bolus doses were used —volunteers received the dose of remifentanil as a fast infusion over 1 min. As would be expected from such an early study, only fit, young, healthy, non-obese adults were enrolled.

Relevance

This paper was one of three articles on the pharmacokinetics of remifentanil published by competing groups in November 1993. The broad findings of this study are generally consistent with those of the other studies. They are also broadly consistent with those of subsequent studies, although Minto later showed that its pharmacokinetics better fit those of a three compartment model. While it shares with the other two publications the distinction of being the first paper on the pharmacokinetics of this agent in humans, it has since received by far the highest number of citations.

Paper 6: Pharmacokinetic model driven infusion of propofol in children

Author details

B Marsh, M White, N Morton, GNC Kenny

Reference

British Journal of Anaesthesia 1991; **67**: 41–8.

Abstract

A computer controlled infusion device for propofol was used to induce and maintain general anaesthesia in 20 children undergoing minor surgical procedures. The device was programmed with an adult pharmacokinetic model for propofol. During and after anaesthesia, blood samples were taken for measurement of propofol concentrations and it was found that the values obtained were systematically overpredicted by the delivery system algorithm. New pharmacokinetic microconstants were derived from our data which reflected more accurately the elimination and distribution of propofol in a prospective study involving another 10 children.

Summary

Although this manuscript is commonly cited as a reference for the 'Marsh' adult pharmacokinetic model for propofol, the manuscript itself is *not* about the pharmacokinetics of propofol in adults, but rather is about the development of a propofol pharmacokinetic for children. The authors first demonstrated that the adult model (a slightly modified version of the Gepts model) performed poorly when used for target-controlled infusion (TCI) in children. They then developed a new paediatric model, also comprising three compartments, and prospectively evaluated the predictive performance of this model. As with other, subsequently published, paediatric models, the new model comprised a larger central compartment volume, faster metabolic and re-distribution clearance than the 'Marsh' adult model. These parameters resulted in improved predictive performance compared with the adult model.

Citation count

623.

Related references

1 Absalom AR, Mani V, Smet De T, *et al*. Pharmacokinetic models for propofol—defining and illuminating the devil in the detail. *Br J Anaesth* 2009; **103**: 26–37.

2 Gepts E, Camu F, Cockshott ID, *et al*. Disposition of propofol administered as constant rate intravenous infusions in humans. *Anesth Analg* 1987; **66**: 1256–63.

3 White M, Kenny GN. Intravenous propofol anaesthesia using a computerised infusion system. *Anaesthesia* 1990; **45**: 204–9.

Key message

Adult pharmacokinetic models perform poorly when used for TCIs in children. The key differences in pharmacokinetics of propofol in children are a larger immediate volume of distribution (central compartment), which requires larger induction doses, and faster metabolism and redistribution clearances, requiring higher maintenance infusion rates.

Strengths

Models were studied in the appropriate patient group (children) and it was a prospective evaluation. Several late (after infusion cessation) blood samples were taken and this is important because they are informative about metabolism and drug clearance.

Weaknesses

Only venous blood samples were used and the timing of the blood samples is not explicitly stated. In addition, there were no early samples, and this is important because it impairs the ability to assess the initial volume of distribution.

Relevance

The paediatric model described in this manuscript is not used and is thus of little clinical relevance. The chief relevance of this paper is that it was the first peer-reviewed publication in which the Marsh (adult) pharmacokinetic parameters for propofol were mentioned (albeit in passing). Although Kenny and White had already published a paper describing a prototype of the TCI system developed in Glasgow, this paper was one of the early papers describing the clinical use of propofol TCI, and certainly novel in that it was the first to describe TCI use in children.

Paper 7: The influence of age on propofol pharmacodynamics

Author details

TW Schnider, CF Minto, SL Shafer, PL Gambus, C Andresen, DB Goodale, EJ Youngs

Reference

Anesthesiology 1999; **90**: 1502–16.

Summary

In a companion article the authors had shown that the pharmacokinetics of propofol are changed with age. In this article they showed that pharmacodynamics are also markedly affected by age. From the semilinear canonical correlation parameter, and also visual inspection of the EEG, they estimated that the time to peak effect after a single propofol bolus is of the order of 1.7 min; and that the k_{eo} for propofol is $0.456\,min^{-1}$.

Citation count

465.

Related references

1 Schnider TW, Minto CF, Gambus PL, *et al*. The influence of method of administration and covariates on the pharmacokinetics of propofol in adult volunteers. *Anesthesiology* 1998; **88**: 1170–182.

2 Schnider TW, Minto CF. Age related changes of the PK-PD of intravenous anaesthetics. *Adv Exp Med Biol* 2003; **523**: 45–56.

3 Absalom AR, Mani V, De ST, *et al*. Pharmacokinetic models for propofol - defining and illuminating the devil in the detail. *Br J Anaesth* 2009; **103**: 26–37.

Key message

Propofol pharmacodynamics are age dependent.

Strengths

This was a scientifically pure approach—these data come from a combined pharmacokinetic–pharmacodynamic study in a single cohort of subjects. Frequent arterial blood samples were taken.

Weaknesses

Only a limited number of subjects (24) were studied. Pharmacodynamic analysis was partly based on the now seldom used EEG parameter. Data analysis of the results after bolus dose excluded the results from patients older than 65. Of the subjects studied there was a limited range of body habitus—few obese volunteers, and no morbidly obese.

Relevance

The k_{eo} from this publication, and the pharmacokinetic model parameters published in the companion publication (involving the same subjects in the same study) form the Schnider model, one of the two most commonly pharmacokinetic models for propofol. In addition, the methodology used is considered by many to be the gold standard, a template which should be used for development of future models.

Paper 8: The pharmacodynamic interaction of propofol and alfentanil during lower abdominal surgery in women

Author details
J Vuyk, T Lim, FHM Engbers, AGL Burm, AA Vletter, JG Bovill

Reference
Anesthesiology 1995; **83**: 8–22.

Summary
In a group of female patients undergoing lower abdominal surgery, the authors studied the pharmacodynamic interaction between propofol and alfentanil for different anaesthetic endpoints. Their study demonstrated a strongly synergistic interaction between the two agents, not only for the ability of the combination to prevent responses to noxious stimuli, but also on the ability of the combination to maintain unconsciousness. It also showed that although it is possible to prevent responses to noxious stimuli with high doses of propofol, the same cannot be achieved with alfentanil alone (i.e. some hypnotic is always required).

Citation count
197.

Related references
1 Vuyk J, Engbers FH, Burm AL *et al.* Pharmacodynamic interaction between propofol and alfentanil when given for induction of anesthesia. *Anesthesiology* 1996; **84**: 288–99.

2 Vuyk J, Mertens MJ, Olofsen E, Burm AG, Bovill JG. Propofol anesthesia and rational opioid selection: determination of optimal EC50-EC95 propofol-opioid concentrations that assure adequate anesthesia and a rapid return of consciousness. *Anesthesiology* 1997; **87**: 1549–62.

3 Bouillon T, Bruhn J, Radu-Radulescu L, Bertaccini E, Park S, Shafer S. Non-steady state analysis of the pharmacokinetic interaction between propofol and remifentanil. *Anesthesiology* 2002; **97**: 1350–62.

4 Mertens MJ, Olofsen E, Engbers FH, *et al.* Propofol reduces perioperative remifentanil requirements in a synergistic manner: response surface modeling of perioperative remifentanil-propofol interactions. *Anesthesiology* 2003; **99**: 347–59.

5 Nieuwenhuijs DJ, Olofsen E, Romberg RR *et al.* Response surface modeling of remifentanil-propofol interaction on cardiorespiratory control and bispectral index. *Anesthesiology* 2003; **98**: 312–22.

6 Bouillon TW, Bruhn J, Radulescu L *et al.* Pharmacodynamic interaction between propofol and remifentanil regarding hypnosis, tolerance of laryngoscopy, bispectral index, and electroencephalographic approximate entropy. *Anesthesiology* 2004; **100**: 1353–72.

Key message
Propofol and alfentanil have a synergistic effect in suppressing responses to intra-abdominal surgical stimuli and consciousness.

Strengths

This was novel methodology—patients were randomized to different propofol doses (target blood concentrations, and then responses to stimuli were assessed at different alfentanil doses). Use of target-controlled infusions of propofol and alfentanil enabled the authors to administer stable plasma (and effect-site) concentrations of both drugs. The measurement of arterial blood concentrations of propofol and alfentanil strongly improved the validity of the results, since use of target blood concentrations is associated with a degree of uncertainty about the actual concentration achieved, particularly when drug combinations are used, resulting in the possibility of pharmacokinetic interactions.

Weaknesses

Again there were only small numbers of subjects in each group. There were also very tight inclusion criteria (only young to middle-aged women, ASA status 1, undergoing lower abdominal laparotomy), and this limits the general applicability of the results.

Relevance

In modern anaesthetic practice, combinations of drugs are almost always used, most commonly a hypnotic with an analgesic. This landmark paper provided a step change in our understanding of the pharmacodynamic interaction between propofol and the opioids during maintenance of anaesthesia. The authors went on to conduct several other important studies on other aspects of pharmacodynamic interactions. For example, they used and adapted their methods to study the interactive effect of hypnotics and opioids on respiratory control, extrapolated their work to other opioids, and used simulations to determine the optimal combinations of propofol and different opioids. A natural extension of their work was also response surface modelling, and this approach has also proven scientifically highly fruitful.

Paper 9: Dynamic and static cerebral autoregulation during isoflurane, desflurane, and propofol anesthesia

Author details

S Strebel, AM Lam, B Matta, TS Mayberg, R Aaslid, DW Newell

Reference

Anesthesiology 1995; **83**: 66–76.

Summary

Autoregulation is maintained with propofol at high doses, whereas with high doses of isoflurane and desflurane autoregulation is impaired.

Citation count

229.

Related references

1 Conti A, Iacopino DG, Fodale V, *et al.* Cerebral haemodynamic changes during propofol-remifentanil or sevoflurane anaesthesia: Transcranial doppler study under bispectral index monitoring. *Br J Anaesth* 2006; **97**: 333–9.

2 Johnston AJ, Steiner LA, Chatfield DA, *et al.* Effects of propofol on cerebral oxygenation and metabolism after head injury. *Br J Anaesth* 2003; **91**: 781–6.

Key message

During neurosurgical procedures, higher doses of propofol can be safely used, whereas use of >1 MAC of inhalational anaesthetics should be avoided.

Strengths

Two clinically relevant doses of each agent were used and both static and dynamic autoregulation were assessed.

Weaknesses

The study used an indirect measurement of cerebral blood flow. Autoregulation is the physiological process by which the brain maintains a constant cerebral blood flow in the face of changing arterial pressure. In this study the authors measured blood *flow velocity* in the middle cerebral artery, rather than *flow rate*, and have measured static and dynamic regulation in flow not velocity. If the middle cerebral artery diameter remains constant despite changes in arterial pressure and anaesthetic dose, then the relative changes in flow and velocity will be identical. The chief weakness of this paper is the assumption that middle cerebral artery diameter is constant, since this assumption is not universally accepted to be true.

A further weakness is the use of nitrous oxide (N_2O). Nitrous oxide exerts an effect on cerebral metabolism and blood flow (on its own it increases both). Since this agent was used in all experimental conditions, it is assumed that it had an equivalent effect for each drug at each dose, and this may or may not be true.

Relevance

This article is one of the reasons why propofol is probably the most popular choice of anaesthetic agent for neurosurgery. It demonstrated that autoregulation was maintained during propofol-based anaesthesia, but not during isoflurane or desflurane-based anaesthesia. Thus, at both low and high doses of propofol, flow-metabolism coupling ensures that proportional changes in cerebral metabolism and blood flow are likely; and this coupling will probably be maintained within the autoregulatory range of blood pressures. The benefits of this are that the reduced blood flow will reduce cerebral blood volume, in turn reducing intracranial pressure thereby improving operating conditions for the surgeon. The matched reduction in flow and metabolism mean that flow remains adequate for the (reduced) metabolic requirements of the brain, and the persistence of autoregulation implies that if the blood pressure increases (or decreases) within the autoregulatory range, then appropriate changes in cerebral vascular tone will maintain the flow at an adequate level for the metabolism.

At low doses of the two volatile agents, some delay in autoregulation was seen, while at higher doses autoregulation was abolished. Thus, at higher doses of isoflurane or desflurane, cerebral blood flow is pressure dependent within the usual (awake) range of autoregulation. If the mean arterial blood pressure increases, the failure of autoregulation (i.e. lack of cerebral vasoconstriction) will result in significant increases in cerebral blood flow, blood volume, and intracranial pressure, and deteriorating operating conditions. Clearly, all of these changes are undesirable during neurosurgical procedures. Since higher anaesthetic higher doses are sometimes required (e.g. for rapid temporary control of systemic hypertension) and so many use this article to argue in favour of propofol for neurosurgery.

Paper 10: Randomized controlled trial of total intravenous anesthesia with propofol versus inhalation anesthesia with isoflurane–nitrous oxide: postoperative nausea and vomiting and economic analysis

Author details

K Visser, EA Hassink, GJ Bonsel, J Moen, CJ Kalkman

Reference

Anesthesiology 2001; **95**: 616–26.

Summary

This randomized controlled trial showed that TIVA reduces the absolute risk of postoperative nausea and vomiting (PONV) by between 15–20% in comparison with isoflurane. At the time of the study, the TIVA technique was in significantly greater use than the isoflurane–nitrous oxide (N$_2$O) technique.

Citation count

141.

Related references

1 Green G, Jonsson L. Nausea – the most important factor determining length of stay after ambulatory anesthesia – a comparative-study of isoflurane and or propofol techniques. *Acta Anaesthesiol Scand* 1993; **37**: 742–6.

2 Smith I, Thwaites AJ. Target-controlled propofol vs. sevoflurane: a double-blind, randomised comparison in day-case anaesthesia. *Anaesthesia* 1999; **54**: 745–52.

Key message

Propofol is associated with a significant reduction in the incidence of postoperative nausea and vomiting.

Strengths

It was a randomized controlled clinical trial and thus has a high level of proof. There was a good explanation of the research question. It was a well-conducted study, with a long period of follow-up, and consideration of most of the financial consequences of PONV.

Weaknesses

There was a high incidence of PONV—apparently because patients were followed-up for longer than in other studies. PONV was not entirely clearly defined, and severity not categorized, when clearly a brief period of mild nausea is less significant than a prolonged period of severe nausea. The conclusions of economic analysis were only valid at the time of publication, when generic versions of propofol were not available (since then prices have fallen by up to 80%).

Relevance

Although most anaesthetists agree that propofol provides a superior recovery from anaesthesia, there are few studies that have rigorously assessed this. One of the chief benefits of using propofol for maintenance of anaesthesia is the low incidence of PONV, and this issue was addressed rigorously in this study. This study provided strong support to the view that propofol provides a superior recovery from anaesthesia and that it is the first choice for maintenance of anaesthesia for patients who are at risk for PONV. The cost analysis is now somewhat irrelevant.

Chapter 5

Monitoring

PS Myles

Introduction

Patient monitoring begins with observation, looking for signs of ill health, and indicators of functional status. Time-honoured traditional monitoring in anaesthesia (still) includes observing skin colour, a finger on the pulse, measurement of blood pressure, and observation of respiration, the latter including the reservoir bag. Developments in technology have progressed at an astounding pace since World War II, such that modern monitoring includes an array of patient and machine variables increasingly being processed via an electronic patient record. Miniaturization and improved computing power have been key to much of this.

Monitoring, underpinned by proper training and vigilance, reduces the risk of undesirable outcomes and so improves patient safety. In 1960, a Special Committee investigating deaths under anaesthesia was sponsored by the New South Wales Government in Australia (Holland, 1970). This attracted worldwide interest and prompted similar efforts elsewhere (Eichhorn et al., 1986; Lunn and Devlin, 1987; Caplan et al., 1990; Holland et al., 1993), culminating in the US Institute of Medicine (2000) report, To err is human, which demonstrated the magnitude of adverse events in the USA. The influence of these reports on the practice of anaesthesia and surgery, and monitoring in particular, is undeniable.

Despite the apparently obvious link between monitoring and improved patient outcomes, efforts to demonstrate such a link were often unsuccessful (Mollet et al., 1993a,b). Most experts agree that this is a credit to the extremely low incidence of serious adverse events attributable to anaesthesia. It was not until 2004 that the first large randomized trial demonstrating effectiveness of patient monitoring, in this case depth of anaesthesia, was published (Myles et al., 2004).

Related references

1 Holland R. Special Committee Investigating Deaths Under Anaesthesia: report on 745 classified cases, 1960–1968. *Med J Aust* 1970; **1**: 573–94.

2 Eichhorn JH, Cooper JB, Cullen DJ, Maier WR, Philip JH, Seeman RG. Standards for patient monitoring during anesthesia at Harvard Medical School. *JAMA* 1986; **256**: 1017–20.

3 Lunn JN, Devlin HB. Lessons from the confidential enquiry into perioperative deaths in three NHS regions. *Lancet* 1987; **2**: 1384–6.

4 Caplan RA, Posner KL, Ward RJ, Cheney FW. Adverse respiratory events in anesthesia: a closed claims analysis. *Anesthesiology* 1990; **72**: 828–33.

5 Holland R, Hains J, Roberts JG, Runciman WB. Symposium: the Australian Incident Monitoring Study. *Anaesth Intensive Care* 1993; **21**: 501–5.

6 Moller JT, Pedersen T, Rasmussen LS et al. Randomized evaluation of pulse oximetry in 20,802 patients: I. Design, demography, pulse oximetry failure rate, and overall complication rate. *Anesthesiology* 1993; **78**: 436–44.

7 Moller JT, Johannessen NW, Espersen K, et al. Randomized evaluation of pulse oximetry in 20,802 patients: II. Perioperative events and postoperative complications. *Anesthesiology* 1993; **78**: 445–53.

8 Committee on Quality of Health Care in America, Institute of Medicine. *To err is human: building a safer health system.* Washington, DC: National Academy Press, USA, 2000.

9 Myles PS, Leslie K, Forbes A, McNeil J, Chan M, for the B-Aware Trial Group. Bispectral index monitoring to prevent awareness during anaesthesia: the B-Aware randomised controlled trial. *Lancet* 2004; **363**: 1757–63.

Paper 1: Electrodes for blood pO$_2$ and pCO$_2$ determination

Author details

JW Severinghaus, AF Bradley

Reference

Journal of Applied Physiology 1958; **13**: 515–20.

Summary

This paper describes the development of the first blood gas machine. The investigators used the principles of the Clarke oxygen (Clark, 1960) and Stowe carbon dioxide (Stow *et al.*, 1957) electrodes to build a device that measured gas tensions in blood and other fluids.

Citation count

735.

Related references

1 Clark LC Jr. Intravascular polarographic and potentiometric electrodes for the study of circulation. *Trans Am Soc Artif Intern Organs* 1960; **6**: 348–54.

2 Severinghaus JW. First electrodes for blood PO$_2$ and PCO$_2$ determination. *J Applied Physiol* 2004; **97**: 1599–600.

3 Stow RW, Baer RF, Randall B. Rapid measurement of the tension of carbon dioxide in blood. *Arch Phys Med Rehabil* 1957; **38**: 646–50.

Key message

The ability to measure arterial blood gases in clinical practice greatly enhanced our understanding of gas exchange and acid–base physiology, and has been a mainstay in the assessment and management of patients undergoing major surgery or those with critical illness. Concepts of buffering, anion gap, and later, hyperchloraemic acidosis and Stewart's quantitative approach to acid–base disorders, have followed.

Strengths

The simply written descriptions of the steps taken to build, test, and evaluate the electrodes are nicely outlined. Attribution to previous inventor-scientists (Clarke and Stow) is clear. The importance of the properties of the semipermeable membranes used, temperature control, and relationship between bicarbonate concentration and carbon dioxide response rate are explored.

Weaknesses

The stability over time, assumptions in the calculations, and responsiveness are all considered but not rigorously tested. No patient data were presented and so demonstration of the clinical utility of such a device had to await later studies.

Relevance

Ready access to accurate measurement of arterial and mixed venous oxygen and carbon dioxide tensions, pH, and base excess have improved patient management in many areas of medicine.

Paper 2: Neuromuscular effects of d-tubocurarine, edrophonium and neostigmine in man

Author details

RL Katz

Reference

Anesthesiology 1967; **28**: 327–36.

Summary

The performance of peripheral and/or abdominal muscle nerve stimulation was evaluated in more than 500 patients, under a variety of anaesthetic techniques and muscle relaxants. These studies documented the wide range in sensitivity to muscle relaxants, justifying monitoring to more reliably determine the extent of neuromuscular block and its recovery. Distinct differences between depolarizing and non-depolarizing muscle relaxants, effects of inhalational anaesthesia, response to single twitch and tetanic stimulation, as well as antagonism with anticholinesterases, were demonstrated.

Citation count

124.

Related references

1 Katz RL, Wolf CE. Neuromuscular and electromyographic studies in man: effects of hyperventilation, carbon dioxide inhalation and d-tubocurarine. *Anesthesiology* 1964; **25**: 781–7.

2 Ali HH, Savarese JJ. Monitoring of neuromuscular function. *Anesthesiology* 1976; **45**: 216–49.

3 Viby-Mogensen J. Clinical assessment of neuromuscular transmission. *Br J Anaesth* 1982; **54**: 209–23.

Key message

Although others had investigated the effects of neuromuscular blockers on muscle function or electromyography, this was the first demonstration of the potential utility of the peripheral nerve stimulator in anaesthesia (Fig. 5.1). Previously, assessment of the extent and recovery of neuromuscular blockade was reliant upon the 'feel' of the anaesthetic reservoir bag and opinion of the surgeon.

Strengths

The diverse range of anaesthetic techniques, testing depolarizing and non-depolarizing relaxants, used at various dosages or via infusion, provided a wealth of information. Efforts were made to standardize blood gases, temperature, and ventilation, with the latter being varied in order to assess its effects. Twitch height was correlated with surgical conditions—the increased sensitivity of monitoring, as opposed to clinical judgement, was highlighted.

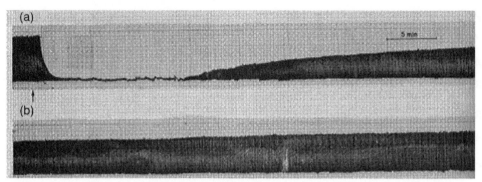

Fig. 5.1 Monitoring of muscle relaxation with the electrical twitch height. (a) At arrow *d*-tubocurarine (0.3 mg kg⁻¹) injected. (b) Continuation of recovery from *d*-tubocurarine. Reproduced from Ronald L. Katz, Comparison of Electrical and Mechanical Recording of Spontaneous and Evoked Muscle Activity: The Clinical Value of Continuous Recording as an Aid to the Rational Use of Muscle Relaxants During Anesthesia. *Anesthesiology*, **26**(2), 204–211, 1965, American Journal of Anaesthesiologists, with permission.

Weaknesses

There was no real attempt to quantify the extent of neuromuscular block and the effects of residual block were not properly considered. Patient disease states were not studied. Patient outcomes attributable to incomplete reversal of block, such as distress, respiratory failure, aspiration or pneumonia, were not reported.

Relevance

The widespread adoption of neuromuscular block monitoring improved our understanding of dose-responsiveness, interaction with medical diseases and other classes of drugs, duration of effect, and reversal. More accurate titration of neuromuscular blockade facilitated tracheal intubation, surgery, and recovery of function.

Paper 3: Stimulus frequency in the detection of neuromuscular block in humans

Author details

HH Ali, JE Utting, C Gray

Reference

British Journal of Anaesthesia 1970; **42**: 967–78.

Abstract

Study of the literature on the physiology of neuromuscular transmission suggested two new methods of assessing the degree of neuromuscular block in the human subject. These were, first, a comparison of the height of the recorded twitch tensions developed in response to repeated single stimuli applied at differing frequencies and, second, examination of the extent of reduction in amplitude of twitch tensions developed in response to a short train of four stimuli. In assessing the first method the use of three frequencies of stimulation was tried (i.e., 0.1 Hz (cps), 0.3 Hz and 1.0 Hz). It was found that as the frequency of stimulation was increased there was reduction in the amplitude of the recorded twitch response in curarized subjects, and that this reduction appeared to depend on the degree of curarization. In assessing the second method a short train of four stimuli at 2 Hz was used, and it was found that there was a progressive fade of successive recorded mechanical twitch responses in curarized subjects which again appeared to depend on the degree of curarization. It is suggested that the amplitude of the twitch response at a higher frequency expressed as a percentage of that at the slower rate, and the last response of the train of four expressed as a percentage of the first may be useful in measuring degree of neuromuscular block in man.

Ali HH, Utting JE, Gray C, 'Stimulus frequency in the detection of neuromuscular block in humans', *British Journal of Anaesthesia*, 1970, 42, 11, pp. 967–978, by permission of Oxford University Press and British Journal of Anaesthesia.

Summary

This group evaluated different patterns of peripheral nerve stimulation in anaesthesia. They found that the ratio of the height of the fourth twitch to that of the first twitch—the train-of-four (TOF)—could be used as a more sensitive measure of neuromuscular blockade.

Citation count

193.

Related references

1 Katz RL, Wolf CE. Neuromuscular and electromyographic studies in man: effects of hyperventilation, carbon dioxide inhalation and d-tubocurarine. *Anesthesiology* 1964; **25**: 781–7.

2 Ali HH, Savarese JJ. Monitoring of neuromuscular function. *Anesthesiology* 1976; **45**: 216–49.

3 Viby-Mogensen J. Clinical assessment of neuromuscular transmission. *Br J Anaesth* 1982; **54**: 209–23.

Key message

The TOF became a standard measure of the degree of neuromuscular block. It was better able to discern residual block, and could be used to compare the relative potency of neuromuscular blockers.

Strengths

The authors compared the known variety of methods of assessing neuromuscular blockade at that time, and clearly identified the superiority of TOF in some situations. Depolarizing (suxamethonium) and non-depolarizing (tubocurarine) drugs were tested in awake and anaesthetized subjects. A correlation between the TOF and clinical signs of muscle weakness including diplopia was noted.

Weaknesses

The potential confounding effects of inhalational anaesthesia, hypothermia, and acid–base and electrolyte disturbance were not evaluated. Statistical comparisons of the different nerve stimulation techniques were not done, and so the reader cannot reliably quantify any differences.

Relevance

The TOF quickly became a routine measure of neuromuscular blockade during and after anaesthesia. There is no need to obtain a baseline (control) measurement, and unlike tetanic stimulation it can be applied in awake patients. It is a more sensitive measure of residual neuromuscular blockade.

Paper 4: Catheterization of heart in man with use of flow-directed balloon-tipped catheter

Author details

HJ Swan, W Ganz, J Forrester, H Marcus, G Diamond, D Chonette

Reference

New England Journal of Medicine 1970; **283**: 447–51.

Summary

A flow-directed balloon-flotation pulmonary artery catheter was developed to enable safe and rapid right heart catheterization in patients with acute myocardial infarction. The effectiveness of right heart and pulmonary artery catheterization without fluoroscopy or catheter manipulation was quickly proven, along with the near absence of arrhythmias.

Citation count

342.

Related references

1 Forrester JS, Ganz W, Diamond G, *et al*. Thermodilution cardiac output determination with a single flow directed catheter for cardiac monitoring. *Am Heart J* 1972; **83**: 306–11.

2 Rao TL, Jacobs KH, El-Etr AA. Reinfarction following anesthesia in patients with myocardial infarction. *Anesthesiology* 1983*;* **59**: 499–505.

3 Iberti TJ, Fischer EP, Leibowitz AB, *et al*. A multicenter study of physician's knowledge of the pulmonary-artery catheter. *JAMA* 1990; **264**: 2928–32.

4 Practice Guidelines for Pulmonary Artery Catheterization. A report by the American Society of Anesthesiologists Task Force. *Anesthesiology* 1993; **78**: 380–94.

5 Connors AF, Speroff T, Dawson NV, *et al*. The effectiveness of right heart catheterization in the initial care of critically ill patients. *JAMA*, 1996; **276**: 889–97.

6 Sandham JD, Hull RD, Brant RF, *et al*. A randomized, controlled trial of the use of pulmonary-artery catheters in high-risk surgical patients. *N Engl J Med* 2003; **348**: 5–14.

7 Shah MR, Hasselblad V, Stevenson LW, *et al*. Implication of the pulmonary artery catheter in critically ill patients: meta-analysis of randomized clinical trials. *JAMA*, 2005; **294**: 1664–70.

Key message

The absence of a need for imaging and near-avoidance of arrhythmias for placement negated risks of right-sided heart catheterization. Better estimation of left-sided filling pressure, and later, cardiac output, provided a rationale basis for the care of critically ill patients during and after surgery. Derived indices such as pulmonary and systemic vascular resistance, and left ventricular stroke work index, could be measured and compared in clinical studies.

Strengths

From a 'eureka' moment on the beach in California, after watching the effectiveness of a spinnaker sail in a calm sea, Swan devised his balloon flotation method. Success in the animal laboratory and then the coronary care unit was readily apparent: ease and speed of placement, much less arrhythmia. Construction of the catheter and its use were clearly outlined.

Weaknesses

The developers of this device had substantial previous experience of central venous and right-heart catheterization—their reported results may not represent practice elsewhere. At this early stage in development there were no convincing clinical outcome data presented. As with all monitoring, better information will not translate into better outcomes unless improvements in therapy can be implemented.

Relevance

The popularly known 'Swan–Ganz' catheter was further developed for measuring cardiac output (by the thermodilution technique), for right atrial and right ventricular pacing, and for measuring right-sided pressures, including pulmonary capillary wedge pressure (Forrester *et al.*, 1972) Infusion ports were later incorporated to facilitate administration of vasoactive and inotropic drugs. The Swan–Ganz catheter became most commonly used in anaesthesia and critical care, to facilitate monitoring and therapy during and after complex surgical procedures.

Paper 5: Neurophysiologic effects of general anesthetics. I. The electroencephalogram and sensory evoked responses in man

Author details

DL Clark, BS Rosner

Reference

Anesthesiology 1973; **38**: 564–82.

Summary

This review paper examined the effects of a variety of general anaesthetics on the electroencephalogram (EEG) and somatosensory evoked responses. The relationship with minimum alveolar concentration (MAC), the concentration which causes unconsciousness (CONC), and the concentration at which a patient responds to commands (MAC awake) were explored. Deepening anaesthesia was associated with an increase in slow wave activity followed by EEG suppression (Fig. 5.2). Subtle differences existed for different anaesthetic agents.

Citation count

286.

Related references

1 Kiersey DK, Bickford RG, Faulconer A. Electro-encephalographic patterns produced by thiopental sodium during surgical operations; description and classification. *Br J Anaesth* 1951; **23**: 141–52.

2 Thornton C, Barrowcliffe MP, Konieczko K, *et al*. The auditory evoked-response as an indicator of awareness. *Br J Anaesth*, 1989; **63**: 113–15.

3 Sigl JC, Chamoun NG. An introduction to bispectral analysis for the EEG. *J Clin Mon* 1994; **10**: 392–404.

4 Myles PS, Leslie K, Forbes A, *et al*. Bispectral index monitoring to prevent awareness during anaesthesia: the B-Aware randomised controlled trial. *Lancet* 2004; **363**: 1757–63.

Key message

Qualitative (but not quantitative) changes in the EEG according to higher concentrations of anaesthetic drug delivery were demonstrated. Different anaesthetic drugs had specific effects on the EEG. The authors noted that the introduction of muscle relaxants exposed patients to the risk of awareness during surgery: EEG and/or evoked responses monitoring may reduce this risk.

Strengths

This comprehensive review, with 114 references including EEG studies dating from the 1930s, identified some specific EEG patterns according to different classes of anaesthetics. The authors highlight the differences between CONC, MAC, and MAC awake, and their lack of continuity on a dose–response curve.

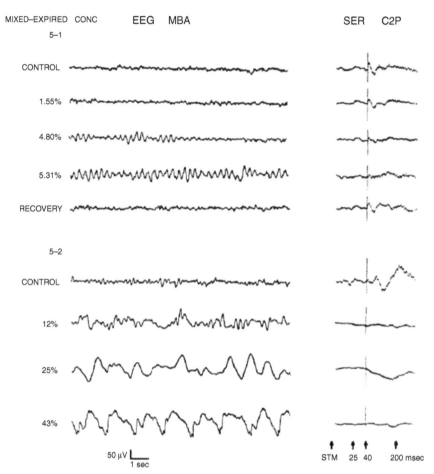

Fig. 5.2 Effects of cyclopropane on the electroencephalogram and somatic evoked responses (SER) of conscious (Subject 5-1) and unconscious (Subject 5-2) man. EEG: monopolar frontal. SER: averaged responses from monopolar recordings at the contralateral post-Rolandic scalp. Fast time base to the left of the vertical bar for evoked responses, slow time base to the right of the bar. Arrows indicate times in ms after stimulus (STIM). Reproduced from D.L. Clark, B.S. Rosner, Neurophysiologic effects of general anesthetics. I. The electroencephalogram and sensory evoked responses in man. *Anesthesiology*, **38**(6), 564–582, 1973, American Journal of Anaesthesiologists, with permission.

Weaknesses

Some of the study findings differed from previous investigators, leaving the reader uncertain as to the particular EEG effects for some anaesthetic agents (or combinations). General EEG patterns were described, but no method of quantifying this according to anaesthetic depth was considered.

Relevance

The EEG effects of general anaesthesia were first studied in the 1950s. Very soon some investigators proposed that the EEG could be used to measure depth of anaesthesia. The relationship between anaesthetic drug administration, anaesthetic depth, and EEG changes were correlated.

Paper 6: Evaluation of pulse oximetry

Author details

M Yelderman, W New Jr

Reference

Anesthesiology 1983; **59**: 349–52.

Summary

Arterial oxygen saturation of haemoglobin can be determined directly and continuously by spectrophotoelectric oximetric techniques. This technique utilizes the wavelength dependence of reduced versus oxyhaemoglobin according to the Lambert–Beer's law. Pulse oximetry uses the light absorbance changes according to arterial pulsation. The authors used a newly developed commercial pulse oximeter to evaluate the accuracy of pulse oximetry over a broad range of arterial saturations. They induced mild degrees of hypoxaemia in volunteers and measured arterial oxygen tension and saturation with laboratory co-oximetry.

Citation count

401.

Related references

1 Hertzman AB. The blood supply of various skin areas as estimated by the photoelectric plethysymograph. *Am J Physiol* 1938; **124**: 328–40.

2 Stephen CR, Slater HM, Johnson AL, *et al.* The oximeter – a technical aid for the anesthesiologist. *Anesthesiology* 1951; **12**: 541–55.

3 Aoyagi T, Kishi M, Yamaguchi K, *et al.* Improvement of an earpiece oximeter. Abstracts, 13th Annual Meeting of the Japan Society of Medical Electronics and Biological Engineering, Osaka, Japan, April 26–27, 1974, pp. 90–1.

4 Catley DM, Thornton C, Jordan C, *et al.* Pronounced, episodic oxygen desaturation in the postoperative period: its association with ventilatory pattern and analgesic regimen. *Anesthesiology*, 1985; **63**: 20–8.

5 Aoyagi T. Pulse oximetry: its invention, theory, and future. *J Anesth* 2003; **17**: 259–66.

6 World Health Organization Global Pulse Oximetry Project. Available at: http://www.safesurg. org/pulse-oximetry.html (accessed 13 November 2009).

Key message

Skin oximetry was first described in the 1930s (Hertzman, 1938), and pulse oximetry was first conceived in 1972 (Stephen *et al.*, 1932). Pulse oximetry rapidly gained widespread popularity, followed by near-universal adoption as a standard of care during anaesthesia. In 2010 the World Health Organization's Global Pulse Oximetry Project was launched to provide affordable pulse oximetry devices for every operating room in the developing world.

Strengths

The authors briefly reviewed the physics underpinning pulse oximetry and then evaluated the performance of a newly-introduced commercial monitor (Fig. 5.3). They reported excellent

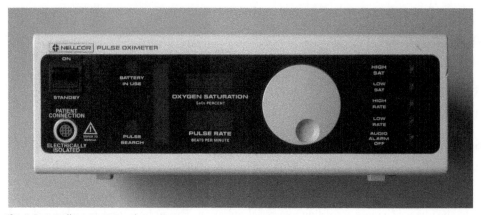

Fig. 5.3 A Nellcor N-100 pulse oximeter.

agreement with standard laboratory measurement of oxygen saturation, and correctly predicted that inaccuracies may occur in situations of poor peripheral perfusion or if dyshaemoglobin species were present.

Weaknesses

The performance of the pulse oximeter for oxygen saturations <70% was not tested, nor were their suggested sources of inaccuracies (poor perfusion, dyshaemoglobin species). The authors intended to measure agreement but used an incorrect method of analysis—linear correlation—rather than intraclass correlation or Bland–Altman agreement. In their analysis they pooled 79 sets of data from five subjects, thus assuming that each measurement was independent. Only one commercial pulse oximeter device was available for testing at that time.

Relevance

Adequate oxygenation is an essential component of safe anaesthesia. Equipment failure, human error, patient comorbidity, and intraoperative incidents threaten tissue oxygenation and so this should be monitored continuously. Relatively cheap, simple-to-use, safe monitoring of tissue oxygenation revolutionized anaesthesia safety.

Paper 7: An analysis of major errors and equipment failures in anesthesia management: considerations for prevention and detection

Author details

JB Cooper, RS Newbower, RJ Kitz

Reference

Anesthesiology 1984; **60**: 34–42.

Summary

A modified critical-incident analysis technique was used in a retrospective examination of the characteristics of human error and equipment failure in anaesthetic practice. The data were used to identify and analyse preventable mishaps. The authors estimate that around 20% (14 of 67) of serious adverse outcomes occurring after anaesthesia probably would have been avoided had oxygen and capnography monitoring been employed.

Citation count

584.

Related references

1 Smith TC. Rapid continuous measurement of mixed expired carbon dioxide concentration. *Anesthesiology* 1968; **29**: 1037–9.

2 Cooper JB, Newbower RS, Long CD, *et al*. Preventable anesthesia mishaps: a study of human factors. *Anesthesiology* 1978; **49**: 399–406.

3 Smalhout B. The importance of monitoring in anesthesia. *Acta Anaesthesiol Belg* 1978; **29**: 45–67.

4 Murray IP, Modell JH. Early detection of endotracheal tube accidents by monitoring carbon dioxide concentration in respiratory gas. *Anesthesiology* 1983; **59**: 344–6.

5 Eichhorn JH, Cooper JB, Cullen DJ, *et al*. Standards for patient monitoring during anesthesia at Harvard Medical School. *JAMA* 1986; **256**: 1017–20.

6 Tinker JH, Dull DL, Caplan RA, *et al*. Role of monitoring devices in prevention of anesthetic mishaps: a closed claims analysis. *Anesthesiology* 1989; **71**: 541–6.

7 Haynes AB, Weiser TG, Berry WR, *et al*. A surgical safety checklist to reduce morbidity and mortality in a global population. *N Engl J Med* 2009; **360**: 491–9.

Key message

Whilst others had promulgated the importance of capnography and oximetry this study was the first to clearly classify and critique the major sources of error and equipment failure in anaesthesia. The most frequent incidents are reproduced in Table 5.1. Human error was very common (82%), with overt equipment failures (14%) and inadequate communication among personnel, haste and distraction also identified. These findings generated great impetus in efforts to improve patient safety around the world, culminating in the recent *Safe Surgery Saves Lives* project (Haynes *et al.*, 2009).

Table 5.1 Distribution of frequent critical incidents

Incident description	Number of incidents
Breathing circuit disconnection during mechanical ventilation	57
Syringe swap	50
Gas flow control technical error	41
Loss of gas supply	32
Intravenous line disconnection	24
Vaporizer off unintentionally	22
Drug ampoule swap	21
Drug overdose (syringe, judgmental)	20
Drug overdose (vaporizer, technical)	20
Breathing circuit leak	19
Unintentional extubation	18
Misplaced tracheal tube	18
Breathing circuit misconnection	18
Inadequate fluid replacement	15
Premature extubation	15
Ventilator malfunction	15
Misuse of blood pressure monitor	15
Breathing-circuit control technical error	15
Wrong choice of airway management technique	13
Laryngoscope malfunction	12
Wrong IV line used	12
Hypoventilation (human error only)	11
Drug overdose (vaporizer, judgmental)	9
Drug overdose (syringe, technical)	8
Wrong choice of drug	7
Total	507*

*Represents 59% of all incidents reported, not including those from directed interviews.

Source: Cooper JB, Newbower RS, Kitz R. An analysis of major errors and equipment failures in anesthesia management: considerations for prevention and detection, *Anesthesiology* 1984; **60**(1): 34–42, with kind permission of the American Society of Anesthesiologists.

Strengths

The inclusion of an investigator from an engineering background, using the technique called critical incident analysis, provided a simple classification system of errors and equipment failure. Voluntary structured reports provided a rich data source. Preventative strategies were then produced.

Weaknesses

This was a retrospective analysis, reliant upon recollections and in many cases self-diagnosis of incidents. Denominator data were not available and so incident rates could not be reliably estimated. The survey technique will tend to collect incidents associated with human factors or equipment failures, with probable under-representation of patient co-morbidity (unavoidable events)—thus the preventable fraction may be spuriously high. The authors acknowledge that there are many ways to classify incident types. Contemporary monitoring practices that include capnography, pulse oximetry and inhalational agent monitoring, and improvements in machine manufacturing, limit relevance to current practice.

Relevance

Additional monitoring was vital, but it must be accompanied by vigilance—the study of human factors in anaesthesia and surgery has since grown. Standards for patient monitoring during anaesthesia at Harvard Medical School were published a few years later (Eichhorn *et al.*, 1986).

Paper 8: Does perioperative myocardial ischemia lead to postoperative myocardial infarction?

Author details

S Slogoff, AS Keats

Reference

Anesthesiology 1985; **62**: 107–14.

Summary

This study found a significant association between intraoperative myocardial ischaemia and PMI. Around 37% of patients had at least one episode of myocardial ischaemia detected, and many such episodes were identified on arrival in the operating room. A difference between anaesthetists suggests perioperative management can reduce this risk.

Citation count

620.

Related references

1 London MJ, Hollenberg M, Wong MG, *et al.* Intraoperative myocardial ischemia: localization by continuous 12-lead electrocardiography. *Anesthesiology* 1988; **69**: 232–41.

2 Mangano DT, Browner WS, Hollenberg M. Association of perioperative myocardial-ischemia with cardiac morbidity and mortality in men undergoing noncardiac surgery. *N Engl J Med* 1990; **323**: 1781–8.

3 Merry AF, Ramage MC, Whitlock RM, *et al.* First-time coronary artery bypass grafting: the anaesthetist as a risk factor. *Br J Anaesth* 1992; **68**: 6–12.

Key message

In the 1980s and early 1990s anaesthetists made great efforts to avoid tachycardia and hypertension, in a belief that this increased myocardial oxygen demand and thus could induce myocardial ischaemia. This was the first study to clearly demonstrate such an effect. But perhaps of greater interest, and certainly the main legacy of the paper, was the identification of one anaesthetist ('anesthesiologist 7') with a threefold higher rate of PMI, and this was correlated with higher rates of tachycardia and hypertension (Table 5.2). Does the anaesthetist affect outcome? A later New Zealand study reported similar findings (Merry *et al.*, 1992).

Strengths

Prospective, standardized measurement of ECG-evidence of myocardial ischaemia optimizes the detection of this adverse event. The criteria for the diagnosis of PMI were predefined. Statistical adjustment of confounding variables identifies ischaemia duration and extent of coronary artery disease as the key risk factors for PMI.

Weaknesses

Individual anaesthetist's practices of perioperative management, in particular administration of usual medications and premedication, were not reported. The number of cases performed by

Table 5.2 Role of anesthesiologists in perioperative myocardial ischemia and postoperative myocardial infarction

Anesthesiologist	No. of patients	Incidence (%)		PMI	During anesthesia		
		Ischemia			Tachycardia	Hypertension	Hypotension
		On arrival	During anesthesia				
1	139	19	29	2.9	19	9	57
2	131	14	22	4.6	21	5	48
3	104	15	26	3.8	23	11	46
4	118	22	38*	5.1	27	14	49
5	138	13	18	5.1	20	8	45
6	129	16	22	3.1	23	4	46
7	64	20	45*	12.5*	48*	17*	38
8	105	26	32	1.9	28	16*	46
9	95	17	26	1.1	24	5	45
Total	1,023	17.8	27.6	4.1	24.3	9.4	47.4
Multiple Chi-square		NS	<0.0005	<0.05	<0.005	<0.01	NS

NS, not significant; PMI, postoperative myocardial infarction.

Source: Slogoff S, Keats AS. Does perioperative myocardial ischemia lead to postoperative myocardial infarction? *Anesthesiology* 1985; **62**(2): 107–114, with kind permission of the American Society of Anesthesiologists.

'anesthesiologist 7' was less than others, such that he/she may have had a few particularly high-risk cases that biased the results. On the other hand, if there were truly a significant effect of the particular anaesthetist's technique, the multivariate discriminant analysis may have missed this if it was co-correlated with the duration of myocardial ischaemia.

Relevance

The association between the haemodynamic changes of tachycardia, hyper- or hypotension, with myocardial ischaemia and PMI, plus the difference in rates in at least one of the anaesthetists, strongly indicate that perioperative management affects outcome. Avoidance of such haemodynamic disturbances, with continuation of usual medical therapies (e.g. β-blockers), premedication to avoid anxiety, and an anaesthetic technique that provided minimal changes in heart rate and blood pressure became core goals of anaesthesia for the cardiac patient. The higher-than-expected rate of myocardial ischaemia emphasizes another issue: that because of the presence of a dedicated observer in the study, and/or automated detection, improved vigilance will detect more events than typically seen in routine practice.

Paper 9: Intraoperative detection of myocardial ischemia in high-risk patients: electrocardiography versus two-dimensional transesophageal echocardiography

Author details

JS Smith, MK Cahalan, DJ Benefiel, BF Byrd, FW Lurz, WA Shapiro, MF Roizen, A Bouchard, NB Schiller

Reference

Circulation 1985; **72**: 1015–21.

Summary

Transoesophageal echocardiography (TOE) was used to detect new SWMAs as early indicators of myocardial ischaemia. About half the patients had new SWMAs; these seem to occur before electrocardiographic evidence of myocardial ischaemia. All three patients with persistent SWMAs were later to be found to have suffered a myocardial infarction.

Citation count

414.

Related references

1 Gewertz BL, Kremser PC, Zarins CK, *et al*. Transesophageal echocardiographic monitoring of myocardial ischemia during vascular surgery. *J Vasc Surg* 1987; **5**: 607–13.

2 Ellis JE, Shah MN, Briller JE, *et al*. A comparison of methods for the detection of myocardial ischemia during noncardiac surgery: automated ST-segment analysis systems, electrocardiography, and transesophageal echocardiography. *Anesth Analg* 1992; **75**: 764–72.

Key message

The detection of perioperative myocardial ischaemia was the focus of much research in the 1980s. This early demonstration of one of the potential benefits of TOE was a forerunner to the eventual near-universal uptake of TOE in cardiac anaesthesia.

Strengths

This was a carefully conducted, prospective study of an at-risk group. Trained observers analysed the TOE data offline.

Weaknesses

The TOE evaluations were not real-time, and so the additional information was not available at the time of surgery—this does not reflect usual anaesthetic practice. The concordance between electrocarddiogram-ischaemia and SWMAs is difficult to verify. Some SWMAs occurred in patients with conduction abnormalities. The proposition that earlier detection may reduce morbidity and mortality has yet to be convincingly demonstrated.

Relevance

Myocardial ischaemia is strongly linked to higher rates of postoperative myocardial infarction. Persistent SWMAs may indicate perioperative myocardial infarction. Earlier detection may facilitate prompt treatment and avoidance of long-term sequelae, plus improve risk stratification and options for postoperative care.

Paper 10: Randomized evaluation of pulse oximetry in 20,802 patients: II. Perioperative events and postoperative complications

Author details

JT Møller, NW Johannessen, K Espersen, O Ravlo, BD Pedersen, PF Jensen, NH Rasmussen, LS Rasmussen, T Pedersen, JB Cooper, JS Gravenstein, B Chraemmer-Jørgensen, M Djernes, F Wiberg-Jørgensen, L Heslet, SH Johansen

Reference

Anesthesiology 1993; **78**: 445–53.

Summary

This Danish study, a randomized trial comparing pulse oximetry with no such monitoring in 20,802 patients, found a higher rate of hypoxaemia in the monitored group. In addition, there was a 19-fold higher rate of respiratory events in the oximetry group in both the operating theatre and recovery room. However, there was no significant difference in major outcomes between the groups. The authors also surveyed the participating anaesthetists to evaluate changes in practice habits and patient care. Anaesthetists indicated that pulse oximetry did in fact avert a small number of serious incidents.

Citation count

238.

Related references

1 Taylor MB, Whitwam JG. The current status of pulse oximetry. Clinical value of continuous noninvasive oxygen saturation monitoring. *Anaesthesia* 1986; **41**: 943–9.

2 Tinker JH, Dull DL, Caplan RA, Ward RJ, Cheney FW. Role of monitoring devices in prevention of anesthetic mishaps: a closed claims analysis. *Anesthesiology* 1989; **71**: 541–6.

3 Moller JT, Pedersen T, Rasmussen LS, *et al*. Randomized evaluation of pulse oximetry in 20,802 patients: I. Design, demography, pulse oximetry failure rate, and overall complication rate. *Anesthesiology*, 1993; **78**: 436–44.

4 Eichhorn JH. Pulse oximetry as a standard of practice in anesthesia. *Anesthesiology* 1993; **78**: 423–6.

Key message

The negative results of this large clinical trial have been over-emphasized by many commentators since its publication. There were some clear benefits of pulse oximetry, and other research plus widespread clinical experience have led to the universal adoption of this monitoring. Issues of study power, a focus on a high risk study cohort (to increase the number of adverse events), and the recognition of the importance of large-scale multicentred trials to identify meaningful improvements in anaesthetic practice have since developed.

Strengths

This study, along with their accompanying design paper (Moller *et al.*, 1993), describes a broad range of patients undergoing many types of surgery. Postoperative complications were predefined. A broad range of process and outcome variables were recorded, allowing a better understanding of the impact of pulse oximetry in routine practice.

Weaknesses

The study was designed to detect a 25% difference between groups. Given the low cost and near absence of any adverse effects of monitoring, plus the enormous number of general anaesthetics given each year around the world, a smaller increment of benefit, say 5%, would be clinically important and lead to a substantial reduction in the number of patients having serious postoperative complications if pulse oximetry was at all beneficial—the study was not powered to detect such an effect. Many critics of this study focus too heavily on P values, rather than the estimates of effect with 95% confidence intervals.

The primary outcome measure was a composite of many events; some of which were unlikely to be affected by oximetry monitoring. There were several 'trends' suggesting a possible reduction in serious complications. For example there were more cases of postoperative coma, 6 vs. 1 (P=0.13). Despite being considered a negative study in many respects, there were suggestions of a lower rate of detected endobronchial intubation, cardiac arrest, bronchospasm, and need for naloxone. Inclusion of a higher risk group would have increased study power. A much larger study was required to reliably identify a beneficial effect of oximetry monitoring in unselected patients. At the time it was seen as unrealistic, but it ought to be remembered that the study was conducted over a 16-month period in five hospitals—perhaps a much larger, multinational effort should have been done?

All complications were treated equally in the composite primary endpoint—hypotension and hypertension should not have been included in this list because it may have diluted a true effect. Also, some of the complications had no rationale for being reduced with pulse oximetry. Higher risk patients (ASA physical status 4) had a higher failure rate of oximetry (7%), denying a possible benefit to many of these subjects. The cluster design was not accounted for in the statistical analysis.

Relevance

Objective, continuous monitoring of tissue oxygenation throughout surgery and the initial recovery period is an essential aim of safe perioperative practice. Anaesthesia is incredibly safe, with serious adverse events being quite rare. However, this makes their detection and elimination that much more important.

Chapter 6

Optimization

MPW Grocott and MG Mythen

Introduction

The observation that patients surviving major surgery exhibited higher values of cardiac output and oxygen delivery than non-survivors was first made in the late 1950s, and has been confirmed many times since. The related hypothesis, that using as goals for all patients the cardiac output and oxygen delivery values exhibited by survivors, would reduce overall mortality, is attributed to Shoemaker. The first paper to directly address this hypothesis was his landmark randomized controlled trial, published in 1988.

Since then, a substantial number of single-centre randomized controlled trials, and a handful of multicentre studies, have been conducted in this area. The unifying theme is the use of a haemodynamic monitor to guide fluid, or fluid and drug (intrope or vasodilator) therapy, to achieve defined augmented haemodynamic goals in comparison to a control group. Consequently, most 'optimization' studies have tested a package of care, rather than varying a single factor between two study groups. The elements of these complex interventions, including the choice of haemodynamic monitor, 'optimization' protocol, fluid and drug therapy, have varied between studies. Furthermore, these studies have been published over a period of more than 20 years, in a variety of different patient groups, limiting direct comparison between studies or synthesis of the data in a systematic review. Notwithstanding these limitations, several published systematic reviews and meta-analyses of this literature show a consistent result: a statistically significant reduction in mortality in the 'optimized' intervention groups (Heyland *et al.*, 1996; Kern and Shoemaker, 2002; Poeze *et al.*, 2005; Hamilton *et al.*, 2011).

It is notable that in established critical illness, the use of blood flow goals to drive resuscitation does not seem to be beneficial. Several studies, including one large multicentre randomized controlled trial (Gattinoni *et al.*, 1995), have failed to demonstrate benefit for patients in the protocol group and in some cases this approach has been associated with harm, with protocol group mortality exceeding control (Hayes *et al.*, 1994). In contrast to these results, use of mixed venous oxygen saturation (SvO_2) obtained from a central venous catheter as the goal of therapy early (recruited in the emergency room) in severe sepsis or septic shock, does seem to result in a significant reduction in mortality (Rivers *et al.*, 2001). This result awaits confirmation by the international multicentre studies currently being conducted. The disparity in effect between 'optimization' in acute injury, for example, the perioperative setting or early in severe sepsis, and established critical illness, highlights fundamental differences in pathophysiology between these two situations that merit further investigation.

Related references

1 Hayes MA, Timmins AC, Yau EH, *et al.* Elevation of systemic oxygen delivery in the treatment of critically ill patients. *N Engl J Med* 1994; **330**: 1717–22.

2 Gattinoni, L. Brazzi L, Pelosi P, *et al.* A trial of goal-oriented hemodynamic therapy in critically ill patients. SvO2 Collaborative Group. *N Engl J Med* 1995; **333**: 1025–32.

3 Heyland DK, Cook DJ, King D, *et al.* Maximizing oxygen delivery in critically ill patients: a methodologic appraisal of the evidence. *Crit Care Med* 1996; **24**: 517–24.

4 Rivers E, Nguyen B, Havstad S, *et al.* Early goal-directed therapy in the treatment of severe sepsis and septic shock. *N Engl J Med* 2001; **345**: 1368–77.

5 Kern JW, Shoemaker WC. Meta-analysis of hemodynamic optimization in high-risk patients. *Crit Care Med* 2002; **30**: 1686–92.

6 Poeze M, Greve JW, Ramsay G. Meta-analysis of hemodynamic optimization: relationship to methodological quality. *Crit Care* 2005; **9**: R771–9.

7 Hamilton MA, Cecconi M, Rhodes A. Systematic review and meta-analysis on the use of preemptive hemodynamic intervention to improve postoperative outcomes in moderate and high-risk surgical patients. *Anesth Analg* 2011; **112**: 1392–402.

Paper 1: Prospective trial of supranormal values of survivors as therapeutic goals in high-risk surgical patients

Author details

WC Shoemaker, PL Appel, HB Kram, K Waxman, TS Lee

Reference

Chest 1988; **94**: 1176–86.

Summary

This is widely regarded as the first of the 'optimization' studies. William Shoemaker, a surgeon from North America, was part of a group that had previously reported a relationship between significantly higher mean cardiac index oxygen delivery and oxygen consumption (CI, DO_2, and VO_2) in survivors of high-risk surgical operations compared to non-survivors. In this study they prospectively tested the hypothesis that deliberately increasing cardiac index and oxygen delivery and oxygen consumption would result in improved outcomes. So-called high-risk surgical patients were studied. The criteria for identifying these patients were based on previous observations. They included severe cardiac and pulmonary disease, extensive ablative surgery for carcinoma, severe trauma, massive blood loss, extremes of age, and renal failure. The expected mortality for the patients based on the group's experience of the previous 7 years was that it would be close to 30%. The paper reports two series. There are 252 patients in the first series that were stratified into those who received pulmonary artery (PA) catheter monitoring in the preoperative period compared to the postoperative period. We will concentrate our discussions on the second series, where the group prospectively randomized the patients into three groups. Thirty patients were randomized into the PA-control group, 28 patients into the PA-protocol, and 30 patients into the CVP-control group. The central venous pressure (CVP) and PA catheter control group had regular routine physiological measurements recorded and standard of care therapy that included the administration of intravenous fluids, blood and inotropic and/or vasodilatory agents according to the team managing the patient. The PA-protocol group received additional fluids and/or blood and/or inotropic agents (mainly dobutamine) to try and achieve the therapeutic goals for supranormal values for cardiac output ($>4.5 l min^{-1} m^{-2}$), oxygen delivery ($>600 ml^{-1} min^{-1} m^{-2}$), and oxygen consumption ($>170 ml min^{-1} m^{-2}$) in both the preoperative and postoperative period. These values were defined empirically from the median values of patients surviving after major surgery. Cardiac output and oxygen transport goals were given priority in the continuing management of these patients as distinct from the control group patients. Haemodynamic variables recorded in the paper show a clear separation of oxygen delivery, cardiac output and oxygen consumption values for the PA-protocol patients when compared to the control patients. There are no differences in other haemodynamic variables, including mean arterial pressure, pulmonary artery pressure and wedge pressure. The mortality rate for the patients in the PA-protocol group was 4% and this was statistically significantly lower than that seen in the PA-control group (33%) and the CVP-control group (23%). The patients in the PA-protocol group also experienced statistically significantly fewer complications when compared to the control groups. In the discussion, the authors highlight that in the environment that there study was conducted, the use of a PA catheter per se makes no difference compared to the use of CVP monitoring, without the use of defined therapeutic goals. Their final conclusion reads: 'Our study suggests that this conservative approach to patients undergoing high-risk surgical procedures is a false economy both fiscally and in terms of patient outcome.'

Citation count

1,285.

Related references

1 Clowes GHJ, Del Guercio LR. Circulatory response to trauma of surgical operations. *Metabolism* 1960; **9**: 67–81.

2 Shoemaker WC. Cardiorespiratory patterns of surviving and nonsurviving postoperative patients. *Surg Gynecol Obstet* 1972; **134**: 810–14.

3 Shoemaker WC, Montgomery ES, Kaplan E, *et al.* Physiologic patterns in surviving and nonsurviving shock patients. Use of sequential cardiorespiratory variables in defining criteria for therapeutic goals and early warning of death. *Arch Surg* 1973; **106**: 630–6.

Key message

Cardiac output and oxygen delivery variables could be augmented by goal-directed perioperative haemodynamic management, and this approach resulted in a reduction in hospital mortality.

Strengths

This was a study from an experienced group with their own historical reference data with a clear rationale for the chosen therapeutic targets. The study includes both emergency and elective surgical patients. Comparative data is provided for both non-randomized patients and a case-series leading up to the randomized control trial. The haemodynamic variables are reported for both control and protocol patients. There is a clear separation between groups for the therapeutic targets, namely cardiac index, oxygen delivery, and oxygen consumption. There is a simple cost analysis, suggesting that it is a false economy not to use the PA-protocol group interventions.

Weaknesses

Weaknesses include the relatively small numbers of patients and concerns regarding blinding (and possible reporting bias). No clear algorithm was described for the haemodynamic management of the control patients. In the control patients, oxygen delivery actually falls in the postoperative period, suggesting there may have been under-treatment of this group.

Relevance

This paper demonstrated for the first time that 'optimization' could improve survival after high-risk major surgery, and led to a large number of studies in the perioperative setting (largely positive) and other situations, including established critical illness and cancer (usually negative).

Paper 2: A randomized clinical trial of the effect of deliberate perioperative increase of oxygen delivery on mortality in high-risk surgical patients

Author details

O Boyd, RM Grounds, ED Bennett

Reference

Journal of the American Medical Association 1993; **270**: 2699–707.

Summary

A single-centre prospective randomized clinical trial from St George's Hospital in London, England on 107 surgical patients who were deemed to be high risk from previously identified criteria (very similar to Shoemaker's study, see paper 1). Patients were randomly assigned to a control group (n=54) and to a protocol group (n=53). The protocol group received additional therapies targeted to an oxygen delivery index of 600 ml min⁻¹ m⁻². Therapy was started preoperatively in many patients and followed through into the postoperative period. Protocol group intervention continued until there was normalization of blood lactate levels. Post-operative care of all patients was provided in an intensive care unit. Both groups were given targets for mean arterial pressure, pulmonary artery occlusion pressure, arterial oxygen saturation, haemoglobin, and urine output. In addition, the protocol group received titrated dopexamine to achieve an oxygen delivery of >600 ml min⁻¹ m⁻². Postoperative complications were recorded from the medical and nursing records. Haemodynamic variables show a clear separation of cardiac index and oxygen delivery between the two groups, but not of oxygen consumption (NB oxygen consumption was not a target for this study). All other haemodynamic variables were similar for the two groups, with the notable exception of heart rate, which is slightly higher in patients receiving dopexamine. Mortality rate for the protocol group was statistically significantly lower at 5.7% vs. 22% for the control group. The biggest difference in mortality was seen in patients who had abdominal surgery as opposed to those who had vascular surgery. Protocol group patients received statistically significantly more fluid in the preoperative period. Protocol group patients experienced statistically significantly fewer postoperative complications and there was a trend towards a shorter length of hospital stay. Follow-up at 15 years showed median survival of 1,107 days in the goal-directed group compared with 674 days for control group patients (p=0.005). Survival was independently associated with age, randomization to the goal-directed study group, and avoidance of significant cardiac complications after surgery.

Citation count

768.

Related references

1 Rhodes A, Cecconi M, Hamilton M, *et al*. Goal-directed therapy in high-risk surgical patients: a 15-year follow-up study. *Intensive Care Med* 2010; **36**: 1327–32.

Key message

Confirmation that the results of the Shoemaker study could be replicated in a different environment (UK compared to USA).

Strengths

Both control group and interventional group received protocolized intervention, the addition of the dopexamine to try and achieve the higher DO_2 being the only difference for the protocol group. Morbid events were clearly defined and bias reduced by using the medical and nursing records as the source for this data. The upper limit of the dose of dopexamine was restricted, guided by heart rate that was not allowed to increase by >20% from baseline.

Weaknesses

This is a small, single-centre study. Some patients were only admitted to the trial in the postoperative period; however, the majority (n=81) were studied from preoperatively through to postoperatively. Study interventions take place in the preoperative and postoperative period but there is no clear information with regards to what happens intraoperatively with regards to haemodynamic variables or treatments received. Mortality rates are rather high for the control group. However, this study did include emergency patients and it is interesting to note that a recently published multicentre randomized control trial from Denmark reported a 5% mortality rate for patients undergoing elective colorectal surgery in ASA grade 1 and 2 patients, whilst a large observational cohort study from the authors of Paper 10 demonstrated a 10% mortality rate for elective surgical patients admitted to ITU in the UK and a 40% mortality rate for patients undergoing emergency surgery.

Relevance

Relevance to modern practice is uncertain in view of the high control group mortality. PAC usage has fallen out of fashion following the Connors paper (see Paper 7) and few centres would now be able to deliver this protocol in this patient group. The results of this study taken together with Shoemaker's results, suggest that the benefits of 'optimization' are not drug specific and support the notion that the haemodynamic goals are the key element of the intervention.

Paper 3: Perioperative plasma volume expansion reduces the incidence of gut mucosal hypoperfusion during cardiac surgery

Author details

MG Mythen, AR Webb

Reference

Archives of Surgery 1995; **130**: 423–9.

Summary

This is a single-centre prospective randomized control trial of 60 patients undergoing cardiac surgery. The objective was to test the hypothesis that perioperative plasma volume expansion would preserve gut mucosal perfusion during elective cardiac surgery. The patients were randomized to standard of care, which included haemodynamic monitoring with invasive arterial pressure and central venous pressure monitoring, or protocol group, where pre- and post-bypass boluses of fluid were administered to achieve maximal stroke volume measured by an oesophageal Doppler probe and monitor. Gut mucosal perfusion was assessed using gastric tonometry. The patients who received the oesophageal Doppler-guided fluid therapy had statistically significantly lower heart rate, higher stroke volume, and higher cardiac output at the end of surgery. This was associated with a marked reduction in the incidence of gut mucosal hypoperfusion as judged by gastric tonometry (7% vs 56%). The patients in the Doppler-guided fluid therapy group experienced fewer complications and had a shorter length of intensive care unit and hospital stay. Only one death occurred and this was in the control group. The protocol group received fewer therapeutic interventions for the treatment of hypotension and oliguria. The difference in the amount of fluid administered between the two groups was relatively modest (in the region of 500 ml) and the increase in stroke volume in the protocol group was only about 17 ml, yet this produced a profound effect on the incidence of gut mucosal hypoperfusion.

Citation count

450.

Related references

1 Mythen MG, Webb AR. Intra-operative gut mucosal hypoperfusion is associated with increased post-operative complications and cost. *Intensive Care Med* 1994; **20**: 99–104.

2 Bennett-Guerrero E, Welsby I, Dunn TJ, *et al.* The use of a postoperative morbidity survey to evaluate patients with prolonged hospitalization after routine, moderate-risk, elective surgery. *Anesth Analg* 1999; **89**: 514–19.

Key message

'Optimization' could be achieved without a PAC and without the use of inotropes or pressors.

Strengths

The study design was based on a previous observational study that reported an association between gut mucosal hypoperfusion (about 50% when defined by abnormal gastric tonometry values) and poor outcome. Sample size was based on this pilot study and, though small, this study was adequately powered for the primary outcome variable (incidence of gut mucosal hypoperfusion). This was the first study to use a surrogate measure of tissue perfusion and thereby provide mechanistic insight into the possible mechanisms of harm in non-optimized patients and benefit from optimization.

Weaknesses

This was a small study of uncertain generalizability due to the use of a non-protocolized 'standard of care' control group. It was not adequately powered for the clinical outcomes. This study of elective, relatively low risk, cardiac surgical patients and may therefore have limited generalizability to non-cardiac surgery. The study had a risk of reporting bias in relation to postoperative complications as a single investigator recorded the intraoperative and postoperative variables. However, ward staff involved in the postoperative management of patients, including discharge from hospital, were blinded to the intraoperative interventions.

Relevance

First study reporting benefit from the use of oesophageal Doppler monitor-guided fluid therapy with no additional inotropes and pressors. Remains applicable to modern practice as Doppler use increases in other contexts.

Paper 4: Intraoperative intravascular volume optimization and length of hospital stay after repair of proximal femoral fracture: randomised controlled trial

Author details

S Sinclair, S James, M Singer

Reference

British Medical Journal 1997; **315**: 909–12.

Abstract

Objectives: To assess whether intraoperative intravascular volume optimization improves outcome and shortens hospital stay after repair of proximal femoral fracture.

Design: Prospective, randomised controlled trial comparing conventional intraoperative fluid management with repeated colloid fluid challenges monitored by oesophageal Doppler ultrasonography to maintain maximal stroke volume throughout the operative period.

Setting: Teaching hospital, London.

Subjects: 40 patients undergoing repair of proximal femoral fracture under general anaesthesia.

Interventions: Patients were randomly assigned to receive either conventional intraoperative fluid management (control patients) or additional repeated colloid fluid challenges with oesophageal Doppler ultrasonography used to maintain maximal stroke volume throughout the operative period (protocol patients).

Main outcome measures: Time declared medically fit for hospital discharge, duration of hospital stay (in acute bed; in acute plus long stay bed), mortality, perioperative haemodynamic changes.

Results: Intraoperative intravascular fluid loading produced significantly greater changes in stroke volume (median 15 ml (95% confidence interval 10 to 21 ml)) and cardiac output (1.2 l/min (0.1 to 2.3 l/min)) than in the conventionally managed group (−5 ml (−10 to 1 ml) and −0.4 l/min (−1.0 to 0.2 l/min)) (P <0.001 and P <0.05, respectively). One protocol patient and two control patients died in hospital. In the survivors, postoperative recovery was significantly faster in the protocol patients, with shorter times to being declared medically fit for discharge (median 10 (9 to 15) days v 15 (11 to 40) days, P <0.05) and a 39% reduction in hospital stay (12 (8 to 13) days v 20 (10 to 61) days, P <0.05).

Conclusions: Proximal femoral fracture repair constitutes surgery in a high risk population. Intraoperative intravascular volume loading to optimal stroke volume resulted in a more rapid postoperative recovery and a significantly reduced hospital stay.

Summary

This was a prospective randomized control trial of 40 patients undergoing repair of proximal femoral fracture under general anaesthesia in a London teaching hospital. Patients were randomly assigned to receive either conventional intraoperative fluid management or additional repeated boluses of fluid guided by oesophageal Doppler to attain maximal stroke volume throughout the operative period. Patients randomized to receive Doppler-guided fluid therapy received statistically significantly more fluid and produced a significantly greater increase in stroke volume (median 15 ml) and cardiac output. One protocol and two control patients died in hospital. The protocol group patients experienced shorter times to be declared medically fit for discharge (median 10 vs 15 days) and an 8-day reduction in hospital stay (12 vs 20).

Citation count

449.

Related references

1 Side CD, Gosling RG. Non-surgical assessment of cardiac function. *Nature* 1971; **232**: 335–6.

Key message

First study of 'optimization' exclusively in patients undergoing emergency surgery.

Strengths

This is one of the few studies evaluating 'optimization' in patients undergoing emergency surgery and was conducted in a patient group that is recognized to have a high mortality and morbidity. Although the study was small, sample size was based on an inhospital audit performed in the years leading up to the study, which demonstrated an anticipated length of stay and hospital mortality similar to that seen in the control group. The fluid algorithm, aside from looking for a rise in stroke volume of 10%, also used the Doppler measured variable of flow time corrected.

Weaknesses

This was a relatively small single-centre trial using the primary outcome variable of declared medically fit for discharge, which is potentially subject to bias. Treatment was not protocolized for the control group.

Relevance

The extensive use of regional anaesthesia for hip fracture surgery results in a high level of awake patients in whom this technique has very limited value. Confirmation that Doppler-guided optimization with fluids alone, with no additional inotropic therapy, could improve clinical outcomes.

Paper 5: Reducing the risk of major elective surgery: randomized controlled trial of preoperative optimization of oxygen delivery

Author details

J Wilson, I Woods, J Fawcett, R Whall, W Dibb, C Morris, E McManus

Reference

British Medical Journal 1999; **318**: 1099–1103.

Abstract

Objectives: To determine whether preoperative optimization of oxygen delivery improves outcome after major elective surgery, and to determine whether the inotropes, adrenaline and dopexamine, used to enhance oxygen delivery influence outcome.

Design: Randomised controlled trial with double blinding between inotrope groups. Setting: York District Hospital, England.

Subjects: 138 patients undergoing major elective surgery who were at risk of developing postoperative complications either because of the surgery or the presence of coexistent medical conditions. Interventions: Patients were randomised into three groups. Two groups received invasive haemodynamic monitoring, fluid, and either adrenaline or dopexamine to increase oxygen delivery. Inotropic support was continued during surgery and for at least 12 hours afterwards. The third group (control) received routine perioperative care.

Main outcome measures: Hospital mortality and morbidity.

Results: Overall, 3/92 (3%) preoptimised patients died compared with 8/46 controls (17%) (P=0.007). There were no differences in mortality between the treatment groups, but 14/46 (30%) patients in the dopexamine group developed complications compared with 24/46 (52%) patients in the adrenaline group (difference 22%, 95% confidence interval 2% to 41%) and 28 patients (61%) in the control group (31%, 11% to 50%). The use of dopexamine was associated with a decreased length of stay in hospital.

Conclusion: Routine preoperative optimization of patients undergoing major elective surgery would be a significant and cost effective improvement in perioperative care.

Summary

This is a single centre randomized control trial of 138 patients undergoing major elective surgery in York District Hospital, England. Patients were deemed to be at risk of developing postoperative complications either because of the type of surgery or the presence of coexistent medical conditions. They were randomized into three groups: two groups received invasive haemodynamic monitoring with a pulmonary artery (PA) catheter and either adrenaline or dopexamine to increase oxygen delivery to predetermined goals whilst a control group received standard of care. Inotropic support was continued during surgery and for at least 12 hours postoperatively. Patients in the two protocolized groups experienced an overall mortality of 3% (3 out of 92) compared to 17% in the control group (8 out of 46; P = 0.007). There was no difference in mortality between the two treatment groups (adrenaline vs dopexamine) but patients treated with dopexamine experienced fewer complications (30% vs 52%) than those treated with adrenaline. The use of dopexamine was also associated with decreased length of hospital stay.

Citation count

428.

Related references

1 Stone MD, Wilson RJ, Cross J, *et al.* Effect of adding dopexamine to intraoperative volume expansion in patients undergoing major elective abdominal surgery. *Br J Anaesth* 2003; **91**: 619–24.

Key message

Despite the passage of time since the earlier studies, adverse outcome remains common after major surgery and optimization improves survival.

Strengths

The administration of the inotropic agents was carried out in a double blind fashion. There is a clear separation in the haemodynamic variables recorded in the two intervention groups, in particular oxygen delivery. Randomization was stratified into three subgroups: vascular surgery, surgery for upper gastrointestinal malignancy, and others.

Weaknesses

The intervention group received a bundle of care that included preoperative admission to an intensive care unit (ICU), fluid optimization and inotrope optimization in the preoperative period and return of the patient to the ICU postoperatively as well as the optimization intervention to try and achieve an increase in oxygen delivery. Although they were receiving standard of care, it has been argued that the control group was relatively under-treated. Mortality was slightly higher than predicted in the control group but much lower than predicted in the two interventional groups. The biggest criticism of this trial has been the issue with regards to the placement of the patients postoperatively. A number of patients in the control group returned to the general ward whereas all patients in the protocolized groups were returned to the ICU. However, whilst this complicated interpretation of this study as a haemodynamic study, we do not believe that this diminishes the overall message that a higher level of care, including targeted fluid and drug administration, seems to produce better results.

Relevance

This study further demonstrated that optimization improves survival in high-risk surgical patients and important reminder that adverse outcome is both common and preventable in this patient group.

Paper 6: A prospective, randomized study of goal-oriented hemodynamic therapy in cardiac surgical patients

Author details

P Pölönen, E Ruokonen, M Hippeläinen, M Pöyhönen, J Takala

Reference

Anesthesia and Analgesia 2000; **90**: 1052–9.

Summary

A prospective randomized study of goal-orientated haemodynamic therapy in cardiac surgical patients. It is a single-centre study of 403 elective cardiac surgical patients, who were randomized to receive goal-directed therapy to maintain a mixed venous oxygen saturation (SvO_2) of >70% and a lactate concentration of <2 mmol l^{-1} from admission to the ICU to up to 8 h postoperatively. The patients receiving this goal-directed therapy had a shorter median length of hospital stay compared to the control group (6 vs 7 days, P <0.05) and patients were discharged from hospital faster (P <0.05). Morbidity was less frequent at the time of hospital discharge in the patients who received goal-directed therapy (1.1% vs 6.1%; P <0.01).

Citation count

283.

Related references

1 Takala J, Meier-Hellmann A, Eddleston J, *et al.* Effect of dopexamine on outcome after major abdominal surgery: a prospective, randomized, controlled multicenter study. European Multicenter Study Group on Dopexamine in Major Abdominal Surgery. *Crit Care Med* 2000; **28**: 3417–23.

Key message

SvO_2 and lactate are useful goals for haemodynamic management which can improve outcomes, at least in this group of patients.

Strengths

The patients were cared for in an intensive care environment with a background of standard care for both groups. Protocolized interventional care for the treatment group was primarily by the administration of dobutamine to achieve a mixed venous saturation of >70% and a lactate of <2 mmol l^{-1}. The dose of dobutamine was limited to 15 µg kg^{-1} min^{-1}.

Weaknesses

Although large, it is a single-centre study. The study reports data from a relatively low-risk group of patients with a low mortality. All patients had a pulmonary artery catheter (PAC) from which SvO_2 data were derived (see paper 7). Although there is a small difference in the length of stay of the patients receiving a PA catheter, as the authors point out, the impact on resources may be substantial. Haemodynamic targets were only met in approximately half of the patients in the protocol group for the SvO_2 and lactate targets.

Relevance

Optimization using goals based on the balance between oxygen delivery and utilization, rather than direct measurement of blood flow and oxygen delivery, result in improved outcomes in these patients. PAC use is more common in cardiac surgery than other clinical contexts so this factor is less of a weakness for this study than some others. The reduction in resource use is impressive.

Paper 7: A randomized, controlled trial of the use of pulmonary-artery catheters in high-risk surgical patients

Author details

JD Sandham, RD Hull, RF Brant, L Knox, GF Pineo CJ Doig, DP Laporta, S Viner, L Passerini, H Devitt, A Kirby, M Jacka; Canadian Critical Care Clinical Trials Group

Reference

New England Journal of Medicine 2003; **348**: 5–14.

Summary

This is a randomized control trial of the use of pulmonary-artery catheters in high risk surgical patients. It is a multicentre study of 3,803 eligible patients, of whom 1,994 underwent randomization into two groups. Overall there was no difference in mortality between patients who were treated with a pulmonary-artery catheter (7.8% mortality) compared to those treated with a central venous pressure line (7.7%). The patients treated with a pulmonary-artery catheter had a higher rate of pulmonary embolism (8 events vs 0 events; P = 0.004). There was a trend towards less renal failure in patients treated with a pulmonary artery catheter. Of note, the expected mortality rate upon which the power calculations were based was 15% in the two groups. All patients were admitted to intensive care in the postoperative period, which was not the standard of care; i.e. both groups underwent a minimum postoperative ICU stay of 24 h. Patients were a mixture of ASA grade III and IV cases, of which the majority were major vascular (around 50%) and abdominal (around 20%). It is interesting to note that the in-hospital mortality rate for ASA class 4 risk patients was around 16.7% to 20.6% and among patients in NYHA class 3 or 4, in-hospital mortality was 13.8% to 18.6%, with a 1-year mortality rate of 29.3% to 35.3%. This is important to note in the context of the relatively high mortality rate reported in the earlier studies of high risk surgical patients.

Citation count

830.

Related references

1 Connors AF Jr, Speroff T, Dawson NV, *et al*. The effectiveness of right heart catheterization in the initial care of critically ill patients. SUPPORT Investigators. *JAMA* 1996; **276**: 889–97.

Key message

The use of pulmonary artery catheters in high-risk surgical patients is not associated with increased mortality.

Strengths

This is a large, multicentre, randomized, pragmatic trial published in a high-profile journal.

Weaknesses

There was a suggestion that this is an optimization study, although the title of the paper talks about it being a study of randomization to PAC or no PAC. The haemodynamic algorithm for the PAC group is a set of suggested interventions, namely the administration of fluid boluses, vasoactive drugs and/or packed red blood cells. Of note, only around 50% of patients received the intervention (inotropic agents or cardioactive drugs or colloids or red blood cells). The haemo-dynamic goals chosen were lower than those reported to produce benefit in previous studies; i.e. they chose a cardiac index goal of $3.5 \, l \, min^{-2}$ and oxygen delivery of $550 \, ml \, min^{-1} \, m^{-2}$ (rather than $600 \, ml \, min^{-1} \, m^{-2}$ used in the earlier studies showing patient benefit). The majority of patients do not achieve the protocol goals in the preoperative and intraoperative period, and only in the postoperative period did more than 50% of patients get above the $550 \, ml \, min^{-1} \, m^{-2}$ for oxygen delivery.

Relevance

Uncertain, this is a very large study published in a high-profile journal and is therefore taken as 'gold standard' in this area. This may be misleading as this study was not originally designed as an 'optimization' study.

Paper 8: Goal-directed intraoperative fluid administration reduces length of hospital stay after major surgery

Author details

TJ Gan, A Soppitt, M Maroof, H el-Moalem, KM Robertson, E Moretti, P Dwane, PS Glass

Reference

Anesthesiology 2002; **97**: 820–6.

Summary

This is a single-centre prospective randomized controlled study of 100 patients undergoing major elective surgery with an anticipated blood loss >500 ml. Patients assigned to a control group that received standard intraoperative care or to a protocol group that in addition received intraoperative plasma volume expansion guided by oesophageal Doppler monitor to maintain maximal stroke volume. The protocol group achieved a significantly higher stroke volume and cardiac output at the end of surgery compared to the control group and these patients in the protocol group had a shorter duration of hospital stay compared to the control group (5 vs 7 days mean and 6 vs 7 days median). The protocol patients also tolerated oral intake of solid food earlier than the control group (a mean of 3 vs 4.7 days and a median of 3 vs 5 days; P = 0.01). Of note, the majority of patients were ASA grade 2 and 1, although there were some ASA grade 3 patients (approximately 20% for each group). There were no deaths in either study group, as would be expected for this type of surgery performed in a teaching centre in the USA. Patients in the protocol group received approximately 600 ml of additional colloid on average and at the end of surgery had a relatively modest mean increase in stroke volume of just 9 ml compared to a reduction of 3 ml seen in the control group, i.e. a difference in stroke volume of 12 ml between the two groups.

Citation count

466.

Key message

Oesophageal Doppler-guided fluid therapy provides an clinical outcome benefit and reduces length of stay in patients undergoing moderate risk surgery.

Strengths

The control group received treatment guided by quite a detailed protocol, which required the administration of fluid for perturbations in heart rate, blood pressure and urine flow. The power of the study was based on a reasonably large observational study from the same institution. The incidence of complications recorded in the control group was consistent with a previous large observational study.

Weaknesses

This was a relatively small single-centre study. There is the potential for bias in the reporting of the outcome variables due to lack of true blinding. Positive outcomes were very much related to return of gastrointestinal tract function yet there was no protocol to challenge the gut. Food and drink seems to have been initiated on return of flatus.

Relevance

This study suggests that 'optimization' can provide benefit in patients at lower risk of adverse outcome following surgery than had previously been demonstrated (there was no postoperative mortality in this study).

Paper 9: Intraoperative oesophageal Doppler guided fluid management shortens postoperative hospital stay after major bowel surgery

Author details

HG Wakeling, MR McFall, CS Jenkins, WG Woods, WF Miles, GR Barclay, SC Fleming

Reference

British Journal of Anaesthesia 2005; **95**: 634–42.

Abstract

Background: Occult hypovolaemia is a key factor in the aetiology of postoperative morbidity and may not be detected by routine heart rate and arterial pressure measurements. Intraoperative gut hypoperfusion during major surgery is associated with increased morbidity and postoperative hospital stay. We assessed whether using intraoperative oesophageal Doppler guided fluid management to minimize hypovolaemia would reduce postoperative hospital stay and the time before return of gut function after colorectal surgery.

Methods: This single centre, blinded, prospective controlled trial randomized 128 consecutive consenting patients undergoing colorectal resection to oesophageal Doppler guided or central venous pressure (CVP)-based (conventional) intraoperative fluid management. The intervention group patients followed a dynamic oesophageal Doppler guided fluid protocol whereas control patients were managed using routine cardiovascular monitoring aiming for a CVP between 12 and 15 mmHg.

Results: The median postoperative stay in the Doppler guided fluid group was 10 vs 11.5 days in the control group P<0.05. The median time to resuming full diet in the Doppler guided fluid group was 6 vs 7 for controls P<0.001. Doppler patients achieved significantly higher cardiac output, stroke volume, and oxygen delivery. Twenty-nine (45.3%) control patients suffered gastrointestinal morbidity compared with nine (14.1%) in the Doppler guided fluid group P<0.001, overall morbidity was also significantly higher in the control group P=0.05.

Conclusions: Intraoperative oesophageal Doppler guided fluid management was associated with a 1.5-day median reduction in postoperative hospital stay. Patients recovered gut function significantly faster and suffered significantly less gastrointestinal and overall morbidity.

Wakeling HG, McFall MR, Jenkins CS, Woods WG, Miles WF, Barclay GR, Fleming SC, 'Intraoperative oesophageal Doppler guided fluid management shortens postoperative hospital stay after major bowel surgery', *British Journal of Anaesthesia*, 2005, 95, 5, pp. 634–642, by permission of Oxford University Press and British Journal of Anaesthesia.

Summary

This is a single-centre, blinded, prospective, controlled randomized trial of 128 consecutive patients undergoing colorectal resection. The patients were randomized to oesophageal Doppler guided or CVP-based intraoperative fluid management. Patients receiving fluid management guided by the oesophageal Doppler had a shorter median postoperative length of stay (10 vs 11.5 days; P <0.05 control). Protocol patients also experienced a shorter time to full diet (6 vs 7 days; P <0.001). Protocol patients also experienced a marked reduction in the number of gastrointestinal morbid events (45.3% vs 14.1%). A treatment algorithm which required boluses of colloid used both CVP and Doppler stroke volume measurement. Additional measures included the determination of 'gut leak' by measurement of a lactulose/mannitol ratio and the measurement of endotoxin and interleukin-6. Of note, there was no difference found between the control group and the stroke volume optimization group in any of these variables.

Citation count

233.

Related references

1 Noblett SE, Snowden CP, Shenton BK, *et al*. Randomized clinical trial assessing the effect of Doppler-optimized fluid management on outcome after elective colorectal resection. *Br J Surg* 2006; **93**: 1069–76.

Key message

The study provided further confirmation that Doppler-guided fluid therapy provides clinical benefit in moderate risk patients.

Strengths

The study describes a homogeneous group of patients (colorectal surgery) with a single surgical operator and single anaesthetist, which helps us to understand what happens in a very controlled environment but does not give us much information about general applicability. The recovery pathway was similar for all patients and was quite tightly controlled, including early challenge of the gastrointestinal tract with water, and a soft diet being introduced at day 3, and early mobilization and restriction of postoperative fluids. Postoperative morbidity was recorded using validated scores, which demonstrated a statistically significant improvement in the quality of recovery score as well as objective morbidity scores. Biological plausibility with cytokine data.

Weaknesses

This was a relatively small, single-centre study. It was conducted prior to the more common use of enhanced recovery, so the lengths of stay for colorectal surgery by current standards would be regarded as relatively long in both groups.

Relevance

Taken together with the Noblett (2006) study, this study provides good evidence that Doppler-guided fluid therapy has value in elective open colorectal surgery. The widespread introduction of enhanced recovery programmes coupled with increasing use of laparoscopic techniques raises questions about the generalizability of these results to current practice in this patient group.

Paper 10: Early goal-directed therapy after major surgery reduces complications and duration of hospital stay. A randomised, controlled trial [ISRCTN38797445]

Author details

R Pearse, D Dawson, J Fawcett, A Rhodes, RM Grounds, ED Bennett

Reference

Critical Care 2005; **9**: R687–93.

Abstract

Introduction: Goal-directed therapy (GDT) has been shown to improve outcome when commenced before surgery. This requires pre-operative admission to the intensive care unit (ICU). In cardiac surgery, GDT has proved effective when commenced after surgery. The aim of this study was to evaluate the effect of post-operative GDT on the incidence of complications and duration of hospital stay in patients undergoing general surgery.

Methods: This was a randomised controlled trial with concealed allocation. High-risk general surgical patients were allocated to post-operative GDT to attain an oxygen delivery index of $600 \, \text{ml min}^{-1} \, \text{m}^{-2}$ or to conventional management. Cardiac output was measured by lithium indicator dilution and pulse power analysis. Patients were followed up for 60 days.

Results: Sixty-two patients were randomised to GDT and 60 patients to control treatment. The GDT group received more intravenous colloid (1,907 SD ± 878 ml versus 1,204 SD ± 898 ml; p <0.0001) and dopexamine (55 patients (89%) versus 1 patient (2%); p <0.0001). Fewer GDT patients developed complications (27 patients (44%) versus 41 patients (68%); p = 0.003, relative risk 0.63; 95% confidence intervals 0.46 to 0.87). The number of complications per patient was also reduced (0.7 SD ± 0.9 per patient versus 1.5 SD ± 1.5 per patient; p = 0.002). The median duration of hospital stay in the GDT group was significantly reduced (11 days (IQR 7 to 15) versus 14 days (IQR 11 to 27); p = 0.001). There was no significant difference in mortality (seven patients (11.3%) versus nine patients (15%); p = 0.59).

Conclusion: Post-operative GDT is associated with reductions in post-operative complications and duration of hospital stay. The beneficial effects of GDT may be achieved while avoiding the difficulties of pre-operative ICU admission.

Summary

This was a single centre, prospective, randomized, controlled trial of goal-directed therapy in the postoperative period. Protocol patients were randomized to goal-directed therapy using fluid and dopexamine to attain an oxygen delivery of $600 \, \text{ml min}^{-1} \, \text{m}^{-2}$. Patients were followed up for 60 days. Treatment was guided by lithium indicator dilution measurement of cardiac output and pulse power analysis. Sixty-two patients were randomized to goal-directed therapy and 60 patients to control. The goal-directed therapy group received more colloid and dopexamine. Complications and length of hospital stay were reduced in the intervention group (44%, 11 days) in comparison to control (68%, 14 days). There was no significant difference in mortality (11% intervention, 15% control).

Citation count

304.

Related references

1 Pearse RM, Ikram K, Barry J. Equipment review: an appraisal of the LiDCO plus method of measuring cardiac output. *Crit Care.* 2004; **8**: 190–5.

Key message

This was the first optimization study using specific oxygen delivery not based on a pulmonary artery catheter (PAC). The combination of the LidCO device for measuring cardiac output and an 'optimization' algorithm incorporating dopexamine resulted in reduced complication and resource use.

Strengths

This was the first study using DO_2 goals based on the LidCO device. It had a clear algorithm in the protocol group involving adding dopexamine on top of fluid therapy which was standardized between groups.

Weaknesses

This was a relatively small, single-centre study. Although the fluid therapy was standardized by protocol between groups, the intervention group still received more fluids.

Relevance

Optimization can be effectively delivered using non-PAC based cardiac output monitoring.

Chapter 7

Complications of anaesthesia

AM Møller

Introduction

During the last few decades the process of anaesthesia has become increasingly safe. Complications directly related to anaesthesia are very rare and general anaesthesia is thought to be a direct cause of mortality in only 1 out of 10,000 operations. Data from perioperative deaths are difficult to analyse as they probably represent a combination of anaesthetic and surgical factors. A confidential enquiry in 1987 into perioperative deaths revealed that very few deaths were actually a direct result of general anaesthesia—0.0007% (Aitkenhead, 2005).

Complications during anaesthesia and in the perioperative period are related to the patient's coexisting disease, to the surgical disease, the surgical procedure, and to anaesthesia. It is very difficult indeed to tell how much each of these factors contributes. Estimates suggest that up to 2% of intensive care unit admissions at any one time are related to anaesthetic problems (Aitkenhead, 2005). Certain medical conditions, such as heart disease, pulmonary disease, endocrine disease and nervous system disease increase the risk of complications from anaesthesia.

This selection of papers aims to describe the incidence and type of complications arising during and after anaesthesia and surgery, and a broad range of interventions aiming at reducing these complications. Though some answers are presented and some interventions proposed, most of these interventions need to be further researched in large clinical high quality trials.

Related references

1 Aitkenhead AR. Injuries associated with anaesthesia. A global perspective. *Br J Anaesth* 2005; **95**: 95–109.

Paper 1: Complications and death following anaesthesia. A prospective study with special reference to the influence of patient-, anaesthesia-, and surgery-related risk factors

Author details

T Pedersen

Reference

Danish Medical Bulletin 1994; **41**: 319–31.

Abstract

The present study describes risk factors, the incidence of complications and mortality in the anaesthetized patient. The aims were further to identify additional patient-, anaesthesia-, technique-, and surgery-related factors associated with cardiopulmonary complications and mortality, to describe the value of preoperative radionuclide cardiography in patients with cardiopulmonary insufficiency, and to evaluate the importance of perioperative manual evaluation of the response to train-of-four nerve stimulation for the occurrence of residual neuromuscular blockade in the recovery room. Complications attributable to anaesthesia-complications caused mainly by the anaesthetic procedure occurred in 0.6% (1:170) of the patients, and mortality attributable to anaesthesia was found to be 0.04% (1:2500). An analysis of the patient data suggests that the seriously ill patients (ASA-class ≥3) were more likely to be affected by errors and a substantial negative outcome such as acute myocardial infarction, irreversible cerebral damage or death, than were more healthy patients (ASA 1-2). One-third of the complications attributable to anaesthesia are judged preventable. Cardiopulmonary complications associated with anaesthesia and surgery and requiring intervention occurred in 1:11 of the anesthetized patients. The cardiopulmonary complications were associated with elderly patients (> or =70 yr), patients with preoperative clinical signs of ischaemic heart disease and recent myocardial infarction, chronic heart failure, and chronic obstructive lung disease, as well as perioperative and emergency procedures involving major abdominal surgery. In patients with severe cardiovascular or pulmonary insufficiency (high-risk patients) preoperative radionuclide cardiography could distinguish between different levels of cardiopulmonary risk in the anaesthetized patient. Patients with a preoperative left ventricular ejection fraction <50% or >70% demonstrated a high incidence of cardiopulmonary complications following anaesthesia (70%). It is recommended that left ventricular ejection fraction be measured in patients referred for major surgery who have an increased risk of cardiopulmonary complications as evidenced clinically by heart failure or severe ischaemic heart disease. Hypotension before anaesthetic induction is associated with a high incidence of cardiopulmonary morbidity and mortality. Postoperative pulmonary complications in comparable groups of patients depend primarily on the type of surgery, as major abdominal surgery was related to the highest incidence of pulmonary complications. Regional anaesthesia may be a superior technique to general anaesthesia, especially in elderly patients with chronic obstructive lung disease admitted to major orthopaedic surgery. Furthermore, in avoidance of postoperative complications such as residual neuromuscular blockade, the choice of muscle relaxant was more decisive than was manual evaluation of the response to train-to-four nerve stimulation.

From 'Complications and death following anaesthesia. A prospective study with special reference to the influence of patient-, anaesthesia-, and surgery-related risk factors', Pedersen T, Danish Medical Bulletin, 1994, 41, pp. 319–331.

Summary

Although rare, one-third of all complications of anaesthesia are considered preventable.

Citation count

82.

Related references

1 Pedersen T, Eliasen K, Henriksen E. A prospective study of risk factors and cardiopulmonary complications associated with anaesthesia and surgery: risk indicators of cardiopulmonary morbidity. *Acta Anaesthesiol Scand* 1990; **34**: 144–55.

2 Pedersen T, Kelbaek H, Munck O. Cardiopulmonary complications in high-risk surgical patients: the value of preoperative radionuclide cardiography. *Acta Anaesthesiol Scand* 1990; **34**: 183–9.

3 Fichtner K, Dick W. The causes of perioperative mortality. A trial of the German "CEPOD study." *Anaesthesist* 1997; **46**: 419–27.

4 Sprung J, Abdelmalak B, Gottlieb A, *et al.* Analysis of risk factors for myocardial infarction and cardiac mortality after major vascular surgery. *Anesthesiology* 2000; **93**: 129–40.

5 honeim MM, Block RI, Haffarnan M, *et al.* Awareness during anesthesia: risk factors, causes and sequelae: a review of reported cases in the literature. *Anesth Analg* 2009; **108**: 527–35.

Key message

Anaesthesia-related mortality was found in 0.04% of the patients and mortality almost exclusively seen in elderly patients with cardiopulmonary disease. Cardiopulmonary complications were seen in 9% of all patients, again primarily in the elderly and those with pre-existing comorbidity. About one-third of the complications were judged preventable.

Strengths

The study includes 7,306 consecutive patients and data were collected prospectively and by the same clinicians, who were not involved in patient care. The size of the study and the prospective design made this study a landmark paper, when it was published. It still remains a basic paper for many papers describing the epidemiology of anaesthesia-related complications.

Weaknesses

The paper has obvious problems distinguishing anaesthesia-related complications from surgery-related complications—merely due to the fact that almost all complications happened in patients with serious comorbidity. The outcomes described in the paper are a mixture of hard and surrogate endpoints—and the importance of each endpoint is variable.

Relevance

Anaesthetic and surgical methods have changed considerably since the paper was published as has the health status and demography of the general population. However, this paper is still relevant as it thoroughly describes a surgical population with a common case-mix over a period of 12 months and with few missing data.

Paper 2: Randomized evaluation of pulse oximetry in 20,802 patients; I. Design, demography, pulse oximetry failure rate, and overall complication rate

Author details

JT Møller, T Pedersen, LS Rasmussen, PF Jensen, BD Pedersen, O Ravlo, NH Rasmussen, K Espersen, NW Johannessen, JB Cooper, JS Gravenstein, B Chraemmer-Jørgensen, F Wiberg-Jørgensen, M Djernes, L Heslet, SH Johansen

Reference

Anesthesiology 1993; **78**: 436–44.

Summary

Although pulse oximetry has a relatively low failure rate, it seems to have a higher failure in those who are more at risk. Its use makes the anaesthetist feel safe but this is a false sense of safety.

Citation count

238.

Related references

1 Cooper JB, Cullen DJ, Nemeskal R, *et al*. Effects of information feedback and pulse oximetry on the incidence of anesthesia complications. *Anesthesiology* 1987; **67**: 686–94.

2 Moller JT, Jensen PF, Johannessen NW, *et al*. Hypoxaemia is reduced by pulse oximetry monitoring in the operating theatre and in the recovery room. *Br J Anaesth* 1992; **68**: 146–50.

Key message

Despite high sensibility for detecting hypoxemia during anaesthesia and recovery, perioperative monitoring with pulse oximetry did not reduce the incidence of postoperative complications. The use of pulse oximetry makes many anaesthetists feel safe.

Strengths

The study is large and methodologically sound. Randomization and allocation concealment were maintained. It has high external validity.

Weaknesses

Even though the study is large it was not large enough to detect any differences in hard outcomes. The outcomes investigated were, for the most part, surrogates. There is multiple testing, but in a non-significant study this probably will not be a problem.

Relevance

This study is one of the few large randomized clinical studies in anaesthesia. No other large study has investigated the impact of a monitoring device in perioperative monitoring. Even though we lack evidence of its effect, most anaesthetists would be reluctant to perform anaesthesia without pulse oximetry today.

Paper 3: Reduction of postoperative mortality and morbidity with epidural or spinal anaesthesia: results from overview of randomised trials

Author details

A Rodgers, N Walker, S Schug, A McKee, H Kehlet, A van Zundert, D Sage, M Futter, G Saville, T Clark, S MacMahon

Reference

British Medical Journal 2000; **321**: 1–12.

Abstract

Objectives: To obtain reliable estimates of the effects of neuraxial blockade with epidural or spinal anaesthesia on postoperative morbidity and mortality.

Design: Systematic review of all trials with randomisation to intraoperative neuraxial blockade or not.

Studies: 141 trials including 9559 patients for which data were available before 1 January 1997. Trials were eligible irrespective of their primary aims, concomitant use of general anaesthesia, publication status, or language. Trials were identified by extensive search methods, and substantial amounts of data were obtained or confirmed by correspondence with trialists.

Main outcome measures: All cause mortality, deep vein thrombosis, pulmonary embolism, myocardial infarction, transfusion requirements, pneumonia, other infections, respiratory depression, and renal failure.

Results: Overall mortality was reduced by about a third in patients allocated to neuraxial blockade (103 deaths/4871 patients versus 144/4688 patients, odds ratio=0.70, 95% confidence interval 0.54 to 0.90, P=0.006). Neuraxial blockade reduced the odds of deep vein thrombosis by 44%, pulmonary embolism by 55%, transfusion requirements by 50%, pneumonia by 39%, and respiratory depression by 59% (all P<0.001). There were also reductions in myocardial infarction and renal failure. Although there was limited power to assess subgroup effects, the proportional reductions in mortality did not clearly differ by surgical group, type of blockade (epidural or spinal), or in those trials in which neuraxial blockade was combined with general anaesthesia compared with trials in which neuraxial blockade was used alone.

Conclusions: Neuraxial blockade reduces postoperative mortality and other serious complications. The size of some of these benefits remains uncertain, and further research is required to determine whether these effects are due solely to benefits of neuraxial blockade or partly to avoidance of general anaesthesia. Nevertheless, these findings support more widespread use of neuraxial blockade.

Summary

Surgery performed using anaesthesia with neuraxial blockade is safer for patients.

Citation count

1229.

Related references

1 Rigg JR, Jamrozik K, Myles PS, *et al*; MASTER Anaethesia Trial Study Group. Epidural anaesthesia and analgesia and outcome of major surgery: a randomised trial. *Lancet* 2002; **359**: 1276–82.

2 Parker MJ, Handoll HH, Griffiths R. Anaesthesia for hip fracture surgery in adults. *Cochrane Database Syst Rev* 2004; **4**: CD000521.

3 Mauermann WJ, Shilling AM, Zuo Z. A comparison of neuraxial block versus general anesthesia for elective total hip replacement: a meta-analysis. *Anesth Analg* 2006; **103**: 1018–25.

4 Choi PT, Beattie WS, Bryson GL, *et al*. Effects of neuraxial blockade may be difficult to study using large randomized controlled trials: the PeriOperative Epidural Trial (POET) Pilot Study. *PLoS One* 2009; **4**(2): e4644.

Key message

The authors found better survival in patients randomized to neuraxial blockade and reductions in risk of venous thromboembolism, myocardial infarction, bleeding complications, pneumonia, respiratory depression, and renal failure. Reduction in mortality did not differ by surgical group, type of blockade, or in trials in which neuraxial blockade was combined with general anaesthesia.

Strengths

The paper deals with an interesting clinical question and looks at relevant outcomes. The methodology is sound, search for relevant papers seems comprehensive, only randomized controlled trials are included and data is analysed on an intention-to-treat basis. Sensitivity analysis was performed in order to evaluate whether the effects on total mortality were dependent upon low-quality trials or type of anaesthesia. However, this did not change the overall result. No publication bias was evident.

Weaknesses

No systematic review or meta-analysis is better than the trials they include. There is a problem for this paper that many of the included trials are old, small, and designed for evaluating other outcomes than the ones in the focus of this review. In 80 out of 141 included trials no events were recorded.

Relevance

This is one of the very first papers to investigate the effect of major anaesthesia interventions on perioperative death and morbidity in a systematic review including meta-analysis. If the results are valid a number-needed-to-treat analysis tells us that for every 100 patients given a neuraxial blockade instead of, or as an addition to general anaesthesia, one death will be avoided. Unfortunately, the results of this systematic review have been challenged by other trials and reviews since its publication.

Paper 4: Drugs for preventing postoperative nausea and vomiting

Author details

JB Carlisle, CA Stevenson

Reference

Cochrane Database of Systematic Reviews 2006; **3**: CD004125.

Summary

Although nausea and vomiting are relatively common after surgery, the drugs used to treat it are not particularly effective if used prophylactically. The risk to benefit profile is therefore marginal at best.

Citation count

89.

Related references

1 Cox F. Systematic review of ondansetron for the prevention and trwatment of postoperative nausea and vomiting in adults. *Br J Theatre Nurs* 1999; **9**: 556–63.

2 Eberhart LHJ, Morin AM, Bothner U, *et al.* Droperidol and 5-HT3-receptor antagonists, alone or in combination, for prophylaxis of postoperative nausea and vomiting. A meta-analysis of randomised controlled trials. *Acta Anaesthesiol Scand* 2000; **44**: 1252–7.

3 Alhashimi D, Alhashimi H, Fedorowicz Z. Antiemetics for reducing vomiting related to acute gastroenteritis in children and adolescents. *Cochrane Database Syst Rev* 2006; **4**: CD005506.

4 Lee A, Fan LT. Stimulation of the wrist acupuncture point P6 for preventing postoperative nausea and vomiting. *Cochrane Database Syst Rev* 2009; **2**: CD003281.

Key message

Eighty per cent of all surgical patients will experience either nausea or vomiting in the postoperative period. If prophylactic antiemetics are given about one-third of all patients would benefit. One to five per cent of patients will experience mild side effects after receiving antiemetics, usually headache or sedation.

Strengths

This study is huge and includes almost every randomized study comparing different antiemetics. The methodology is according to Cochrane review standards and is thus very good, which makes the conclusions reliable.

Weaknesses

This review is almost too big and individual comparisons are difficult to find.

Relevance

The review contains updated and relevant information regarding postoperative nausea and/or vomiting.

Paper 5: Org 25969 (sugammadex), a selective relaxant binding agent for antagonism of prolonged rocuronium-induced neuromuscular block

Author details

M Shields, M Giovannelli, RK Mirakhur, I Moppett, J Adams, Y Hermens

Reference

British Journal of Anaesthesia 2006; **96**: 36–43.

Abstract

Background: Org 25969 is a cyclodextrin compound designed to reverse a rocuronium-induced neuromuscular block. The aim of this study was to explore the efficacy, dose–response relation and safety of Org 25969 for reversal of a prolonged rocuronium-induced neuromuscular block.

Methods: Thirty anaesthetized adult patients received rocuronium 0.6 mg kg^{-1} as an initial dose followed by increments to maintain a deep block at a level of <10 PTCs (post-tetanic counts) recorded every 6 min. Neuromuscular monitoring was carried out using accelerometry, in a train-of-four (TOF) mode using TOF-Watch®SX. At recovery of T_2, following at least 2 h of neuromuscular block, patients received their randomly assigned dose of 0.5, 1.0, 2.0, 4.0 or 6.0 mg kg^{-1} of Org 25969. Anaesthesia and neuromuscular monitoring were continued for a minimum period of 30 min after Org 25969 administration. The main end-point of the study was the time to achieve a sustained recovery of TOF ratio to 0.9. Patients were followed up for 7 days after anaesthesia.

Results: The results showed a dose-related decrease in the average time taken to attain a TOF ratio of 0.9 from 6:49 (mins) with the 0.5 mg kg^{-1} dose to 1:22 with the 4.0 mg kg^{-1} dose. Weighted non-linear regression analysis showed the fastest achievable time to TOF ratio of 0.9 to be 1:35. Org 25969 produced no major adverse effects.

Conclusion: Org 25969 effectively reversed a deep and prolonged neuromuscular block induced by rocuronium. The effective reversal dose appears to be 2–4 mg kg^{-1}.

Summary

A new class of neuromuscular blocking reversal agents is described.

Citation count

97.

Related references

1 Flockton EA, Mastronardi P, Hunter JM *et al.* Reversal of rocuronium-induced neuromuscular block with sugammadex is faster than reversal of cisatracurium-induced block with neostigmine. *Br J Anaesth* 2008; **100**: 622–30.

2 Staals LM, Snoeck MM, Driessen JJ, et al. Multicentre, parallel-group, comparative trial evaluating the efficacy and safety of sugammadex in patients with end-stage renal failure or normal renal function. *Br J Anaesth* 2008; **101**: 492–7.

3 de Boer HD. Neuromuscular transmission: new concepts and agents. *J Crit Care* 2009; **24**: 36–42.

4 Caldwell JE, Miller RD. Clinical implications of sugammadex. *Anaesthesia* 2009; **64**(Suppl 1): 66–72.

5 Duvaldestin P, Kuizenga K, Saldien V *et al.* A randomized, dose-response study of sugammadex given for the reversal of deep rocuronium- or vecuronium-induced neuromuscular blockade under sevoflurane anesthesia. *Anesth Analg* 2010; **110**: 74–82.

Key message

Sugammadex was effective in reversing a deep and prolonged neuromuscular block induced by rocuronium. The effective reversal dose was 2–4 mg.

Strengths

This paper is very well written and explains the biological background for the effect of sugammadex very well. The study is well performed and well presented.

Weaknesses

Five different doses of sugammadex are compared; however, there is no control (placebo) group. One of the doses, for example, the 6-mg dose, could have been replaced with a placebo group. It is not clear whether this is an industry-initiated or researcher-initiated study and conflicts of interest are not clearly stated. The study is underpowered to evaluate adverse effects and safety.

Relevance

The development of sugammadex is one of the most important interventions directly related to anaesthesia and complications related to anaesthesia that has happened in decades. This paper is just one of several high-quality papers published on this topic in recent years.

Paper 6: Effect of perioperative beta blockade in patients with diabetes undergoing major non-cardiac surgery: randomised placebo controlled, blinded multicentre trial

Author details

AB Juul, J Wetterslev, C Gluud, A Kofoed-Enevoldsen, G Jensen, T Callesen, P Nørgaard, K Fruergaard, M Bestle, R Vedelsdal, A Miran, J Jacobsen, J Roed, MB Mortensen, L Jørgensen, J Jørgensen, ML Rovsing, PL Petersen, F Pott, M Haas, R Albret, LL Nielsen, G Johansson, P Stjernholm, Y Mølgaard, NB Foss, J Elkjaer, B Dehlie, K Boysen, D Zaric, A Munksgaard, JB Madsen, B Øberg, B Khanykin, T Blemmer, S Yndgaard, G Perko, LP Wang, P Winkel, J Hilden, P Jensen, N Salas; DIPOM Trial Group

Reference

British Medical Journal 2006; **332**: 1482.

Abstract

Objectives: To evaluate the long term effects of perioperative beta blockade on mortality and cardiac morbidity in patients with diabetes undergoing major non-cardiac surgery.

Design: Randomised placebo controlled and blinded multicentre trial. Analyses were by intention to treat.

Setting: University anaesthesia and surgical centres and one coordinating centre.

Participants: 921 patients aged >39 scheduled for major non-cardiac surgery.

Interventions: 100 mg metoprolol controlled and extended release or placebo administered from the day before surgery to a maximum of eight perioperative days.

Main outcome measures: The composite primary outcome measure was time to all cause mortality, acute myocardial infarction, unstable angina, or congestive heart failure. Secondary outcome measures were time to all cause mortality, cardiac mortality, and non-fatal cardiac morbidity.

Results: Mean duration of intervention was 4.6 days in the metoprolol group and 4.9 days in the placebo group. Metoprolol significantly reduced the mean heart rate by 11% (95% confidence interval 9% to 13%) and mean blood pressure by 3% (1% to 5%). The primary outcome occurred in 99 of 462 patients in the metoprolol group (21%) and 93 of 459 patients in the placebo group (20%) (hazard ratio 1.06, 0.80 to 1.41) during a median follow-up of 18 months (range 6–30). All cause mortality was 16% (74/462) in the metoprolol group and 16% (72/459) in the placebo group (1.03, 0.74 to 1.42). The difference in risk for the proportion of patients with serious adverse events was 2.4% (−0.8% to 5.6%).

Conclusions: Perioperative metoprolol did not significantly affect mortality and cardiac morbidity in these patients with diabetes. Confidence intervals, however, were wide, and the issue needs reassessment.

Summary

The use of beta adrenoceptor blockers in the perioperative period was not associated with a mortality benefit in diabetic patients undergoing non-cardiac surgery.

Citation count

211.

Related references

1 Mangano DT, Layug EL, Wallace A, *et al*. Effect of atenolol on mortality and cardiovascular morbidity after noncardiac surgery. Multicenter Study of Perioperative Ischemia Research Group. *N Engl J Med* 1996; **335**: 1713–20.

2 Poldermans D, Boersma E, Bax JJ, *et al*. The effect of bisoprolol on perioperative mortality and myocardial infarction in high-risk patients undergoing vascular surgery. Dutch Echocardiographic Cardiac Risk Evaluation Applying Stress Echocardiography Study Group. *N Engl J Med* 1999; **341**: 1789–94.

3 Brady AR, Gibbs JS, Greenhalgh RM, *et al*; POBBLE trial investigators. Perioperative beta-blockade (POBBLE) for patients undergoing infrarenal vascular surgery: results of a randomized double-blind controlled trial. *J Vasc Surg* 2005; **41**: 602–9.

4 Devereaux PJ, Yang H, Guyatt GH, *et al*. Rationale, design, and organization of the PeriOperative ISchemic Evaluation (POISE) trial: a randomized controlled trial of metoprolol versus placebo in patients undergoing noncardiac surgery. POISE Trial Investigators. *Am Heart J* 2006; **152**: 223–30.

5 Bangalore S, Wetterslev J, Pranesh S, *et al*. Perioperative beta blockers in patients having non-cardiac surgery: a meta-analysis. *Lancet* 2008; **372**: 1962–76.

6 Devereaux PJ, Yang H, Yusuf S, *et al*. Effects of extended-release metoprolol succinate in patients undergoing non-cardiac surgery (POISE trial): a randomised controlled trial. POISE Study Group. *Lancet* 2008; **371**: 1839–47.

Key message

In this trial there was no effect of metoprolol on cardiac morbidity or mortality in patients with diabetes undergoing major non-cardiac surgery.

Strengths

The trial is randomized, blinded, and placebo controlled—including 921 patients from 13 centres. Adequate methods were used for securing allocation concealment and methodologically the research protocol was generally strict and the study is of high internal and external validity. It is highly clinically relevant.

Weaknesses

The composite primary outcome (mortality, myocardial infarction, unstable angina, and congestive heart failure) can be difficult to interpret. The decrease in heart rate caused by metoprolol may partly have compromised blinding of the randomization code.

Relevance

This high-quality trial is an important element in the ongoing discussion of the effects of periop-erative beta blockade on mortality and cardiac morbidity. Even if conclusive evidence is not yet available, the high-quality trial questions the ongoing use of perioperative beta blockade.

Paper 7: Effect of high perioperative oxygen fraction on surgical site infection and pulmonary complications after abdominal surgery: the PROXI randomized clinical trial

Author details

CS Meyhoff, J Wetterslev, LN Jorgensen, SW Henneberg, C Høgdall, L Lundvall, PE Svendsen, H Mollerup, TH Lunn, I Simonsen, KR Martinsen, T Pulawska, L Bundgaard, L Bugge, EG Hansen, C Riber, P Gocht-Jensen, LR Walker, A Bendtsen, G Johansson, N Skovgaard, K Heltø, A Poukinski, A Korshin, A Walli, M Bulut, PS Carlsson, SA Rodt, LB Lundbech, H Rask, N Buch, SK Perdawid, J Reza, KV Jensen, CG Carlsen, FS Jensen, LS Rasmussen; PROXI Trial Group

Reference

Journal of the American Medical Association 2009; **302**: 1543–50.

Summary

This was a large trial of 1,400 patients undergoing abdominal surgery randomized to either 30% or 80% oxygen during surgery and for 2 h afterwards. It was found that there was no difference in infections at the site of surgery between those patients receiving 30% and those receiving 80% oxygen.

Citation count

52.

Related references

1 Greif R, Akça O, Horn EP, *et al.* Supplemental perioperative oxygen to reduce the incidence of surgical-wound infection. Outcomes Research Group. *N Engl J Med* 2000; **342**: 161–7.

2 Pryor KO, Fahey TJ 3rd, Lien CA, *et al.* Surgical site infection and the routine use of perioperative hyperoxia in a general surgical population: a randomized controlled trial. *JAMA* 2004; **291**: 79–87.

3 Belda FJ, Aguilera L, García de la Asunción J, *et al.* Supplemental perioperative oxygen and the risk of surgical wound infection: a randomized controlled trial. Spanish Reduccion de la Tasa de Infeccion Quirurgica Group. *JAMA* 2005; **294**: 2035–42.

4 Meyhoff CS, Wetterslev J, Jorgensen LN, *et al.* Perioperative oxygen fraction - effect on surgical site infection and pulmonary complications after abdominal surgery: a randomized clinical trial. Rationale and design of the PROXI-Trial. PROXI Trial Group. *Trials* 2008; **9**: 58.

Key message

Administration of 80% oxygen during surgery and 2 h postoperatively compared to 30% oxygen does not affect the surgical site infection rate. There was no difference in the incidence of pulmonary complications or adverse events.

Strengths

The trial is large, including 1,400 patients from 14 centres in Denmark. It is a randomized, blinded, clinical trial of high methodological quality. Follow-up was thorough with a low rate of missing data.

Weaknesses

The trial included patients undergoing many different types of surgery and though this results in a high external validity, it may also conceal an effect on some subgroup of patients, e.g. colorectal surgery. There may be differences between centres concerning type of anaesthesia and other factors, but randomization was stratified to take this into account.

Relevance

During the last 10 years several trials have been published on the topic of perioperative oxygen fraction with differing results. The trials have been of varying quality and rather heterogeneous. This well-performed, high-quality trial plays an important part in the discussion.

Paper 8: Effects of intravenous fluid restriction on postoperative complications: comparison of two perioperative fluid regimens: a randomized assessor-blinded multicenter trial

Author details

B Brandstrup, H Tønnesen, R Beier-Holgersen, E Hjortsø, H Ørding, K Lindorff-Larsen, MS Rasmussen, C Lanng, L Wallin, LH Iversen, CS Gramkow, M Okholm, T Blemmer, PE Svendsen, HH Rottensten, B Thage, J Riis, IS Jeppesen, D Teilum, AM Christensen, B Graungaard, F Pott; The Danish Study Group on Perioperative Fluid Therapy

Reference

Annals of Surgery 2003; **238**: 641–8.

Summary

There is much debate about optimization of patients' physiology before surgery. This paper concludes that a restricted fluid replacement regimen was not associated with an adverse outcome over a more liberal policy. In fact complications were reduced in this group of patients.

Citation count

526.

Related references

1 MacKay G, Fearon K, McConnachie A, *et al*. Randomized clinical trial of the effect of postoperative intravenous fluid restriction on recovery after elective colorectal surgery. *Br J Surg* 2006; **93**: 1469–74.

2 Holte K, Foss NB, Andersen J, *et al*. Liberal or restrictive fluid administration in fast-track colonic surgery: a randomized, double-blind study. *Br J Anaesth* 2007; **99**: 500–8.

3 de Aguilar-Nascimento JE, Diniz BN, do Carmo AV, *et al*. Clinical benefits after the implementation of a protocol of restricted perioperative intravenous crystalloid fluids in major abdominal operations. *World J Surg* 2009; **33**: 925–30.

4 Vermeulen H, Hofland J, Legemate DA, *et al*. Intravenous fluid restriction after major abdominal surgery: a randomized blinded clinical trial. *Trials* 2009; **10**: 50.

Key message

Fluid restriction during and after colorectal surgery reduces complication rate.

Strengths

This randomized clinical trial used adequate methods for generation of allocation sequence and concealment. Blinded assessment of outcome measures was used.

Weaknesses

The study is not blinded and this may have been difficult anyway. The patient sample was not fully consecutive. The patient numbers are relatively small, and small numbers may give rise to unequal distribution of important prognostic factors. In addition the number of patients currently smoking and the level of colonic anastomoses both favoured the restricted group.

Relevance

Reducing complications after abdominal surgery remains a clinically important issue. The results of this trial challenges clinical practice in a field that has been much debated but little researched for a long time.

Paper 9: Avoidance of nitrous oxide for patients undergoing major surgery: a randomized controlled trial

Author details

PS Myles, K Leslie, MT Chan, A Forbes, MJ Paech, P Peyton, BS Silbert, E Pascoe; ENIGMA Trial Group

Reference

Anesthesiology 2007; **107**: 221–31.

Summary

When nitrous oxide is avoided in inhalational anaesthesia there is a decrease in complication rate.

Citation count

123.

Related references

1 Shorrab AA, Atallah MM. Total intravenous anaesthesia with ketamine-midazolam versus halothane-nitrous oxide-oxygen anaesthesia for prolonged abdominal surgery. *Eur J Anaesthesiol* 2003; **20**: 925–31.

2 Fleischmann E, Lenhardt R, Kurz A, *et al.* Nitrous oxide and risk of surgical wound infection: a randomised trial. *Lancet* 2005; **366**: 1101–7.

3 Leslie K, Myles PS, Chan MT, *et al.* Risk factors for severe postoperative nausea and vomiting in a randomized trial of nitrous oxide-based vs nitrous oxide-free anaesthesia. ENIGMA Trial Group. *Br J Anaesth* 2008; **101**: 498–505.

4 Myles PS, Chan MT, Kaye DM, *et al.* Effect of nitrous oxide anesthesia on plasma homocysteine and endothelial function. *Anesthesiology* 2008; **109**: 657–63.

5 Myles PS, Leslie K, Peyton P, *et al.* Nitrous oxide and perioperative cardiac morbidity (ENIGMA-II) Trial: rationale and design. ANZCA Trials Group. *Am Heart J* 2009; **157**: 488–94.

Key message

Omitting nitrous oxide from anaesthesia decreases the incidence of complications after major surgery as well as the incidence of severe postoperative nausea and vomiting. No difference in length of stay was found.

Strengths

The trial included 2,050 patients in 19 centres worldwide. Patients were adequately randomized and stratified according to centre and elective/emergency status.

Weaknesses

No primary outcome is defined. Sample size was calculated from a reduction in length of stay from 4 days to 3.5 days. The question of whether it was a decrease in nitrous oxide or increase in oxygen that had the effect is not explored.

Relevance

Many anaesthetists favour using nitrous oxide as a supplement to general anaesthesia. The debate about the pros and cons concerning this has been based on empirical data for a long time. This paper helps to obtain evidence-based decision-making on this topic.

Paper 10: Effects of a perioperative smoking cessation intervention on postoperative complications: a randomized trial

Author details

D Lindström, O Sadr Azodi, A Wladis, H Tønnesen, S LinderH, Nåsell, S Ponzer, J Adami

Reference

Annals of Surgery 2008; **248**: 739–45.

Summary

Cessation of smoking within 4 weeks of elective surgery is associated with benefits although the effect was not statistically significant.

Citation count

81.

Related references

1 Møller AM, Villebro N, Pedersen T, *et al.* Effect of preoperative smoking intervention on postoperative complications: a randomised clinical trial. *Lancet* 2002; **359**: 114–17.

2 Møller AM, Pedersen T, Villebro N, *et al.* Impact of lifestyle on perioperative smoking cessation and postoperative complication rate. *Prev Med* 2003; **36**: 704–9.

3 Sørensen LT, Jørgensen T. Short-term pre-operative smoking cessation intervention does not affect postoperative complications in colorectal surgery: a randomized clinical trial. *Colorectal Dis* 2003; **5**: 347–52.

4 Barrera R, Shi W, Amar D, *et al.* Smoking and timing of cessation: impact on pulmonary complications after thoracotomy. *Chest* 2005; **127**: 1977–83.

5 Møller A, Villebro N. Interventions for preoperative smoking cessation. *Cochrane Database Syst Rev* 2005; **3**: CD002294.

6 Thomsen T, Tønnesen H, Møller AM. Effect of preoperative smoking cessation interventions on postoperative complications and smoking cessation. *Br J Surg* 2009; **96**: 451–61.

Key message

Smoking cessation intervention 4 weeks before surgery effectively reduces the postoperative complication rate.

Strengths

The intervention intended to keep the patients smoke-free for an 8-week period—as opposed to other studies where patients have been allowed to just cut down on their smoking. Furthermore the patients are very well described according to their smoking habits and degree of dependency.

Weaknesses

The patients studied in this trial underwent a wide range of different surgical procedures. While improving the external validity, this also makes the patients a very heterogeneous group. The postoperative complications registered were not predefined; giving way to potential outcome reporting bias.

Relevance

As preoperative smoking intervention seems to be effective in reducing perioperative complications, this is an intervention that is very relevant to daily clinical practice. Smoking cessation intervention should be an option in any surgical setting worldwide.

Chapter 8

Mechanisms of anaesthesia

A Jenkins

Introduction

This chapter will focus on ten papers that have revolutionized our understanding of how general anaesthetics alter the ability of the brain to perceive and interpret the world around us. These papers have each made a specific advance that either at the time, or in hindsight, has contributed directly to our understanding of where and how general anaesthetics exert their effects in the nervous system. Therefore, the focus of this chapter will be on the molecular pharmacology of anaesthetic drugs and the ways in which they alter neurophysiological function. It would be wrong of course to say that general anaesthetic drugs selectively target the nervous system. In addition to their neurological effects, general anaesthetic drugs directly modulate cardiac, vascular, and pulmonary systems and understanding all of these actions is critical to a full understanding of the anesthetized state. However, in this chapter I have chosen to consider only those studies that focus mainly on the neuronal actions of these drugs, with a view to understanding what is arguably the most profound effect of anaesthetics: how they reversibly remove awareness and consciousness.

In writing this chapter I asked many colleagues to share their views on which papers have had the greatest impact on our understanding of the molecular mechanisms of general anaesthetics. The work of Overton and Meyer was mentioned by many but I have chosen not to include their famous papers of the late 19th century. Their independent observations on the correlation between hydrophobicity and anaesthetic or narcotizing potency were certainly groundbreaking and to this day, viable theories of anaesthetic action must take their findings into account. It may be argued by some that the 'Meyer–Overton' correlations were in fact the first description of a general anaesthetic 'structure–activity relationship'. Unfortunately, the molecular data were limited and the theories of anaesthetic action that grew from their findings were simply not congruent with the laws of thermodynamics and principles of pharmacology.

An epiphany in the study of molecular anaesthetic mechanisms transpired upon the discovery of proteins that act as anaesthetic receptors. The description of soluble, membrane-free anaesthetic-sensitive proteins was quickly followed by the discovery of anaesthetic-sensitive, membrane-bound proteins in neurones whose function is to control neuronal excitability. Over the last 25 years, the full weight of pharmacology, physiology, and biophysics have been brought to bear on the study of anaesthetic–protein interactions, yielding many striking results. Most importantly, these studies have generated a rational theory for the mechanisms of general anaesthesia. This chapter will focus mainly on the actions of anaesthetics on one of these proteins, the gamma-aminobutyric acid A (GABA$_A$) receptor. The papers I have selected depict how this receptor was identified as perhaps the most common and important anaesthetic target site, how this hypothesis was tested and verified and how these molecular events integrate within the nervous system to produce sedation and loss of consciousness.

We now know that general anaesthetics modulate the function of several ion channels and it would be disingenuous for me to not to say clearly that the anaesthetized state is generated by a combination of anaesthetic actions at a variety of receptors and ion channels. For example, xenon and ketamine anaesthesia is mediated by the blockade of excitatory N-methyl-D-aspartate (NMDA) receptors and volatile anaesthetics have strong actions on both GABA$_A$ receptors and 2P-domain potassium channels. Nevertheless, the majority of agents used to induce and maintain general anaesthesia act at the GABA$_A$ receptor, the most common fast inhibitory ligand-gated ion channel in the central nervous system.

Paper 1: Structural basis for the inhibition of firefly luciferase by a general anesthetic

Author details

NP Franks, A Jenkins, E Conti, WR Lieb, P Brick

Reference

Biophysics Journal 1998; **75**: 2205–11.

Abstract

The firefly luciferase enzyme from *Photinus pyralis* is probably the best-characterized model system for studying anesthetic-protein interactions. It binds a diverse range of general anesthetics over a large potency range, displays a sensitivity to anesthetics that is very similar to that found in animals, and has an anesthetic sensitivity that can be modulated by one of its substrates (ATP). In this paper we describe the properties of bromoform acting as a general anesthetic (in *Rana temporaria* tadpoles) and as an inhibitor of the firefly luciferase enzyme at high and low ATP concentrations. In addition, we describe the crystal structure of the low-ATP form of the luciferase enzyme in the presence of bromoform at 2.2-Å resolution. These results provide a structural basis for understanding the anesthetic inhibition of the enzyme, as well as an explanation for the ATP modulation of its anesthetic sensitivity.

Summary

This paper demonstrated that bromoform (a halogenated alkane: $CHBr_3$) acted as a general anaesthetic and inhibited the function of the luciferase enzyme with a square dependence on bromoform concentration at low substrate concentrations. More importantly, the authors soaked crystals of recombinant luciferase with a solution containing bromoform, froze them at 100 K and recorded the diffraction pattern generated when they were illuminated with synchrotron radiation. These images were used to determine the co-ordinates of the anaesthetic–protein complex. The authors found that two molecules of bromoform simply occupied the luciferin binding site, without inducing any changes in secondary structure. While occupying the anaesthetic binding pocket, the molecules interacted with backbone carbonyls, polar and apolar components of the pocket and local water molecules.

Citation count

134.

Related references

1 Franks NP, Lieb WR. Mapping of general anaesthetic target sites provides a molecular basis for cutoff effects. *Nature* 1985; **316**: 349–51.

2 Moss GW, Curry S, Franks NP, *et al*. Mapping the polarity profiles of general anesthetic target sites using n-alkane-(alpha, omega)-diols. *Biochemistry* 1991; **30**: 10551–7.

3 Bhattacharya AA, Curry S, Franks NP. Binding of the general anesthetics propofol and halothane to human serum albumin. High resolution crystal structures. *J Biol Chem* 2000; **275**: 38731–8.

4 Baenziger JE, Corringer PJ. 3D structure and allosteric modulation of the transmembrane domain of pentameric ligand-gated ion channels. *Neuropharmacology* 2011; **60**: 116–25.

Key message

Anaesthetics modulate protein function by binding to pre-formed water-containing amphiphilic pockets. While bound, they interact with polar and apolar components of the pocket, but they do not induce large changes in protein structure.

Strengths

This paper used model systems with predictable and well-understood kinetics. The data are unambiguous and are consistent with the previous work on luciferase. The structure of the anaesthetic–protein complex accounted for the observed functional data perfectly.

Weaknesses

The authors used non-mammalian model systems and a non-clinical drug. This study would have been even more impressive had the protein been a GABA$_A$ receptor and the drug propofol or isoflurane.

Relevance

This paper elegantly demonstrates how the function of a large protein can be altered by a handful of low energy interactions with a small promiscuous molecule. As a result of this interaction, the binding of the anaesthetic does not induce large conformational changes in protein structure. Instead, the anaesthetic molecule simply alters the balance between the different states in which the protein (and in this case, substrate) can exist. In recent years, it has become apparent that this is how general anaesthetics alter the function of receptors in the nervous system.

Paper 2: Minimum alveolar anesthetic concentration: a standard of anesthetic potency

Author details

EI Eger II, LJ Saidman, B Brandstater

Reference

Anesthesiology 1965; **26**: 756–63.

Summary

In this seminal pharmacological study, the authors measured the ability of different partial pressures of halothane to block movement in response to a set of noxious stimuli (tail clamp, facial electrodes, movement of the endotracheal tube, 20-cm incision and paw clamp). The clamp was a crushing stimulus generated by a 10-inch arterial forcep closed around the paw or tail until the ratchet locked closed. The authors were careful to standardize their anaesthetic regimen, using only a single agent, and throughout the procedure, were able to record temperature, blood pressure, alveolar anaesthetic concentration, carbon dioxide (CO_2) concentration and arterial blood gas PO_2 and PCO_2.

They found that a response to a mild stimulus (e.g. paw clamp) could be blocked with half of the amount of anaesthetic that was required to block a very painful stimulus (e.g. tail clamp). However, the amount of anaesthetic needed to block the response to the same stimulus between different animals was constant. In addition, the amount of anaesthetic required to block the response to the tail clamp remained constant over the 500-min duration of the experiment. With the exception of severe hypoxia, they found that MAC remained relatively stable in response to changes in blood pH or end-tidal CO_2.

Citation count

701.

Related references

1 Antognini JF, Schwartz K. Exaggerated anesthetic requirements in the preferentially anesthetized brain. *Anesthesiology* 1993; **79**: 1244–9.

Key message

MAC is a useful means for the determination of anaesthetic potency. As such, MAC appears to be a useful standard by which all inhalation anaesthetics can be compared.

Strengths

This study established a benchmark concentration of drug that can be used to achieve general anaesthesia. By conducting their *in vitro* experiments at MAC, investigators were able to ensure for the first time, that their experiments used clinically relevant amounts of anaesthetic. Much of the early literature on anaesthetic mechanisms contains descriptions of experiments performed at concentrations much higher than MAC. The results of many of these studies therefore really have no meaningful bearing on our understanding of anaesthetic action (although perhaps they have some bearing on understanding the toxic or pathological effects of anaesthetics). In addition, the standardization of anaesthetic dose permitted the measurement of anaesthetic effects on other aspects of physiology, for example, cardiac output or vascular tone. The establishment of a standardized concentration–response relationship placed the understanding of anaesthetic action firmly in the realm of rational and classical pharmacology.

Weaknesses

The report, as with many that utilize large mammals, suffers from a low number of replicates. Also, the datasets only extend to three times the time constant for some of the effects described, slightly limiting the resolution of the study. Finally, the neurocircuitry that controls the tail clamp response is located within the spinal cord. These circuits are very different from those that maintain awareness and consciousness in the cerebrum. Therefore, this study was more relevant to understanding drug mechanisms in the spinal cord, but perhaps less informative on drug action in other regions of the central nervous system.

Relevance

At the time when this manuscript was published, the general consensus was 'there was a wide range of susceptibility to an anaesthetic agent'. This paper overturned this misunderstanding, instead demonstrating that anaesthetic requirement remains constant during surgery and remains constant between individuals. The authors also state that the constant partial pressure in the lungs results in a constant partial pressure in the brain (or in their case, the spinal cord).

Paper 3: Selective action of anesthetics on synapses and axons in mammalian sympathetic ganglia

Author details

MG Larrabee, JM Posternak

Reference

Journal of Neurophysiology 1952; **15**: 91–114.

Summary

The authors measured the effects of general anaesthetics on the transmission of neural signals through the cat stellate ganglion. They utilized the fact that there are two parallel signal pathways through the ganglion: one passes directly though the ganglion, the other pathway contains a synapse. First the authors demonstrated that signalling via the direct pathway could be blocked by high concentrations of anaesthetics. In addition, myelination of the fibres did not alter the effect of anaesthetics on the height of the propagated action potentials. In contrast, pentobarbital selectively blocked the synaptic pathway, in a dose-dependent manner. At concentrations where the action potential height was still close to 100% of the control value, the postsynaptic response had been blocked by more than 80%. They repeated this with three more agents (chloretone, chloroform, and octanol) and found that the synaptic pathway was usually approximately 2–10 times more sensitive than the direct path. In contrast, they found that other alcohols exhibited no selectivity and that urethane had a selectivity that was inverted from the other selective agents (the direct path was more sensitive than was the synaptic pathway). Finally, the authors demonstrated that the molecular weight of the anaesthetics were positively correlated with narcotizing concentrations.

Citation count

332.

Key message

Synapses are more sensitive to general anaesthetics than are nerve fibres. The authors predicted that 'this could result from a selective action . . . on some structures associated with . . . post-synaptic cell bodies'.

Strengths

The authors were able to simultaneously record the effect of anaesthetics on neural transmission, without having to worry about differences in effect-site concentration, or preparation-to-preparation variability. They were able to show clear and unambiguous differences in how different anaesthetics modulated the transmission of information through the nervous system.

Weaknesses

The authors do report changes in action potential size, but these generally occur at concentrations higher than those needed to change synaptic transmission. There continues to this day, a debate concerning how large a molecular or cellular anaesthetic effect needs to be in order for it to play a role in generating the anaesthetized state. Given the confusion surrounding the anaesthetic EC_{50} (half maximal effective concentration) at the time, the authors did well to emphasize the importance of the synaptic effects discovered here.

Relevance

These findings critically drove a wedge between the older 'non-specific' theories of general anaesthesia. Instead the authors hypothesized that anaesthetics were selective for certain structures in the nervous system and that these structures were critically located on post-synaptic membranes.

Paper 4: General anesthetics modulate GABA receptor channel complex in rat dorsal root ganglion neurons

Author details

M Nakahiro, JZ Yeh, E Brunner, T Narahashi

Reference

Federation of American Societies for Experimental Biology Journal 1989; **3**: 1850–4.

Summary

Isoflurane, enflurane, and halothane all enhanced the function of GABA$_A$ receptors in cultured dorsal root ganglion neurones when activated by low concentrations of GABA. When receptors were activated by high concentrations of GABA over a long period of time, the response desensitized. Enflurane briefly reversed and then enhanced this desensitization.

Citation count

145.

Related references

1 Harrison NL, Simmonds MA. Modulation of the GABA receptor complex by a steroid anaesthetic. *Brain Res* 1984; **323**: 287–92.

2 MacIver MB, Tanelian DL, Mody I. Two mechanisms for anesthetic-induced enhancement of GABAA-mediated neuronal inhibition. *Ann N Y Acad Sci* 1991; **625**: 91–6.

3 Jones MV, Brooks PA, Harrison NL. Enhancement of gamma-aminobutyric acid-activated Cl- currents in cultured rat hippocampal neurones by three volatile anaesthetics. *J Physiol* 1992; **449**: 279–93.

Key message

Inhaled anaesthetics enhance the function of inhibitory GABA$_A$ receptors expressed on the surface of dorsal root ganglion cells.

Strengths

A major strength of this manuscript was the use of the relatively new whole-cell patch-clamp electrophysiological technique. It provided the investigators with unprecedented control of the receptors being investigated. This technique has since become the standard recording technique for measuring the action of anaesthetics in neuronal preparations.

Weaknesses

The concentrations of anaesthetic used in this study are high. The authors claim to be working in the clinical range, but the micromolar concentrations of isoflurane, halothane, and enflurane used here are 3–4 times MAC. We have subsequently learned that MAC-equivalent concentrations also produce robust GABA$_A$ receptor modulation.

Relevance

The authors reported that the bidirectional effects of the anaesthetics on receptor kinetics are strong evidence for the direct and specific interaction of anaesthetic molecules with neuronal ion channels. By doing so, they refuted the non-specific theories that were still popular at the time.

This paper was one of several at this time that demonstrated that inhaled anaesthetics modulated ion channel function. By so doing, the authors helped bring the study of anaesthetic mechanisms out of the non-specific realm, and into the fields of rational molecular pharmacology and neurophysiology.

Paper 5: Inducing anesthesia with a GABA analog, THIP

Author details

SC Cheng, EA Brunner

Reference

Anesthesiology 1985; **63**: 147–51.

Summary

In this simple but profound study, the authors injected the novel chemical THIP and other compounds that were known to be anaesthetics (midazolam, thiopental and gamma-hydroxybutyrate) into the tail veins of six rats or mice. After administration, they recorded several measures of anaesthesia, behaviour, and sedation. These included tail pinch, radiant tail-flick test, spontaneous exploration, respiratory rate, and a graded righting reflex. All of the animals became anaesthetized, but the authors noticed that THIP produced a more long-lived anaesthetized state. They found that THIP was equipotent with thiopental for inducing anaesthesia.

Citation count

40.

Related references

1 Chandra D, Jia F, Liang J, *et al.* $GABA_A$ receptor a4 subunits mediate extrasynaptic inhibition in thalamus and dentate gyrus and the action of gaboxadol. *Proc Natl Acad Sci USA* 2006; **103**: 15230–5.

Key message

General anaesthesia can be achieved when a membrane-permeable analogue of the inhibitory neurotransmitter GABA is injected into the bloodstream of rats.

Strengths

A very clear demonstration that the prolonged activation of $GABA_A$ receptors is a central component of generating sedation and general anaesthesia

Weaknesses

The authors did not know or appreciate at which $GABA_A$ receptors THIP was acting. Also, it would have been interesting to see THIP and anaesthetics administered simultaneously; if a profoundly synergistic effect had occurred, it would have further confirmed the importance of $GABA_A$ receptors in defining the anaesthetized state.

Relevance

THIP, better known now as gaboxadol, was subsequently investigated in clinical trials for use as a sleep-aid. More recently, it has been discovered that THIP is highly active at extra-synaptic $GABA_A$ receptors. It inhibits the function of the nervous system by prolonging synaptic transmission (synaptic spill-over), and by generating an 'inhibitory shunt', or leak current, on neuronal cell bodies. In this way, its action is analogous to volatile anaesthetics activating 2P-domain potassium channels. The importance of this leak current in defining the anaesthetized state was not fully appreciated until after the work of Faulkner *et al.* (discussed later in this chapter in Paper 10).

However, the most striking and most commonly overlooked finding of this study is that prolonged GABA$_A$ receptor activation can render an animal unconscious.

Paper 6: Stereoselective effects of etomidate optical isomers on gamma-aminobutyric acid type A receptors and animals

Author details

SL Tomlin, A Jenkins, WR Lieb, NP Franks

Reference

Anesthesiology 1998; **88**: 708–17.

Summary

Before the revolution of gene cloning, heterologous expression of neuronal genes and site directed mutagenesis, investigators had to use different strategies to demonstrate that anaesthetic binding sites were structurally constrained and therefore capable of differentiating between molecules with very similar structures and identical physical properties. In this study, Tomlin *et al.* utilized the two optical isomers of etomidate to demonstrate that the more potent anaesthetic enantiomer also had the greatest efficacy for modulating $GABA_A R$ function. Using the loss of righting reflex in tadpole, the authors established that the R(+) isomer was almost 10-fold more potent an anaesthetic than the S(−) isomer. They also showed that the R(+) isomer was 6–10 times more effective at potentiating the function of $GABA_A Rs$ expressed in PA3 cells. Finally, the authors showed that the two isomers were equally effective at disrupting the structure of lipid bilayers.

Citation count

110.

Related references

1 Franks NP, Lieb WR. Stereospecific effects of inhalational general anesthetic optical isomers on nerve ion channels. *Science* 1991; **254**: 427–30.

2 Hall AC, Lieb WR, Franks NP. Stereoselective and non-stereoselective actions of isoflurane on the $GABA_A$ receptor. *Br J Pharmacol* 1994; **112**: 906–10.

Key message

General anaesthetic binding sites are highly discriminatory and are capable of detecting subtle differences in the molecules that enter them. These subtle differences produce different effects on receptor function and are preserved as they propagate up through the nervous system, revealing the same selectivity on whole animal behaviour.

Strengths

When a pair of isomers with different anaesthetic potencies has equal effects on the structure of lipids, but different effects on a neuronal protein (with the same selectivity as the anaesthetic effects), it is impossible for a lipid-based mechanism of anaesthesia to account for the differences seen in the whole animal. This study was probably the final nail in the coffin for the lipid hypothesis of anaesthesia action.

Weaknesses

This study utilized β1-containing receptors that have been reported to be relatively insensitive to etomidate, although that does not appear to be the case here. In fact, the elevated sensitivity of β2 or β3 containing receptors is likely to reveal a greater degree of selectivity.

Relevance

This report is supported by an earlier and equally important study of the optical isomers of isoflurane acting on molluscan potassium channels and cholinergic receptors and was followed-up with a study with three barbiturate anaesthetics. In all three cases, the difference in anaesthetic potency was matched by the difference in the ability of the anaesthetic to modulate the function of the critical receptor or ion channel. These reports all highlight the opportunity in the future for designing highly selective drugs that will perhaps discriminate between different subunits of the same receptor family, yielding fewer deleterious side effects.

Paper 7: Sites of alcohol and volatile anaesthetic action on GABA$_A$ and glycine receptors

Author details

SJ Mihic, Q Ye, MJ Wick, VV Koltchine, MD Krasowski, SE Finn, MP Mascia, CF Valenzuela, KK Hanson, EP Greenblatt, RA Harris, NL Harrison

Reference

Nature 1997; **389**: 385–9.

Abstract

Volatile anaesthetics have historically been considered to act in a nonspecific manner on the central nervous system. More recent studies, however, have revealed that the receptors for inhibitory neurotransmitters such as gamma-aminobutyric acid (GABA) and glycine are sensitive to clinically relevant concentrations of inhaled anaesthetics. The function of GABA$_A$ and glycine receptors is enhanced by a number of anaesthetics and alcohols, whereas activity of the related GABA rho1 receptor is reduced. We have used this difference in pharmacology to investigate the molecular basis for modulation of these receptors by anaesthetics and alcohols. By using chimaeric receptor constructs, we have identified a region of 45 amino-acid residues that is both necessary and sufficient for the enhancement of receptor function. Within this region, two specific amino-acid residues in transmembrane domains 2 and 3 are critical for allosteric modulation of both GABA$_A$ and glycine receptors by alcohols and two volatile anaesthetics. These observations support the idea that anaesthetics exert a specific effect on these ion-channel proteins, and allow for the future testing of specific hypotheses of the action of anaesthetics.

Summary

This paper was the first to demonstrate that a single amino acid residue can control the structure of the anaesthetic binding site in the GABA$_A$ receptor. When it was mutated, the receptor became anaesthetic-insensitive. Three laboratories, led by Harris, Greenblatt, and Harrison had all independently noted that while the functions of GABA$_A$ and glycine receptors were enhanced by general anaesthetics, a closely related family member, the 'GABA$_C$' receptor was insensitive. By studying differences in the amino acid sequences of the three proteins and by splicing together mixtures of the insensitive and sensitive subunits, they were able to identify two transmembrane domains that were essential for conferring anaesthetic sensitivity.

In a second round of experiments, the authors focused on the handful of differences within this region and discovered that site directed mutagenesis at two conserved positions (a serine in the second transmembrane domain and an alanine in the third transmembrane domain) to the homologous residue in the GABA$_C$ receptor r1 subunit (an isoleucine and tryptophan respectively) rendered the mutated receptors insensitive to enflurane and ethanol.

Citation count

870.

Related references

1 Belelli D, Lambert JJ, Peters JA, *et al*. The interaction of the general anesthetic etomidate with the gamma-aminobutyric acid type A receptor is influenced by a single amino acid. *Proc Natl Acad Sci USA* 1997; **94**: 11031–6.

2 Mascia MP, Trudell JR, Harris RA. Specific binding sites for alcohols and anesthetics on ligand-gated ion channels. *Proc Natl Acad Sci USA* 2000; **97**: 9305–10.

3 Jenkins A, Greenblatt EP, Faulkner HJ, *et al*. Evidence for a common binding cavity for three general anesthetics within the GABAA receptor. *J Neurosci* 2001; **21**: RC136.

Key message

Inhaled anaesthetics make specific interactions with a small number of residues on two inhibitory neurotransmitter-activated ion channels.

Strengths

This study was the first to use site-directed mutagenesis to alter the anaesthetic pharmacology of an anaesthetic target protein. It inferred that the drug–receptor interaction was highly selective and as such, it presented extremely strong evidence against a non-specific theory of anaesthetic action. Finally, it was also a great example of the benefits of multi-laboratory collaborations.

Weaknesses

While abolishing the sensitivity of $GABA_A$ and glycine receptors to anaesthetics, this study did not show that an isoleucine-to-serine or tryptophan-to-alanine switch was able to confer anaesthetic sensitivity to the $GABA_C$ receptor.

Relevance

This paper demonstrates that general anaesthetic mechanisms are little different from any other pharmacological effect: specific drug–protein interactions occur that alter the normal function of the target protein and that these specific interactions can be disrupted with specific mutations. This paper spawned many other studies duplicating these findings in other subunits and extending the original finding to other parts of the subunits studies here. Subsequent studies also extended the original finding to predict the physical nature of the anaesthetic binding site. Perhaps of greatest importance, the methodology and findings of this paper were verified in a critical study by Jurd *et al*. (Paper 8) that revealed that critical point mutations, when incorporated into the genome of an animal, render it resistant to the effects of some general anaesthetics.

Paper 8: General anesthetic actions *in vivo* strongly attenuated by a point mutation in the GABA$_A$ receptor β3 subunit

Author details

R Jurd, M Arras, S Lambert, B Drexler, R Siegwart, F Crestani, M Zaugg, KE Vogt, B Ledermann, B Antkowiak, U Rudolph U

Reference

Federation of American Societies for Experimental Biology Journal 2003; **17**: 250–2.

Summary

This paper was the first to report the introduction of a point mutation into a mouse gene that subsequently altered the sensitivity of the animal to two intravenous general anaesthetics. It had previously been reported that β1 containing GABA$_A$ receptors had a reduced sensitivity to propofol and etomidate as compared to β2 and β3 containing receptors. It was subsequently shown that substitution of an asparagine for a methionine (at the position homologous to the conserved serine reported in Mihic *et al.*) reduced the effect of intravenous agents in β3 containing receptors. Armed with this knowledge, Jurd *et al.* targeted exon 8 of the mouse GABA$_A$R β3 gene, introducing a N265M mutation and a floxed neomycin resistance cassette. After neomycin selection, the cassette was removed by crossed breeding with a cre-mouse line, leaving an intronic LoxP site and the single mutant methionine codon. This mutation had only modest effect on the spatial expression of the β3 subunit and no obvious effect on the relative expression of other GABA$_A$R subunits. The mutant animals had normal motor activity and normal sensitivity to painful heat stimuli. However, the mutation dramatically reduced the loss of righting reflex time and virtually abolished the latency for the hindpaw withdrawal reflex for both propofol and etomidate. The mutant mice had become highly resistant to the anaesthetic actions of two intravenous anaesthetics. Strikingly, this was not the case for the steroid anaesthetic alphaxalone, which is thought to act elsewhere on the GABA$_A$ receptor.

Citation count

317.

Related references

1 Zeller A, Arras M, Jurd R, *et al.* Mapping the contribution of beta3-containing GABA$_A$ receptors to volatile and intravenous general anesthetic actions. *BMC Pharmacol* 2007; **7**: 2.

Key message

In mice, propofol and etomidate make specific interactions with a residue in the GABA$_A$ β3 subunit. This leads to the general anaesthetic effect of these two drugs. When this residue is replaced with another, the receptor loses its anaesthetic binding site and the drugs can no longer anaesthetize the mutant animal.

Strengths

This paper successfully links the molecular events that occur within the general anaesthetic binding sites in the GABA$_A$ receptor, to the simultaneous effects in the intact animal. This paper verifies the importance and relevance of *in vitro* experiments and underscores just how selective general anaesthetics are in their interactions with neuronal proteins.

Weaknesses

Subsequent studies have shown that the mutation results in subtle changes in receptor expression and gating. Mutant animals can compensate for these effects. Therefore, the results are not as clean as may appear at first glance. However, these small effects should not detract from what is a highly impressive experiment; an anaesthetic insensitive animal was produced.

Relevance

This paper demonstrates the critical role the $GABA_AR$ β subunit has in defining the anaesthetized state. By better understanding the temporal and spatial expression of the different $GABA_AR$ subunits in the brain, we will certainly gain a better understanding of how these molecular events integrate to alter pain sensation, awareness and consciousness.

Paper 9: The sedative component of anesthesia is mediated by GABA$_A$ receptors in an endogenous sleep pathway

Author details

LE Nelson, TZ Guo, J Lu, CB Saper, NP Franks, M Maze

Reference

Nature Neuroscience 2002; **5**: 979–84.

Abstract

We investigated the role of regionally discrete GABA (gamma-aminobutyric acid) receptors in the sedative response to pharmacological agents that act on GABA$_A$ receptors (muscimol, propofol and pentobarbital; 'GABAergic agents') and to ketamine, a general anaesthetic that does not affect GABA$_A$ receptors. Behavioral studies in rats showed that the sedative response to centrally administered GABAergic agents was attenuated by the GABA$_A$ receptor antagonist gabazine (systemically administered). The sedative response to ketamine, by contrast, was unaffected by gabazine. Using c-Fos as a marker of neuronal activation, we identified a possible role for the tuberomammillary nucleus (TMN): when gabazine was microinjected directly into the TMN, it attenuated the sedative response to GABAergic agents. Furthermore, the GABA$_A$ receptor agonist muscimol produced a dose-dependent sedation when it was administered into the TMN. We conclude that the TMN is a discrete neural locus that has a key role in the sedative response to GABAergic anaesthetics.

Summary

The authors induced loss of righting reflex in rats via intracerebroventricular injection of the GABA agonist muscimol, two GABAergic anaesthetics (propofol and pentobarbital) and an NMDAergic anaesthetic ketamine. They successfully attenuated the effect of the three GABAergic compounds with a subcutaneous injection of the GABA antagonist gabazine, but not ketamine. Using c-Fos expression as a marker for neurones that had recently been active, they showed that the GABAergic agents simultaneously increased activity in the ventrolateral preoptic nucleus and decreased activity in the TMN, two brain regions critical for determining wakefulness. Finally, discrete injection of the antagonist gabazine into the TMN reduced the sedative actions of propofol and pentobarbital.

Citation count

280.

Related references

1 Zecharia AY, Nelson LE, Gent TC, *et al.* The involvement of hypothalamic sleep pathways in general anesthesia: testing the hypothesis using the GABAA receptor beta3N265M knock-in mouse. *J Neurosci* 2009; **29**: 2177–87.

Key message

General anaesthetics produce sedation by enhancing the function of $GABA_A$ receptors located in a small nucleus of the sleep-arousal system. While the action of almost all $GABA_A$ receptors are enhanced during anaesthesia, contributing to immobility, amnesia and antinociception, it is the effects in the TMN that cause patients to 'go to sleep' during anaesthesia.

Strengths

The authors used complementary techniques to pinpoint the sedative effects of anaesthetics on a small region of the brain. They demonstrate that the different components of anaesthesia are readily separable.

Weaknesses

The therapeutics used here are not purely GABAergic and do have effects on other ion channels and receptors at clinically relevant concentrations. Also, it is technically almost impossible to prevent spread of drug to surrounding brain areas.

Relevance

This paper explains how during normal wakefulness, the ventrolateral preoptic nucleus is held inactive by noradrenergic input from the locus coeruleus. This means that the ventrolateral preoptic nucleus is unable to release GABA into the TMN, its target nucleus. Therefore during wakefulness, the TMN does not receive GABAergic inhibition from the ventrolateral preoptic nucleus and continues its function of releasing stimulating histamine into the cortex. During the induction of anaesthesia, inhibition of the locus coeruleus allows the ventrolateral preoptic nucleus to become active, inhibiting the effect of the TMN on the cortex, resulting in a non-REM sleeplike state.

This paper shows that anaesthesia is not a non-specific or generalized effect on the whole nervous system or an emergent property of global modulation. General anaesthetics are selective for different receptors at the molecular level. Different brain nuclei express differing arrays of receptors, and are, therefore, differentially modulated by anaesthetic drugs. This observation, coupled with the different ways in which these nuclei are electrically coupled, mean that during anaesthesia, some nuclei are silent, while others are critically active.

Paper 10: Disruption of synchronous gamma oscillations in the rat hippocampal slice: a common mechanism of anaesthetic drug action

Author details

HJ Faulkner, RD Traub, MA Whittington

Reference

British Journal of Pharmacology 1998; **125**: 483–92.

Summary

The authors took slices of rat hippocampus and maintained them under physiological conditions in the lab. They electrically excited each slice at two different positions, in the *stratum oriens* at either end of the CA1 region. After the stimulation was complete, the authors would 'listen' to the electrical activity of two groups of neurones in the *stratum pyrimidale*. Due to the innate connectivity and biophysical properties of the slice, the incoming excitation, or information, causes the two groups of neurones to oscillate together, mirroring each other's activity. More specifically, the neurones in the two areas reciprocally inhibit each other, via a GABAergic mechanism, allowing incoming signals to entrain activity at both sites. At high frequencies, this kind of brain connectivity has been shown to be involved in controlling awareness and cognition. The authors repeated these measurements in the presence of three different sedatives: thiopental, diazepam, and morphine (five different concentrations of each). What the authors were able to show was that with thiopental, the ability of the two brain areas to oscillate or work together simply collapsed when the concentration of anaesthetic was at or above the concentration needed to maintain general anaesthesia. Perhaps paradoxically, diazepam which also acts at the $GABA_A$ receptor, albeit via quite a different mechanism, did not collapse the reciprocal or synchronous activity. Morphine had a more complex group of behaviours. Computer models of electrical activity in this brain region predicted that this kind of effect could only occur if the drug was simultaneously enhancing synaptic inhibition and increasing a low level and constant generalized inhibition in the two areas.

Citation count

84.

Related references

1 Sebel PS, Lang E, Rampil IJ, *et al.* A multicenter study of bispectral electroencephalogram analysis for monitoring anesthetic effect. *Anesth Analg* 1997; **84**: 891–9.

Key message

Normal brain function is dependent on finely tuned circuits functioning together, constantly handshaking information from one region to another. Much as you would find with a radio set tuned into a specific radio station, different brain regions and patterns of information are tuned to one another for optimal function. An essential component in the timing or tuning of these circuits is the $GABA_A$ receptor. Anaesthetics that alter the strength or duration of inhibition at these receptors cause the circuits to no longer be in tune. The result is that information can now no longer pass freely and optimally through the brain.

Strengths

This was the first paper to emphasize the importance of anaesthetics acting at synapses and at other inhibitory sites in the nervous system. This was only possible through the gathering of data using a very difficult electrophysiological preparation and the use of extremely powerful numerical modelling techniques. In this case, the total is very much greater than the sum of the parts. This complex study successfully integrated the two methods to take our understanding of anaesthetic pharmacology out of the test tube and into specific brain regions.

Weaknesses

Synchronicity in other bands of frequencies are also important for controlling wakefulness and these were not studied here. The results would have been even more striking had the authors used more selective agents such as etomidate (purely GABAergic) and ketamine (predominantly NMDAergic). As it stands, thiopental is rather a 'dirty' drug, and modulates the function of several ion channels.

Relevance

When this study was published, reductionist studies, such as those described in this chapter, had clearly demonstrated that $GABA_A$ receptors were sensitive to clinically relevant concentrations of anaesthetics. However, no one had truly bridged the gap between a molecular mechanism, and the integrated effects of anaesthetics in the neurocircuitry of the brain. The authors of this paper successfully transcended this knowledge gap, demonstrating that as the concentration of the anaesthetic around hippocampal $GABA_A$ receptors reached the EC_{50} for anaesthesia, so the ability of the brain to transmit information from one place to another simply ceased.

Chapter 9

Local anaesthesia

HBJ Fischer

Introduction

Local anaesthesia covers a wide spectrum of anaesthetic practice, from local infiltration to central neuraxial and major peripheral nerve blockade and is used for surgical anaesthesia and a variety of pain management systems—acute postoperative and non-surgical pain, chronic pain, and palliative care.

Many major developments in local anaesthesia have been described in the last 30 years or so and the recent introduction of ultrasound guidance for some peripheral and central neuraxial blocks has resulted in a significant increase in its use. This is in marked contrast to the situation that prevailed between the 1950s and the 1970s when local anaesthesia was scarcely used in many countries. From its 'discovery' by Carl Koller in 1884 until the 1940s, local anaesthesia was seen as a safer and more effective alternative to the general anaesthetics of the era. However, its use declined as a result of improvements in the safety and effectiveness of general anaesthesia and concerns about the potential for serious neurological injury (especially with spinal anaesthesia).

Local anaesthesia is a practical skill—the ability to place the correct volume and concentration of drug close to the selected nerve structure(s) so as to maximize benefit and minimize risk. This is reflected in the published literature, in four main categories of publication.

1 Descriptions of original nerve block techniques.
2 A much larger body of work describing multiple modifications of the original techniques claiming a variety of benefits for the new technique—greater efficacy, improved safety, quicker onset, longer duration or any combination thereof.
3 Complications, side effects, and serious adverse outcomes.
4 Case series, observational studies, and randomized trials that produce a specific endpoint when compared to another local anaesthetic technique, general anaesthesia, or systemic analgesia.

Many claims have been made in support of the beneficial effects of local anaesthesia compared to general anaesthesia over the last 30 years, some of which have been confirmed. Other benefits, such as reduced mortality/morbidity and improved outcome from surgery are more difficult to confirm with evidence both in favour and against; as surgical and anaesthetic practice improve, the balance of risks and benefits of local anaesthesia continues to evolve. So what criteria are required for selection as a landmark paper?

The ten selected papers cover the progress of local anaesthesia from Koller's original description (Paper 1) up to the impact of ultrasound-guided regional anaesthesia (USGRA) (Papers 9 and 10) in approximately chronological order. The purist may say that local anaesthesia is limited to the use of local anaesthetic drugs, which cause reversible sodium channel blockade (Paper 4). However, the discovery of opioid receptors and their role in producing segmental analgesia at a spinal cord level has had a profound effect on the way in which we use regional techniques; Paper 5 is included for that reason. Otherwise, I have selected papers that have advanced our technical knowledge and changed our clinical practice (Papers 2, 3, and 6) and papers that attempt to interrogate the best of the published randomized controlled studies to provide evidence of the important benefits and risks of local anaesthesia (Papers 7 and 8).

Paper 1: Carl Koller (1857–1944) and the introduction of cocaine into anesthetic practice

Author details

JAW Wildsmith

Reference

Regional Anesthesia 1984; **9**: 161–4.

Summary

This Special Article was written to mark the centenary of the first published description of the local anaesthetic effects of cocaine. It summarizes the early animal experiments of its toxic and systemic effects and the clinical use of cocaine, as a cure for sore throats and treatment of morphine addiction. Carl Koller was a young trainee ophthalmologist, with a growing reputation for his research work, when he discovered the local anaesthetic effects of cocaine by instilling cocaine powder firstly into the eye of a guinea pig and then into his own eye. His hand-written preliminary communication was read out to a medical audience in Heidelberg on 15 September 1884, marking the scientific origins of local anaesthesia.

Citation count

5.

Related references

1 Brown DL, Fink BR. The history of neural blockade and pain management. In: Cousins MJ, Bridenbaugh PO (eds) *Neural blockade in clinical anesthesia and management of pain*, 3rd edn., pp. 3–27. Philadephia, PA: Lippincott-Raven, 1998.

2 Reutsch YA, Boni T, Borgeat A. From cocaine to ropivacaine: the history of local anaesthetic drugs. *Curr Top Med Chem* 2001; **1**: 175–82.

3 Grzybowski A. Cocaine and the eye: a historical overview. *Ophthalmologica* 2008; **222**: 296–301.

Key message

Cocaine was already familiar to physicians in the 19th century and its ability to produce localized numbness was understood. Koller was 26 years old when he recognized the clinical implications of what others had missed and changed the course of anaesthesia.

Strengths

This is a very readable account of Koller's discovery, drawing on published work of the time and other material. Its strength lies in the author's access to private memorabilia loaned to him by Koller's daughter, Hortense Becker, which gives a unique insight into this remarkable man.

Weaknesses

There is controversy concerning Koller's role as the first person to use cocaine for local anaesthesia. As a derivative of erythroxylum coca, a plant endemic to South America and widely used by the indigenous peoples, claims have been made of cocaine being used clinically on that continent before Koller's description. To date, however, there is no published literature to support the use of cocaine as a local anaesthetic for surgery prior to 1884.

Relevance

While cocaine has gained a notorious reputation in recent years as a highly addictive drug of abuse, it has paved the way for many advances in anaesthesia and surgery. This paper describes the introduction of the first local anaesthetic drug and also gives an insight into the medico-political world of 19th century Europe; why a colleague presented Koller's work to the world rather than Koller himself, the speed with which cocaine entered clinical use throughout Europe and North America, and why Koller was forced to leave Vienna (challenging a colleague to a duel might have had something to do with it!).

Paper 2: The subclavian perivascular technique of brachial plexus anesthesia

Author details
AP Winnie, VJ Collins

Reference
Anesthesiology 1964; **25**: 353–63.

Summary
Anatomical and radio-opaque contrast studies demonstrate the continuity of the perivascular brachial plexus sheath from its origins on the transverse processes of the cervical vertebrae to the mid-humeral area. The injection technique is described in detail and the sensory and motor effects of injecting different volumes (50 and 25 ml) of local anaesthetic at the axillary and subclavian perivascular levels are compared. A success rate of 98% is recorded using paraesthesia, compared to 88% when no paraesthesiae are elicited.

Citation count
189.

Related references
1 Neal JM, Gerancher JC, Hebl JR, *et al.* Upper extremity regional anesthesia: essentials of our current understanding, 2008. *Reg Anesth Pain Med* 2009; **34**: 134–70.

Key message
Understanding the anatomical relations of the brachial plexus sheath makes it possible to predict the extent of the sensory and motor block and the success rate of the block, depending on the site of injection and volume of local anaesthetic injected.

Strengths
Using anatomical dissection and X-ray contrast studies, this paper rejects the accepted wisdom of the time, with regard to supraclavicular brachial plexus blocks, and describes a more logical approach to the plexus. It sets the benchmark for future research and developments in upper limb peripheral nerve blockade.

Weaknesses
Although the basic principles of the perivascular sheath concept remain true, subsequent research has refined our knowledge and rendered some of Winnie's findings redundant. Multiple neuro-stimulation/injection techniques and ultrasound guidance, using smaller volume injections have replaced large volume, single injections with paresthesiae/fascial clicks. Few clinicians would now wish to produce interscalene blockade via the axillary route.

Relevance

Although published over 40 years ago, this paper sets the standard for modern regional anaesthetic practice—the use of imaging techniques to complement anatomical knowledge, informative diagrams, illustrated technique instructions, data collection in a comparative study, and assessment of potential complications. It even mentions the ease of perineural catheter insertion as an aside, long before they became a routine part of regional anaesthesia practice.

Paper 3: The Psoas compartment block

Author details

D Chayen, H Nathan, M Chayen

Reference

Anesthesiology 1976; **45**: 95–9.

Summary

The anatomy of the lumbar plexus and surrounding muscles is described in detail; in particular, between the fourth and fifth lumbar transverse processes, the five nerves supplying the proximal part of the lower limb are close together in an area, the authors term the psoas compartment. They study the best technique for needle insertion in 60 cadavers, including X-ray contrast studies and describe a clinical trial of 100 patients undergoing a variety of lower limb surgical procedures.

Citation count

202.

Related references

1 Winnie AP, Ramamurthy S, Durrani Z. The inguinal paravascular technic of lumbar plexus anesthesia. "The 3 in 1 block". *Anesth Analg* 1973; **52**: 989–96.

2 Farny J, Drolet P, Girard M. Anatomy of the posterior approach to the lumbar plexus block. *Can J Anesth* 1994; **41**: 480–5.

3 Capdevila X, Macaire P, Dadure C, *et al*. Continuous psoas compartment block for postoperative analgesia after total hip arthroplasty: new landmarks, technical guidelines and clinical evaluation. *Anesth Analg* 2002, **94**: 1606–13.

4 Fischer HB, Simanski CJ. A procedure-specific systematic review and consensus recommendations for analgesia after total hip replacement. *Anaesthesia* 2005; **60**: 1189–202.

Key message

An injection of 30 ml of local anaesthetic into the psoas compartment, situated between the quadratus lumborum and the psoas major muscles at the interspace of the fourth and fifth lumbar transverse processes, provides regional analgesia of the thigh and may be used in combination with a sciatic nerve block for more extensive blockade of the lower limb.

Strengths

A new peripheral nerve block technique is developed from a detailed anatomical examination of the origins and distribution of the lumbar plexus and its relations with the surrounding muscles and bony structures. The clinical study of 100 patients achieves a 90% success rate and the failures are analysed in some detail; two complications are noted.

Weaknesses

The technique described depends on the loss of resistance to air to indicate entry into the psoas compartment – a technique few, if any, would now still use. The space identified is intermuscular (between psoas and quadratus lumborum) and the terminal nerves of the plexus have already left the psoas muscle. Injecting into this space may allow the local anaesthetic to diffuse towards the paravertebral space, so the site of nerve block may not be limited to the psoas compartment. Details of the clinical study are sketchy; the local anaesthetic(s) used and their concentrations are lacking and there is no data regarding the assessment of sensory or motor block.

Relevance

This is possibly the last completely original description of a major peripheral nerve block published. Although its use was not widespread initially, it has become the standard peripheral nerve block for total hip replacement postoperative analgesia. New imaging technology (ultrasound, magnetic resonance imaging, computed tomography) has refined our understanding of the anatomy and given rise to alternative terminology for the block (psoas sheath, posterior lumbar plexus). Many modifications of the landmarks and endpoints have been described to improve success rates and minimize complications but the original concept remains intact—the ability to provide widespread lumbosacral analgesia of the proximal lower limb with a single peripheral nerve injection.

Paper 4: Molecular mechanisms of local anesthesia: a review

Author details
JF Butterworth IV, GR Strichartz

Reference
Anesthesiology 1990; **72**: 711–34.

Summary
Local anaesthetics reversibly block neuronal impulses by inhibition of voltage gated Na^+ channels. This inhibition affects the conformational changes that occur in the structure of the Na^+ channel during the activation process—the transformation of the channel from the closed resting state to the open conducting state. These changes account for almost all the inhibition; physical occlusion of the channel by the LA molecule contributes little to the prevention of conduction. The specific site of LA binding with the Na^+ channel is most likely to be within the protein subunits of the channel wall; LAs enter the membrane and reversibly bind with the receptor, according to their structure and physico-chemical properties. The affinity of LAs for the Na^+ channel receptor increases with the frequency of nerve stimulation—'phasic block'. Tonic block is the term for low frequency (<0.5 Hz) block.

Citation count
583.

Related references
1 Marban E, Yamagishi T, Tomaselli GF. Structure and function of voltage gated sodium channels. *J Physiol* 1998; **503**: 647–57.

2 Lipkind GM, Fozzard HA. Molecular modeling of local anesthetic drug binding by voltage-gated sodium channels. *Mol Pharmacol* 2005; **68**: 1611–22.

3 Strichartz GR. Novel ideas of local anaesthetic actions on various ion channels to ameliorate postoperative pain. *Br J Anaesth* 2008; **101**: 45–7.

Key message
Local anaesthetic drugs act on the protein subunits of Na^+ channels by inhibiting conformational change, probably by molecular electrostatic charge; the speed of onset, intensity of the block, and duration are governed by the physico-chemical properties of the drug and the frequency of nerve stimulation.

Strengths
The model proposed in this review is speculative but offers an alternative and credible explanation for the mechanism of action of LAs compared to the previously held view that they worked by open channel blocking on a mechanical basis. New information about the structure and function of the Na^+ and other ion voltage-gated channels has become available but the model of LA action proposed in this review remains valid and is a cornerstone of our understanding of how local anaesthetics work.

Weaknesses

The science of how local anaesthetics react with Na^+ channels is derived from isolated cells and tissues and although the hypothesis withstands critical analysis, it remains largely theoretical. Whether all the clinical actions of local anaesthetics can be explained by this mechanism remains speculative at the present time. In particular, a short infusion of lidocaine, only sufficient to produce a low plasma concentration, is known to produce a sustained, clinically significant, period of analgesia in some chronic pain conditions. The kinetics of lidocaine Na^+ channel blockade are not enough to fully explain the mode of action, so further research is needed.

Relevance

Understanding how local anaesthetic drugs produce their clinical benefits and their toxic side effects is fundamental to the way in which we use them safely and effectively. The basic sciences of molecular chemistry, pharmacology and neurophysiology can be difficult to understand but this paper manages to distil all the important basic scientific principles into a clinically important context, which nearly 20 years on, still remains relevant.

Paper 5: The rational use of intrathecal and extradural opioids

Author details

M Morgan

Reference

British Journal of Anaesthesia 1989; **63**: 165–88.

Summary

This review examines the impact of intrathecal and extradural opioids on clinical practice in the decade following their introduction. The author poses five key questions as a basis to interrogate the published data.

1 Could the use of spinal opioids deliver the advantages predicted by the laboratory research?

2 What comparative data were there for the opioids available?

3 What were the merits of the extradural compared with the intrathecal route of administration?

4 What data were there to compare spinal opioids with other methods of analgesia?

5 What were the nature, incidence and severity of the complications of spinal opioids?

   This review achieves those objectives and makes recommendations for the more rational use of spinal opioids.

Citation count

181.

Related references

1 Yaksh TL and Rudy TA. Analgesia mediated by a direct spinal action of narcotics. *Science* 1976; **192**: 1357–8.

2 Cousins MJ, Mather LE. Intrathecal and epidural administration of opioids. *Anesthesiology* 1984; **61**: 276–310.

Key message

The main conclusions are: (1) lipophilic opioids are a more logical choice for spinal use than morphine because of the greater incidence of complications seen with morphine, (2) a fixed dose of spinal opioids provides adequate analgesia for the majority of patients, (3) intrathecal administration is a more logical choice than epidural but the greater risk of complications and the difficulties of repeat administration make the epidural route the more practical option, (4) close observation of the patient for at least 24 h is necessary to avoid the potential for delayed respiratory depression, especially if morphine is used.

Strengths

This is an authoritative account of the first decade of clinical use of neuraxial opioids. Initial reports of human use caused considerable excitement and led to a rapid growth in research publications and routine clinical use. By today's standards, the clinical research and clinical application might be judged to be uncontrolled and haphazard. This review restores objectivity and caution to counterbalance the initial enthusiasm and provides a scientific basis for future research and the development of clinical guidelines for safer, more effective use.

Weaknesses

Since its publication there have been major developments in the use of spinal opioids, some of which could have been foreseen in the article. The combination of opioids with low concentrations of local anaesthetic was already widespread at that time and would merit some discussion. Many of the opioids studied in this review are no longer in widespread use and therefore some may feel that the review is of largely historical interest.

Relevance

The discovery of opioid receptors in the brain and spinal cord in a variety of animal models during the 1970s led to a rapid translation of laboratory work into clinical practice. The introduction of central neuraxial opioids transformed the way in which local anaesthetic spinal and epidural techniques would be used in future. Studies of small groups of terminally ill cancer patients confirmed that the bolus administration of morphine via the epidural and spinal routes provided effective pain relief at a spinal cord level. Soon, central neuraxial opioids were being used to treat postoperative pain and for labour and obstetric surgery. Chronic pain and palliative care also saw a rapid growth in their use. The speed at which laboratory research was applied in the clinical setting was remarkable—'never before had sophisticated laboratory research moved so rapidly into the clinical field', and probably will not do so again. The reason being that both the drugs and the injection techniques were already familiar to anaesthetists—it was only the combination of both that was novel.

Paper 6: A prospective, randomised comparison of preoperative and continuous balanced epidural or paravertebral bupivacaine on post-thoracotomy pain, pulmonary function and stress responses

Author details

J Richardson, S Sabanathan, J Jones, RD Shah, S Cheema, AJ Mearns

Reference

British Journal of Anaesthesia 1999; **83**: 387–92.

Abstract

Both epidural and paravertebral blocks are effective in controlling post-thoractomy pain, but comparison of preoperative and balanced techniques, measuring pulmonary function and stress responses, has not been undertaken previously. We studied 100 adult patients, premedicated with morphine and diclofenac, allocated randomly to receive thoracic epidural bupivacaine or thoracic paravertebral bupivacaine as preoperative bolus doses followed by continuous infusions. All patients also received diclofenac and patient-controlled morphine. Significantly lower visual analogue pain scores at rest and on coughing were found in the paravertebral group and patient-controlled morphine requirements were less. Pulmonary function was significantly better preserved in the paravertebral group who has higher oxygen saturations and less postoperative morbidity. There was a significant increase in plasma concentrations of cortisol from baselines in both the epidural and paravertebral groups and in plasma glucose in the epidural group, but no significant change from baseline in plasma glucose in the paravertebral group. Areas under the plasma concentration vs time curves for cortisol and glucose were significantly lower in the paravertebral group. Side effects, especially nausea, vomiting and hypotension, were troublesome only in the epidural group. We conclude that with these regimens, paravertebral block was superior to epidural bupivacaine.

Summary

Thoracic epidural and thoracic paravertebral infusions of local anaesthetic are effective at controlling post-thoractomy pain. This study also looks at the influence of each technique on respiratory function and the stress response to surgery, within the context of a perioperative, multimodal analgesia regimen. Boluses of bupivacaine were administered prior to induction of anaesthesia and infusions commenced postoperatively and continued for 5 days. The paravertebral group showed lower pain scores, less rescue analgesia requirements, better preservation of pulmonary function, lower neuroendocrine stress response, and fewer side effects.

Citation count

177.

Related references

1 Davies RG, Myles PS, Graham JM. A comparison of the analgesia efficacy and side-effects of paravertebral vs epidural blockade for thoracotomy – a systematic review and meta-analysis of randomised trials. *Br J Anesth* 2006; **96**: 418–26.

2 Joshi GP, Bonnet F, Shah R, *et al.* A systematic review of randomised trials evaluating regional techniques for postthoracotomy analgesia. *Anesth Analg* 2008; **107**: 1026–40.

Key message

Thoracic paravertebral local anaesthetic infusions offer a quality of post-thoracotomy analgesia equivalent to, or better than thoracic epidural infusions. Paravertebral infusions also have a superior protective effect on postoperative pulmonary function and the surgical stress response and fewer postoperative side effects.

Strengths

This is a well-conducted, prospective randomized controlled trial comparing the two major regional analgesia techniques for thoracotomy. It is also one of the earliest studies to consider the importance of balanced analgesia within the perioperative pathway.

Weaknesses

The study avoided the use of local anaesthetic–opioid mixtures for logistical reasons, using intravenous patient-controlled analgesia morphine as rescue medication. The study also used different and relatively high concentrations of bupivacaine for the epidural (10–15-ml boluses of 0.25% bupivacaine and an infusion of 0.25% at $0.1\,\mathrm{ml\,kg^{-1}h^{-1}}$) and the paravertebral (20-ml bolus of 0.5% bupivacaine and an infusion of 0.5% at $0.1\,\mathrm{ml\,kg^{-1}h^{-1}}$), which may account for the relatively high rate of hypotension in the epidural group. There was a twofold difference between the groups for bupivacaine usage and although plasma bupivacaine levels were not measured, this may account for the higher number of confused patients in the paravertebral group.

Relevance

Current practice with epidural infusions is to use a combination of low concentration local anaesthetic with an opioid, with a recommended maximum duration of up to 72 h. Similarly, paravertebral infusions now comprise lower concentrations of local anaesthetic, even without an added opioid. So there are differences between this study and current practice. Nevertheless, the results of the study are important and have been borne out by subsequent studies and systematic reviews and this remains an important contribution to our knowledge on paravertebral and epidural analgesia.

Paper 7: Reduction of postoperative mortality and morbidity with epidural or spinal anaesthesia: results from overview of randomised trials

Author details

A Rodgers, N Walker, S Schug, A McKee, H Kehlet, A van Zundert, D Sage, M Futter, G Saville, T Clark, S MacMahon

Reference

British Medical Journal 2000; **321**: 1–12.

Abstract

Objectives: To obtain reliable estimates of the effects of neuraxial blockade with epidural or spinal anaesthesia on postoperative morbidity and mortality.

Design: Systematic review of all trials with randomisation to intraoperative neuraxial blockade or not.

Studies: 141 trials including 9559 patients for which data were available before 1 January 1997. Trials were eligible irrespective of their primary aims, concomitant use of general anaesthesia, publication status, or language. Trials were identified by extensive search methods and substantial amounts of data were obtained or confirmed by correspondence with trialists.

Main outcome measures: All cause mortality, deep vein thrombosis, pulmonary embolus, myocardial infarction, transfusion requirements, pneumonia, other infections, respiratory depression, and renal failure.

Results: Overall mortality was reduced by about a third in patients allocated to neuraxial blockade (103 deaths /4871 patients versus 144/4688 patients, odds ratio = 0.70, confidence interval 0.54 to 0.90, P= 0.0006). Neuraxial blockade reduced the odds of deep vein thrombosis by 44%, pulmonary embolism by 55%, transfusion requirements by 50%, pneumonia by 39% and respiratory depression by 59% (all $P<0.0001$). There were also reductions in myocardial infarction and renal failure. Although there was limited power to assess subgroup effects, the proportional reductions in mortality did not clearly differ by surgical group, type of blockade (epidural or spinal), or in those trials in which neuraxial blockade was combined with general anaesthesia compared with trials in which neuraxial blockade was used alone.

Conclusion: Neuraxial blockade reduces postoperative mortality and other serious complications. The size of some of these benefits remains uncertain and further research is required to determine whether these effects are due solely to benefits of neuraxial blockade or partly to the avoidance of general anaesthesia. Nevertheless, these findings support more widespread use of neuraxial blockade.

Summary

This is the first systematic review of the beneficial effects of central neuraxial blockade on outcome from surgery, as measured by the relative risk reduction in eight major causes of postoperative morbidity and mortality. Over 9,500 patients in 141 trials are included in the study. Meta-analysis reveals a reduction in the risk of all-cause mortality of about one-third with reductions in risk for the individual major causes of morbidity and mortality ranging from 59% reduction (respiratory depression) to 39% (pneumonia). Smaller reductions in the risk of postoperative myocardial infarction and renal failure were also noted. Central neuraxial blockade, either as the sole anaesthetic technique or in combination with general anaesthesia, offered a significant reduction in mortality and morbidity compared to matched patient groups who received only a general anaesthetic.

Citation count

1229.

Related references

1 Yeager MP, Glass DD, Neff RK, *et al*. Epidural anesthesia and analgesia in high-risk surgical patients. *Anesthesiology* 1987; **66**: 729–36.

2 Ballantyne JC, Carr DB, deFerranti S, *et al*. The comparative effects of postoperative analgesic therapies on pulmonary outcome: cumulative meta-analyses of randomized, controlled trials. *Anesth Analg* 1998; **86**: 598–612.

3 Beattie WS, Badner NH, Choi P. Epidural analgesia reduces postoperative myocardial infarction: a meta-analysis. *Anesth Analg* 2001; **93**: 853–8.

Key message

Central neuraxial blockade offers a significant reduction in the risk of postoperative all-cause mortality and in the risks of individual causes of morbidity. Reduction in mortality did not differ by surgical subgroup, the type of blockade used or in trials where the regional technique was used as the sole technique compared to in combination with a general anaesthetic.

Strengths

The large number of studies and patients included in the review represent a substantial database to interrogate and the headline findings are impressive. This study caused a great deal of interest from both medical professionals and the general public when it was published. Whether used as the sole anaesthetic technique, or in combination with a general anaesthetic technique, spinal and epidural blockade appear to confer a protective benefit to patients undergoing major surgery, compared to patients who receive only a general anaesthetic.

Weaknesses

The paper was criticized on a number of grounds soon after its publication, particularly when subsequent large randomized studies failed to confirm its findings. Some of the problems are inherent meta-analytical weaknesses; failure to control publication bias and heterogeneity, the inclusion of data from studies of outmoded surgical and anaesthetic practice. Changing practice, in particular the routine use of thromboprophylaxis and the introduction of new anaesthetic and surgical practices, has also reduced the risks to patients whether general anaesthesia or regional anaesthesia is used. Subgroup meta-analysis highlighted specific mortality reduction in surgery for fractured hip surgery and vascular surgery but these studies were small, had high mortality and mainly pre-dated later improvements in perioperative care for these high risk patient groups.

Relevance

This paper was the first (and remains the largest) systematic review to examine the influence of regional anaesthesia on postoperative morbidity and mortality. Despite the limitations of the paper, it stands out as a landmark paper; it has a strong message, has encouraged others to confirm or refute its data, and has stimulated research into how outcome from surgery can be influenced by improvements in preoperative assessment, changes in anaesthetic and surgical practice, and better postoperative care and rehabilitation.

Paper 8: Major complications of central neuraxial block: report on the third National Audit Project of the Royal College of Anaesthetists

Author details

TM Cook, D Counsell, JAW Wildsmith

Reference

British Journal of Anaesthesia 2009; **102**: 179–90.

Abstract

Background: Serious complications of central neuraxial block (CNB) are rare. Limited information on their incidence and impact impedes clinical decision-making and patient consent. The Royal College of Anaesthetists Third National Audit Project was designed to inform this situation.

Methods: A 2 week national census estimated the number of CNB procedures performed annually in the UK National Health Service. All major complications of CNBs performed over 1 yr (vertebral canal abscess or haematoma, meningitis, nerve injury, spinal cord ischaemia, fatal cardio-vascular collapse, and wrong route errors) were reported. Each case was reviewed by an expert panel to assess causation, severity, and outcome. 'Permanent' injury was defined as symptoms persisting for more than 6 months. Efforts were made to validate denominator (procedures performed) and numerator (complications) data through national databases.

Results: The census phase produced a denominator of 707, 455 CNB. Eighty-four major complications were reported, of which 52 met the inclusion criteria at the time they were reported. Data were interpreted 'pessimistically' and 'optimistically'. 'Pessimistically' there were 30 permanent injuries and 'optimistically' 14. The incidence of permanent injury due to CNB (expressed per 100 000 cases) was 'pessimistically' 4.2 (95% confidence interval 2.9–6.1) and 'optimistically' 2.0 (1.1–3.3). 'Pessimistically' there were 13 deaths or paraplegias, 'optimistically' five. The incidence of paraplegia or death was 'pessimistically' 1.8 per 100 000 (1.0–3.1) and 'optimistically' 0.7 (0–1.6). Two-thirds of initially disabling injuries resolved fully.

Conclusions: The data are reassuring and suggest that CNB has a low incidence of major complications, many of which resolve within 6 months.

Summary

The prospective national audit establishes, as accurately as possible, the number and incidence of serious complications of CNB in the UK. The 2-week national census produced a denominator of 707,455 central neuraxial blocks and 84 serious complications were notified during the 12-month reporting period. Fifty-two cases met the criteria for inclusion in the study, giving an overall incidence of between 2.0 (optimistically) and 4.2 (pessimistically) per 100,000. Deaths and paraplegia directly related to CNB were between 0.7 and 1.8 per 100,000. Two-thirds of the patients who had disabling injuries recovered during the study period and follow-up period. The data for the UK are reassuring and the risks of serious adverse events associated with CNB are as good as, or better than those reported in other major studies.

Citation count

121.

Related references

1 Aromaa U, Lahdensuu M, Cozanitis DA. Severe complication associated with epidural and spinal anaesthesia in Finland 1987-1993. A study based on patient insurance claims. *Acta Anaesthesiol Scand* 1997; **41**: 445–52.

2 Auroy Y, Benhamou D, Bargues L, *et al.* Major complications of regional anaesthesia in france; the SOS regional anesthesia hotline service. *Anesthesiology* 2002; **97**: 1274–80.

3 Moen V, Dahlgren N, Irestedt L. Severe Neurological Complications after Central Neuraxial Blockades in Sweden 1990-1999. *Anesthesiology* 2004; **101**: 950–9.

Key message

The National Audit Project provides an accurate estimate of how many spinals, epidurals, and caudals are performed per year in the UK. More importantly, we also have a record of both the absolute numbers and the incidence of serious adverse events associated with central neuraxial blockade. The incidence is similar to, or better than, the published findings of other large retrospective studies and allows anaesthetists to have confidence in the estimates of risk when discussing central neuraxial blocks with patients. The greatest risks are associated with perioperative epidural infusions, especially in the elderly undergoing major cancer surgery. The rates of complication for obstetrics, paediatrics, and chronic pain are extremely low.

Strengths

The project achieved a high response rate for the census period (100% with 92% accuracy of data gathering) and detailed reporting and follow-up of all the cases included in the final analysis. Analysing the causal relationship between CNB and any serious adverse event is complex; this is taken into account by the study methodology, resulting in the use of the optimistic and pessimistic range of incidences. The results were validated against any data held by external bodies and large retrospective studies in Sweden and Finland.

Weaknesses

In any voluntary reporting system the data are subject to both clinical and statistical uncertainty. The clinical case reports are subject to variation in the amount of detail supplied by the referring hospital and the progress and ultimate outcome of every case is not always certain before the end of the study. In some cases the relationship between the CNB and any adverse event may be casual rather than causal. Statistical accuracy is also difficult to guarantee in any study of rare events especially where zero or very few numerators are reported in some subgroups. These uncertainties are discussed in some detail in the paper and the authors are reassured by the narrow confidence intervals for the major determinants of injury.

Relevance

This is the largest prospective study of the major risks of CNB. The data is robust and specific for both the main CNB techniques and the major clinical specialties. Any discussion with patients about the risks and benefits of CNB can now be undertaken with more confidence. The data also helps inform medico-legal and clinical governance discussions in a more objective way than was previously possible.

Paper 9: Ultrasonographic guidance improves sensory block and onset time of three in one blocks

Author details

P Marhofer, K Schrogendorfer, H Koinig, S Kapral, C Weinstabl, N Nayer

Reference

Anesthesia and Analgesia 1997; **85**: 854–7.

Summary

Two groups of 20 patients were prospectively randomized to receive a 3-in-1 block for preoperative analgesia for fractured hip repair using either US or NS to locate the femoral nerve. The US group showed reduced onset time, improved quality of sensory block and a lower risk of adverse incidents, compared to the NS group. Failure rates were not different between the groups.

Citation count

285.

Related references

1 Marhofer P, Schrogendorfer K, Wallner T, *et al.* Ultrasonographic guidance reduces the amount of local anaesthetic for 3 in 1 blocks. *Reg Anesth Pain Med* 1998; **23**: 584–8.

2 Domingo-Triado V, Selfa S, Martinez F, *et al.* Ultrasound guidance for lateral midfemoral sciatic nerve block: a prospective, comparative, randomized study. *Anesth Analg* 2007; **104**: 1270–4.

Key message

Ultrasound-guided nerve location provides quicker onset and better quality sensory blockade of the femoral, obturator, and lateral cutaneous nerve of the thigh compared to a peripheral nerve stimulator technique.

Strengths

This is an early randomized controlled trial comparing NS and US when used to identify the femoral nerve. Onset of sensory blockade is plotted separately for each nerve, allowing assessment of both individual and overall block failure rates. The incidence of complete failure and 2-in-1 blocks was not significant between the groups but the overall success rate was in favour of US.

Weaknesses

There is no detail about the randomization or blinding methods and no assessment of the onset time, intensity and duration of motor blockade. There was a failure to visualize the femoral nerve in three out of the 20 patients in the US group but no difference in failed blocks between the groups.

Relevance

This is one of the earliest randomized controlled trials in which ultrasound is compared against the standard nerve location technology. This paper marks an important point in the evolution of ultrasound-guided regional anaesthesia (USGRA)—the move from enthusiastic acceptance of a new technology to objective comparison with the accepted standard of the day.

Paper 10: Ultrasound-guided regional anesthesia and analgesia, a qualitative systematic review

Author details

SS Liu, JE Ngeow, JT YaDeau

Reference

Regional Anesthesia and Pain Medicine 2009; **34**: 47–59.

Summary

As with all new medical technologies, it is important to examine the evidence of any superior risk/benefits for ultrasound guided regional anaesthesia (USGRA) compared to existing nerve location technology. The review examines the data for upper limb nerve blocks, lower limb blocks, and epidural (pre-puncture scanning only). The study concludes that USGRA reduces block performance time, with fewer needle passes and patient discomfort and reduces block onset time, compared to peripheral nerve stimulator techniques, for upper and lower limb blocks. There is no difference in block success rates in terms of quality of surgical anaesthesia or conversion to general anaesthesia rates. Due to the rarity of serious adverse events, it is not possible to show any advantage in favour of USGRA for toxic systemic reactions or nerve injury.

Citation count

69.

Related references

1 Koscielniak-Nielsen ZJ. Ultrasound-guided peripheral nerve blocks: what are the benefits? *Acta Anaesthesiologica Scand* 2008; **52**: 727–37.

2 Walker KJ, McGrattan K, Aas-Eng K, *et al*. Ultrasound guidance for peripheral nerve blockade (Review). *Cochrane Database Syst Rev* 2009; **4**: CD006459.

Key message

USGRA is an important development in regional anaesthesia. For peripheral nerve blocks, USGRA significantly reduces the time to perform blocks and reduces the number of needle passes required to locate the nerve. It also reduces the onset time for sensory block in some studies. USGRA has a more limited role in improving the performance of central neuraxial blocks, particularly for obstetric epidural analgesia.

Strengths

Only RCTs and large prospective case series (>100 patients) are analysed, thus avoiding possible publication bias from observational studies, retrospective comparative studies, and small case series.

Weaknesses

The RCTs showed inconsistency in the control groups; most used neurostimulation as the comparator but some used surface landmarks, fascial pops or transarterial approaches and USGRA + nerve stimulator. Some RCTs used multiple injections; others used single injection techniques.

Heterogeneity may therefore be a confounding factor. Only three RCTs were identified for lower limb blocks in adults, so the small study populations may influence the results. The majority of studies are from a small number of departments with expertise in the field of USGRA, so extrapolation to wider clinical practice may be of limited relevance.

Relevance

Since the first description of Doppler ultrasound guidance in 1978, USGRA has been developed by small groups of experts to the point where it has been widely adopted by other practitioners and clinical utility has preceded the confirmation of potential benefits. Without good data, claims of unproven advantage and benefit of USGRA over other nerve location techniques might be accepted without question. Some of the early claims of benefit were not going to be achieved, as reflected in this review and it is an important tool in highlighting areas of current uncertainty and thereby targeting future research in a more focussed direction. Currently, the benefits over neuro-stimulation are marginal and in particular there appears to be no sign of a reduction in the risks of complications. As more practitioners become skilled in its use and developments in ultrasound technology improve the utility of the equipment, other benefits may become apparent.

Chapter 10

Perioperative cardioprotection

ML Riess and JR Kersten

Introduction

Patients with coronary artery disease are at an increased risk for developing perioperative myocardial infarction. Myocardial ischaemia and reperfusion is an almost inevitable consequence of many cardiac procedures including percutaneous coronary intervention, cardiac valve replacement, coronary artery bypass grafting, and heart transplantation. In addition, a substantial number of patients undergoing non-cardiac surgery are at risk for myocardial ischaemia and reperfusion injury. Various therapeutic approaches to the problem have been suggested and these focus either on decreasing the incidence of perioperative ischaemic events or, if ischaemia does occur, attenuating the deleterious consequences on cardiac function and viability. Preoperative treatment of patients undergoing high-risk surgery with beta-receptor antagonists and HMG-CoA (3-hydroxy-3-methyl-glutaryl-CoA) reductase inhibitors ('statins') has been demonstrated to protect against myocardial infarction. Interestingly, a growing body of evidence suggests that enhancing endogenous cardioprotective pathways with pre- and postconditioning (after the ischaemic event) strategies may represent a promising approach to attenuating the severity of ischaemia and reperfusion injury. This chapter describes seminal original papers in the area of perioperative cardioprotection highlighting the potential efficacy of several different pharmacological approaches to improving cardiovascular outcome in patients with coronary artery disease.

Ten key investigations that highlight the progress in basic and clinical science in the area of perioperative cardioprotection are presented. In the last 10–15 years, a growing body of evidence has indicated that a variety of pharmacological approaches to decrease cardiovascular risk in patients with coronary artery disease exist including pre- and postconditioning with volatile anaesthetics; the use of noble gases to trigger endogenous cardioprotective signalling without producing loss of consciousness or hypotension; statin therapy to favourably modulate cardiovascular biology that may be both dependent and independent of cholesterol lowering; and judicious use of beta-blockers titrated to achieve maximum efficacy, but with a low risk for adverse effects. A large number of investigations have demonstrated that disease states such as diabetes and hyperglycaemia impair cardioprotective signalling. Conversely, moderate control of blood glucose concentrations in patients at risk for myocardial ischaemia may improve patient outcomes. Great progress has been made in elucidating mechanisms of myocardial ischaemia and reperfusion injury. However, the work done to date likely represents only the tip of the iceberg. Additional strategies to improve outcome in patients with cardiovascular disease continue to be urgently required.

Paper 1: Isoflurane mimics ischemic preconditioning via activation of K_{ATP} channels: reduction of myocardial infarct size with an acute memory phase

Author details

JR Kersten, TJ Schmeling, PS Pagel, GJ Gross, DC Warltier

Reference

Anesthesiology 1997; **87**: 361–70.

Summary

In the 1980s, volatile anaesthetics were demonstrated to increase tolerance of myocardium to ischaemic injury and to enhance functional recovery of myocardium (Murray *et al.*, 1986). These actions were largely attributed to anaesthetic effects on major determinants of myocardial oxygen consumption (e.g. negative inotropic effects and decreased ventricular loading conditions). In this landmark paper, Kersten *et al.* showed that: (1) isoflurane elicits an intracellular cardioprotective memory effect that outlasts its administration, similarly to ischaemic preconditioning (Warltier *et al.*, 1988), and (2) that anaesthetic-induced cardiovascular depression was *not* a contributing factor during cardiac preconditioning. In the same year, the findings of this study on anaesthetic preconditioning in dogs were corroborated by Cason *et al.* (1997) in rabbits.

Citation count

395.

Related references

1 Murry CE, Jennings RB, Reimer KA. Preconditioning with ischemia: a delay of lethal cell injury in ischemic myocardium. *Circulation* 1986; **74**: 1124–36.

2 Warltier DC, al-Wathiqui MH, Kampine JP, *et al.* Recovery of contractile function of stunned myocardium in chronically instrumented dogs is enhanced by halothane or isoflurane. *Anesthesiology* 1988; **69**: 552–65.

3 Cason BA, Gamperl AK, Slocum RE, *et al.* Anesthetic-induced preconditioning: previous administration of isoflurane decreases myocardial infarct size in rabbits. *Anesthesiology* 1997; **87**: 1182–90.

Key message

A clinically relevant concentration of the volatile anaesthetic isoflurane attenuated myocardial infarct size in an *in vivo* model by eliciting a cardioprotective memory effect that outlasted its administration. The beneficial effect of isoflurane to protect against infarction was mediated by opening of K_{ATP} channels and was abolished by the K_{ATP} channel antagonist glyburide, an oral antidiabetic drug.

Strengths

This investigation was conducted in a relevant canine model and was the first study to show that volatile anaesthetics trigger a memory effect unrelated to changes in myocardial energy metabolism. The results were also the first evidence of the involvement of K_{ATP} channels during anaesthetic preconditioning.

Weaknesses

As is typical of most *in vivo* myocardial infarction studies, the degree of cardioprotection could only be assessed with changes in infarct size, and not by changes in functional outcome. Evidence for K_{ATP} channel involvement was obtained solely by pharmacological antagonism with glyburide. Glyburide is a non-specific antagonist and the contribution of mitochondrial versus sarcolemmal K_{ATP} channels could not be evaluated during this investigation.

Relevance

'Preconditioning' with ischaemia was described over two decades ago and refers to a phenomenon in which a brief period of myocardial ischaemia protects the heart against injury during a subsequent more prolonged period of coronary artery occlusion and reperfusion. A defining attribute of ischaemic preconditioning is the presence of a memory period during which myocardium remains resistant to infarction even in the absence of an ongoing preconditioning stimulus. This investigation demonstrated that volatile anaesthetics are also capable of preconditioning myocardium. Since this paper's publication more than a decade ago, the work has become a foundation for many more basic science and clinical investigations evaluating the efficacy and mechanisms of anaesthetic cardioprotection. In addition, the finding that the oral antidiabetic drug glyburide abolished cardioprotection by isoflurane added to the increasing awareness that diabetes and its treatment may interfere with cardioprotective signalling.

Paper 2: Halothane reduces reperfusion injury after regional ischaemia in the rabbit heart *in vivo*

Author details

W Schlack, B Preckel, H Barthel, D Obal, V Thämer

Reference

British Journal of Anaesthesia 1997; **79**: 88–96.

Abstract

In addition to having anti-ischaemic effects, halothane can protect isolated rat hearts and isolated cardiomyocytes against reperfusion injury of the "oxygen paradox" type. The aim of this study was to investigate if halothane can also protect against myocardial reperfusion injury in vivo. Twenty-two rabbits anaesthetized with alpha-chloralose underwent 30 min of occlusion of a major coronary artery and 2 h of subsequent reperfusion. Seven animals received 1 MAC of halothane for the first 15 min of reperfusion (halothane group), and eight animals served as untreated controls (controls group). In seven additional animals, the haemodynamic effects of halothane were antagonized by an i.v. infusion of noradrenaline (halothane-noradrenaline group). We measured cardiac output (CO) by an ultrasonic flow probe around the ascending aorta, left ventricular pressure (LVP) by a tip manometer and infarct size by triphenyltetrazolium staining. Baseline LVP was mean 92 (SEM 4) mmHg and CO was 289 (16) ml min^{-1}. During coronary occlusion, LVP was reduced to 86 (4)% of baseline and CO to 84 (4)% (similar in all groups). During halothane administration at reperfusion, LVP declined further to 55 (6)% of baseline and CO to 66 (9)% (P <0.05 halothane group vs control group). Noradrenaline prevented the reduction in LVP (halothane–noradrenaline group 87 (5)% of baseline, control group 84 (6)% and reduction in CO (halothane-noradrenaline group 89 (5)%, control group 83 (6)%. Infarct size was 49 (6)% of the area at risk in controls and was reduced markedly by administration of halothane to 32 (3)% in the halothane group (P <0.05) and to 30 (3)% in the halothane-noradrenaline group (P <0.05). Treatment with halothane during the early reperfusion period after myocardial ischaemia protected the myocardium against infarction *in vivo*, independent of the haemodynamic effect of halothane.

Summary

Ischaemic 'postconditioning' was originally used to describe the phenomenon during which several brief periods of coronary artery re-occlusion performed to produce 'stuttered' reperfusion (Zhao *et al.*, 2003) decreased the magnitude of reperfusion injury. Subsequently, volatile anaesthetics administered during the first few minutes of reperfusion *after* prolonged ischaemia (Chiari *et al.*, 2005) were also shown to protect against myocardial infarction and this action was termed 'anaesthetic postconditioning'. This investigation by Schlack *et al.* was actually the first to demonstrate that anaesthetics postcondition myocardium against reperfusion injury *in vivo*.

Citation count

40.

Related references

1 Zhao ZQ, Corvera JS, Halkos ME, *et al*. Inhibition of myocardial injury by ischemic postconditioning during reperfusion: comparison with ischemic preconditioning. *Am J Physiol Heart Circ Physiol* 2003; **285**: H579–H588.

2 Chiari PC, Bienengraeber MW, Pagel PS, *et al*. Isoflurane protects against myocardial infarction during early reperfusion by activation of phosphatidylinositol-3-kinase signal transduction: evidence for anesthetic-induced postconditioning in rabbits. *Anesthesiology* 2005; **102**: 102–9.

Key message

The volatile anaesthetic halothane protected against myocardial ischaemia and reperfusion injury even when administered after the ischaemic event.

Strengths

Anaesthetic postconditioning was first demonstrated in this relevant *in vivo* model of myocardial infarction. Halothane was known to significantly decrease the haemodynamic determinants of myocardial oxygen consumption; however, concurrent administration of norepinephrine during halothane failed to abolish the cardioprotective effects of this volatile anaesthetic. These findings refuted the contention that the haemodynamic effects of halothane were primarily responsible for reductions of myocardial infarct size during anaesthetic administration.

Weaknesses

This early study of anaesthetic postconditioning did not specifically examine mechanisms whereby halothane protected against reperfusion injury.

Relevance

During cardiac *pre*conditioning any pharmacological or mechanical (e.g. coronary artery occlusion and reperfusion to produce ischaemic preconditioning) intervention must be implemented *before* the onset of prolonged myocardial ischaemia if it is to be effective to decrease the extent of injury. Such a strategy could be achieved during cardiac surgery in which the timing of an ischaemic event is often predictable. However, during non-cardiac surgery the presence of myocardial ischaemia is frequently unpredictable. Thus, an intervention such as anaesthetic postconditioning that does not require foreknowledge of an ischaemic event is likely to be more clinically relevant. The results of this study suggested that anaesthetics might be useful to treat the consequences of myocardial ischaemia and reperfusion after the inciting event.

Paper 3: Effects of propofol, desflurane, and sevoflurane on recovery of myocardial function after coronary surgery in elderly high-risk patients

Author details

SG De Hert, S Cromheecke, PW ten Broecke, E Mertens, IG De Blier, BA Stockman, IE Rodrigus, PJ Van der Linden

Reference

Anesthesiology 2003; **99**: 314–23.

Summary

Although many basic science investigations have conclusively demonstrated the cardioprotective effects of preconditioning by volatile anaesthetics, there remains only limited *clinical* evidence that choosing a volatile anaesthetic over an intravenous technique produces greater protection of myocardium against the deleterious effects of ischaemia and reperfusion injury. In this study, De Hert *et al.* confirmed that volatile anaesthetics are indeed cardioprotective in patients and that this is true even in elderly, high-risk patients undergoing coronary artery bypass graft surgery. Interestingly, volatile anaesthetics were administered *throughout* the surgery, and were not given only before (preconditioning) or after (postconditioning) cardiopulmonary bypass. The method of administering volatile anaesthetics during cardiac surgery was subsequently shown to impact effectiveness at reducing myocardial ischaemia and reperfusion injury (De Hert *et al.*, 2004).

Citation count

159.

Related references

1 De Hert SG, Van der Linden PJ, Cromheecke S, et al. Cardioprotective properties of sevoflurane in patients undergoing coronary surgery with cardiopulmonary bypass are related to the modalities of its administration. *Anesthesiology* 2004; **101**: 299–310.

Key message

In contrast to the intravenous anaesthetic propofol, the volatile anaesthetics sevoflurane and desflurane administered throughout surgery were more efficacious to preserve cardiac function after cardiopulmonary bypass in high-risk coronary artery surgery patients and to decrease myocardial damage postoperatively.

Strengths

This investigation was among the first to show that volatile anaesthetics were superior to intravenous anaesthesia with regard to cardioprotection after coronary artery bypass graft surgery. Concentrations of troponin I, a marker for cardiac injury, were decreased and myocardial performance was improved by volatile anaesthetics.

Weaknesses

This investigation was not sufficiently powered to evaluate more robust markers of outcome such as postoperative myocardial infarction or survival, a limitation that has plagued many clinical studies of anaesthetic cardioprotection. Volatile anaesthetic agents were given throughout surgery; therefore, the independent contributions of anaesthetics to produce pre- or postconditioning effects could not be evaluated.

Relevance

This is one of the earliest and important positive studies demonstrating that volatile anaesthetics are superior to intravenous techniques in patients undergoing cardiac surgery, although the overall evidence is limited. The results also suggested that the effects of volatile anaesthetics to decrease myocardial ischaemia and reperfusion injury after cardiac surgery in humans may represent a class effect of volatile anaesthetics.

Paper 4: Preconditioning by sevoflurane decreases biochemical markers for myocardial and renal dysfunction in coronary artery bypass graft surgery: a double-blinded, placebo-controlled, multicenter study

Author details

K Julier, R da Silva, C Garcia, L Bestmann, P Frascarolo, A Zollinger, PG Chassot, ER Schmid, MI Turina, LK von Segesser, T Pasch, DR Spahn, M Zaugg

Reference

Anesthesiology 2003; **98**: 1315–27.

Summary

After a smaller single-centre study by Belhomme *et al.* (1999) this investigation presented the results of the first larger double-blinded, placebo-controlled, multicenter trial of the use of anaesthetic preconditioning to improve outcome in patients after cardiac surgery. Seventy-two patients (in contrast to only 20 in the Belhomme study) were assigned to anaesthetic preconditioning or placebo, during concurrent intravenous anaesthesia with propofol, for coronary artery bypass graft surgery. Anaesthetic preconditioning was achieved by administering sevoflurane for a limited time (10 min) followed by washout, and at a concentration high enough (4 %) to elicit a strong preconditioning stimulus. Haemodynamic stability despite this high concentration (equivalent to 2 minimum alveolar concentration [MAC]) was maintained by concurrent cardiopulmonary bypass (CPB) and significant vasopressor support. Postoperative levels of classic biochemical markers for cardiac necrosis (total creatine kinase [CK], CK-MB, and troponin T) were *not* different between the groups except for a lower N-terminal pro-brain natriuretic peptide (NT-proBNP) in the preconditioning group (a marker for less myocardial dysfunction). Holter monitoring did not show any differences in ST-segment changes or arrhythmias in the preconditioning vs the placebo group, although, the study was largely underpowered to discover significant differences in many of the measured parameters. In addition, patients assigned to the sevoflurane group may have had more preoperative ischaemic episodes compared to the placebo group. The 2 positive findings were: (1) reduced postoperative serum levels of cystatin C, an indicator of preserved postoperative renal function, and (2) translocation of protein kinase C delta and epsilon isoforms in atrial tissue after preconditioning. The latter has been described as a pivotal step in the trigger phase of anaesthetic preconditioning (Zaugg *et al.*, 2002). Of additional significance, patients were followed for one year after surgery and a decreased incidence of late cardiac events was observed in the preconditioning compared to the placebo group (3% vs 17%) (Garcia *et al.*, 2005). The findings constituted the first evidence that anaesthetic preconditioning might improve long term outcome in patients.

Citation count

229.

Related references

1 Belhomme D, Peynet J, Louzy M, *et al.* Evidence for preconditioning by isoflurane in coronary artery bypass graft surgery. *Circulation* 1999; **100**(suppl 2): 340–4.

2 Zaugg M, Lucchinetti E, Spahn DR, *et al.* Volatile anesthetics mimic cardiac preconditioning by priming the activation of mitochondrial K_{ATP} channels via multiple signaling pathways. *Anesthesiology* 2002; **97**: 4–14.

3 Garcia C, Julier K, Bestmann L, *et al.* Preconditioning with sevoflurane decreases PECAM-1 expression and improves one-year cardiovascular outcome in coronary artery bypass graft surgery. *Br J Anaesth* 2005; **94**: 159–65.

Key message

A 10-min exposure to a high concentration of sevoflurane preconditioned myocardium before coronary artery bypass grafting as evidenced by decreased postoperative NT-proBNP.

Strengths

This was a relatively large, double-blinded, placebo-controlled, multicentre trial to investigate the efficacy of anaesthetic preconditioning on short- and long-term outcome. It also directly demonstrated protein kinase C translocation to subcellular targets in human myocardium in response to sevoflurane administration.

Weaknesses

Although the study may have been sufficiently powered to demonstrate changes in BNP, other markers of ischaemic injury were not found to be different between groups and this may have resulted, in part, from a lack of statistical power. Indices of postoperative ventricular function were not reported. Administration of high doses of sevoflurane and vasopressors required to support blood pressure during anaesthetic preconditioning could have limited the efficacy of this intervention.

Relevance

This was a seminal investigation of both short- and long-term outcome (Zaugg *et al.*, 2002) in patients subjected to a true cardiac preconditioning stimulus with a volatile anaesthetic before coronary artery bypass grafting.

Paper 5: The effects of interrupted or continuous administration of sevoflurane on preconditioning before cardio-pulmonary bypass in coronary artery surgery: comparison with continuous propofol

Author details

B Bein, J Renner, D Caliebe, R Hanss, M Bauer, S Fraund, J Scholz

Reference

Anaesthesia 2008; **63**: 1046–55.

Abstract

Volatile anaesthetics have been shown to exert cardioprotective properties in experimental and clinical studies. However, the mode of administration may influence these cardioprotective effects. The present study was designed to compare the effect of interrupted administration of sevoflurane before cardiopulmonary bypass with continuous sevoflurane administration and with propofol-only anaesthesia, on cardioprotection as assessed by left ventricular performance and myocardial cell damage during coronary artery bypass grafting. Forty-two patients scheduled for coronary bypass surgery were randomly assigned to one of three groups: propofol-only (P; n = 14), continuous (SevoC; n = 14) and interrupted sevoflurane administration (SevoI; n = 14). Myocardial cell damage as assessed by Troponin T (cTNT) and creatine kinase MB (CK-MB) were chosen as the primary endpoints and echocardiographic myocardial performance index (MPI) measurements were also performed. Up to 48 h postoperatively, in group SevoI, postoperative cTNT values (mean (SD) 0.13 (0.04) ng ml^{-1}) were significantly (p <0.05) lower than both the P (0.26 (0.31) ng ml^{-1}) and SevoC (0.25 (0.17) ng ml^{-1}) groups. CK-MB levels were also significantly (p <0.05) lower in the SevoI group at 24 h after surgery and MPI significantly improved compared with both the P and SevoC groups. There was, however, no difference with respect to cytokine release and length of stay in either the intensive care unit or in the hospital. We conclude that prior interrupted sevoflurane administration confers some cardioprotection as compared with continuous sevoflurane administration or propofol-based anaesthesia.

Summary

Although volatile anaesthetics appear to be a robust stimulus to induce cardiac preconditioning in animal models, their efficacy in humans appears to be somewhat more limited (Piriou *et al.*, 2007). In this study, Bein *et al.* provided evidence that preconditioning with anaesthetics, analogous to ischaemic preconditioning (Sandhu *et al.*, 1997), requires *interrupted* administration to decrease myocardial injury as assessed with troponin T and CK-MB. This study confirmed previous evidence from the laboratory (Riess *et al.*, 2004) and provided additional insight as to why some clinical studies of anaesthetic preconditioning may have failed to demonstrate improvement in patient outcomes. More recently, the findings were corroborated by Frassdorf *et al.* (2009) who demonstrated that troponin C levels were decreased when administration of 1 MAC sevoflurane was interrupted for 5 min in cardiac surgical patients.

Citation count

25.

Related references

1 Sandhu R, Diaz RJ, Mao GD, *et al.* Ischemic preconditioning: differences in protection and susceptibility to blockade with single-cycle versus multicycle transient ischemia. *Circulation* 1997; **96**: 984–95.

2 Riess ML, Kevin LG, Camara AK, *et al.* Dual exposure to sevoflurane improves anesthetic preconditioning in intact hearts. *Anesthesiology* 2004; **100**: 569–74.

3 Piriou V, Mantz J, Goldfarb G, *et al.* Sevoflurane preconditioning at 1 MAC only provides limited protection in patients undergoing coronary artery bypass surgery: a randomized bi-centre trial. *Br J Anaesth* 2007; **99**: 624–31.

4 Frassdorf J, Borowski A, Ebel D, *et al.* Impact of preconditioning protocol on anesthetic-induced cardioprotection in patients having coronary artery bypass surgery. *J Thorac Cardiovasc Surg* 2009; **137**: 1436–42.

Key message

Preconditioning by interrupted sevoflurane administration was shown to produce a greater degree of cardioprotection as compared to continuous administration of volatile anaesthetic, or to propofol infusion, in patients undergoing coronary artery bypass grafting.

Strengths

The investigators translated a laboratory finding to clinical practice and advanced understanding of how the mode of administration might impact the clinical efficacy of anaesthetic preconditioning.

Weaknesses

Similar to other clinical investigations of this type, the trial was not sufficiently powered to detect differences in long-term outcomes between groups and it lacked mechanistic insights that might explain how cardioprotective signalling is altered by interrupted anaesthetic administration in humans.

Relevance

This study is an important step forward in the bench-to-bedside translation of anaesthetic cardioprotection.

Paper 6: Isoflurane-induced preconditioning is attenuated by diabetes

Author details

K Tanaka, F Kehl, W Gu, JG Krolikowski, PS Pagel, DC Warltier, JR Kersten

Reference

American Journal of Physiology: Heart and Circulation Physiology 2002; **282**: H2018–23.

Abstract

Volatile anesthetics stimulate, but hyperglycemia attenuates, the activity of mitochondrial ATP-regulated K^+ channels. We tested the hypothesis that diabetes mellitus interferes with isoflurane-induced preconditioning. Acutely instrumented, barbiturate-anesthetized dogs were randomly assigned to receive 0, 0.32, or 0.64% end-tidal concentrations of isoflurane in the absence or presence of diabetes (3 wk after administration of alloxan and streptozotocin) in six experimental groups. All dogs were subjected to a 60-min left anterior descending coronary artery occlusion followed by 3 h of reperfusion. Myocardial infarct size (triphenyltetrazolium staining) was $29 \pm 3\%$ (n = 8) of the left ventricular area at risk in control experiments. Isoflurane reduced infarct size (15 ± 2 and $13 \pm 1\%$ during 0.32 and 0.64% concentrations; n = 8 and 7 dogs, respectively). Diabetes alone did not alter infarct size ($30 \pm 3\%$; n = 8) but blocked the protective effects of 0.32% ($27 \pm 2\%$; n = 7) and not 0.64% isoflurane ($18 \pm 3\%$; n = 7). Infarct size was directly related to blood glucose concentrations in diabetic dogs, but this relationship was abolished by higher concentrations of isoflurane. The results indicate that blood glucose and end-tidal isoflurane concentrations are important determinants of infarct size during anesthetic-induced preconditioning.

Summary

Increases in blood glucose concentration produced by diabetes attenuated anaesthetic preconditioning against myocardial infarction, analogous to findings that diabetes and acute hyperglycaemia 'dose'-dependently abolished ischaemic preconditioning (Kersten *et al.*, 2000). Lower blood glucose levels and higher isoflurane concentrations correlated with less myocardial necrosis, and the results were consistent with the interpretation that volatile anaesthetics stimulated, whereas, elevated glucose concentrations inhibited K_{ATP} channel activity *in vivo*. The findings highlighted the potential importance of optimizing perioperative glucose control in the context of promoting pharmacological cardioprotection (Armour and Kersten, 2008).

Citation count

57.

Related references

1 Kersten, JR, Toller WG, Gross ER, *et al.* Diabetes abolishes ischemic preconditioning: role of glucose, insulin, and osmolality. *Am J Physiol Heart Circ Physiol* 2000; **278**: H1218–H1224.

2 Amour J, Kersten JR. Diabetic cardiomyopathy and anesthesia: bench to bedside. *Anesthesiology* 2008; **108**: 524–30.

Key message

Diabetes attenuated cardioprotection by isoflurane preconditioning in a relevant model of myocardial infarction. The extent of infarction was directly related to blood glucose and inversely proportional to volatile anaesthetic concentrations.

Strengths

This study was one of the first to evaluate the impact of diabetes on cardioprotective signalling with volatile anaesthetics.

Weaknesses

Myocardial oxygen consumption was not measured, and differences in myocardial metabolism during the administration of isoflurane in the presence or absence of diabetes that might account for impaired anaesthetic preconditioning could not be evaluated. Relatively low isoflurane concentrations (comparable to 0.25 and 0.5 MAC) were used and blood glucose concentrations observed in diabetic animals varied between $200-400\,\mathrm{mg\,dl^{-1}}$. The study conditions may not have reflected surgical planes of anaesthesia or the presence of severe hyperglycaemia.

Relevance

This investigation demonstrated that a disease state, such as diabetes, could impair anaesthetic cardioprotection and supported earlier findings that K_{ATP} channel activation was adversely modulated by diabetes and hyperglycaemia in a 'glucose'-dependent fashion. The findings served as an impetus for further evaluation of the mechanisms whereby diabetes and hyperglycaemia interfere with cardioprotective signalling, and supported the search for strategies to restore anaesthetic preconditioning during hyperglycaemia.

Paper 7: Continuous perioperative insulin infusion decreases major cardiovascular events in patients undergoing vascular surgery: a prospective, randomized trial

Author details

B Subramaniam, PJ Panzica, V Novack, F Mahmood, R Matyal, JD Mitchell, E Sundar, R Bose, F Pomposelli, JR Kersten, DS Talmor

Reference

Anesthesiology 2009; **110**: 970–7.

Summary

In a seminal, but controversial investigation, Van den Berghe *et al.* (2001) demonstrated that tight glycaemic control of critically ill (predominantly cardiac surgical) patients in the intensive care unit (ICU) improved outcomes. In contrast, no studies had previously evaluated the efficacy of perioperative glucose control in patients undergoing vascular surgery without ICU admission. In this study, perioperative glycaemic control with *continuous* intravenous insulin infusion was demonstrated to improve outcome compared with an *intermittent* insulin bolus technique. All-cause mortality, myocardial infarction and congestive cardiac failure were significantly decreased in the continuous group and continuous insulin infusion was a negative predictor for adverse cardiac events. Continuous intravenous insulin therapy resulted in lower blood glucose levels, and possibly less postoperative glucose variability, actions that might have been responsible for the improved outcome observed in these patients. Although the incidence of hypoglycaemia was not statistically different between groups, hypoglycaemia is a potentially harmful side effect of insulin therapy (Lipshutz and Gropper, 2009) that could mitigate the beneficial effects of decreasing blood glucose concentration.

Citation count

28.

Related references

1 Van den Berghe G, Wouters P, Weekers F, *et al.* Intensive insulin therapy in the critically ill patients. *N Engl J Med* 2001; **345**: 1359–67.

2 Lipshutz AK, Gropper MA. Perioperative glycemic control: an evidence-based review. *Anesthesiology* 2009; **110**: 408–21.

Key message

Continuous insulin infusion to achieve blood glucose levels between 100–150 mg dl^{-1} reduces the incidence of perioperative myocardial infarction in vascular surgery patients.

Strengths

This study addresses an important question that controlling blood glucose concentration with a clinically relevant, insulin administration strategy improves outcome in a high-risk population of vascular surgical patients.

Weaknesses

The study was unblinded, and the continuous infusion group was subjected to more frequent monitoring of initial blood glucose concentrations as compared with the intermittent bolus group. This difference in frequency could conceivably have introduced study bias and could, in part, be responsible for the substantial risk reduction observed. A major weakness of the study was that the study was prematurely discontinued after 236 of 993 planned patients were recruited because of changes in surgical volume resulting in slow recruitment. As a result, the investigation lacked sufficient statistical power to detect differences in important outcomes such as postoperative wound infections, renal failure, and overall mortality.

Relevance

The results of this investigation support the contention that moderate control of blood glucose concentrations with perioperative continuous insulin infusion may improve outcomes in vascular surgical patients without substantially increasing the risk of hypoglycaemia.

Paper 8: Xenon administration during early reperfusion reduces infarct size after regional ischemia in the rabbit heart *in vivo*

Author details

B Preckel, J Müllenheim, A Moloschavij, V Thämer, W Schlack

Reference

Anesthesia and Analgesia 2000; **91**: 1327–32.

Summary

Preckel *et al.* demonstrated for the first time that the noble gas xenon postconditioned the heart against myocardial ischaemia and reperfusion injury. This group later showed that xenon also produced a preconditioning effect (Weber *et al.*, 2005), and other investigations confirmed that several non-anaesthetic noble gases such as helium, neon and argon were also cardioprotective (Pagel *et al.*, 2007). Despite the absence of chemical reactivity, xenon has been shown to interact with receptors and ion channels that are critical elements in cardioprotective signal transduction, similarly, to what has been observed with volatile anaesthetic agents. Interestingly, neither haemodynamic effects nor subsequent changes in myocardial oxygen supply and demand relations appeared to be necessary to elicit the cardioprotective effect of xenon.

Citation count

80.

Related references

1 Weber NC, Toma O, Wolter JI, *et al.* The noble gas xenon induces pharmacological preconditioning in the rat heart in vivo via induction of PKC-epsilon and p38 MAPK. *Br J Pharmacol* 2005; **144**: 123–32.

2 Pagel PS, Krolikowski JG, Shim YH, *et al.* Noble gases without anesthetic properties protect myocardium against infarction by activating prosurvival signaling kinases and inhibiting mitochondrial permeability transition in vivo. *Anesth Analg* 2007; **105**: 562–9.

Key message

The noble gas xenon reduced myocardial infarction when given upon reperfusion.

Strengths

This was the first study to demonstrate that a noble gas could exert a postconditioning effect when given at reperfusion.

Weaknesses

The study used only one 'subanaesthetic' concentration of xenon. In addition, specific mechanisms responsible for the cardioprotective effects of xenon were not investigated.

Relevance

This landmark study provided evidence that a potentially non-anaesthetic noble gas devoid of haemodynamic effects could substantially decrease myocardial ischaemia and reperfusion injury. These findings suggested that the therapeutic application of noble gases to protect against myocardial injury could be relevant in a variety of different clinical situations during which changes in consciousness and hypotension might represent serious limitations to the use of alternative drugs such as volatile anaesthetic agents.

Paper 9: Statins are associated with a reduced incidence of perioperative mortality after coronary artery bypass graft surgery

Author details

W Pan, T Pintar, J Anton, V-V Lee, WK Vaughn, CD Collard

Reference

Circulation 2004; **110**: II-45–9.

Summary

This large retrospective cohort study demonstrated that statin therapy improved outcomes after primary coronary artery bypass graft surgery. Statins have been widely prescribed to decrease low-density lipoprotein (LDL) cholesterol and a growing body of evidence indicated that statins have cardioprotective effects independent of reductions in LDL cholesterol (Lefer *et al.*, 2001). Statins have been shown to modulate and improve endothelial function by increasing nitric oxide production, and these drugs attenuated leucocyte–endothelium interactions, and decreased platelet aggregation (Lefer *et al.*, 1999). Statins scavenged reactive oxygen species, decreased endothelial cell apoptosis, and produced antithrombotic effects. Their anti-inflammatory effects contributed to atherosclerotic plaque stability. The direct cardioprotective effects of statins might be particularly important in diseases such as diabetes mellitus where endogenous signal transduction responsible for normal protection against ischaemic injury was impaired (Gu *et al.*, 2008). Although treatment with statins appeared to improve patient outcomes, the duration of preoperative treatment that produced risk reduction was unclear. A small risk of rhabdomyolysis (Pasternak *et al.*, 2002) may have been present in patients in whom statins were continued perioperatively, however, acute withdrawal of these drugs has also been shown to increase cardiovascular risk (Heeschen *et al.*, 2002) by increasing oxidative stress and enhancing endothelial dysfunction (Vecchione and Brandes, 2002). Although the study failed to show that statin therapy was independently associated with a decreased risk of MI, cardiac arrhythmias, stroke, or renal dysfunction, a 50% reduction in 30-day all-cause mortality was observed in patients on preoperative statin therapy and this finding persisted even after adjusting for selection bias and comorbidities using propensity score matching.

Citation count

133.

Related references

1 Lefer AM, Campbell B, Shin YK, *et al.* Simvastatin preserves the ischemic-reperfused myocardium in normocholesterolemic rat hearts. *Circulation* 1999; **100**: 178–84.

2 Dotani MI, Elnicki DM, Jain AC, *et al.* Effect of preoperative statin therapy and cardiac outcomes after coronary artery bypass grafting. *Am J Cardiol* 2000; **86**: 1128–30, A6.

3 Lefer AM, Scalia R, Lefer DJ. Vascular effects of HMG CoA-reductase inhibitors (statins) unrelated to cholesterol lowering: New concepts for cardiovascular disease. *Cardiovasc Res* 2001; **49**: 281–7.

4 Heeschen C, Hamm CW, Laufs U, *et al.* Withdrawal of statins increases event rates in patients with acute coronary syndromes. *Circulation* 2002; **105**: 1446–52.

5 Pasternak RC, Smith SC Jr, Bairey-Merz CN, *et al.* ACC/AHA/NHLBI clinical advisory on the use and safety of statins. *Circulation* 2002; **106**: 1024–8.

6 Vecchione C, Brandes RP. Withdrawal of 3-hydroxy-3-methylglutaryl coenzyme A reductase inhibitors elicits oxidative stress and induces endothelial dysfunction in mice. *Circ Res* 2002; **91**: 173–9.

7 Poldermans D, Bax JJ, Kertai MD, *et al.* Statins are associated with a reduced incidence of perioperative mortality in patients undergoing major noncardiac vascular surgery. *Circulation* 2003; **107**: 1848–51.

8 Gu W, Kehl F, Krolikowski JG, *et al.* Simvastatin restores ischemic preconditioning in the presence of hyperglycemia through a nitric oxide-mediated mechanism. *Anesthesiology* 2008; **108**: 634–42.

Key message

Preoperative statin therapy prior to coronary artery bypass graft surgery reduced the risk of postoperative mortality and stroke.

Strengths

Following a case-control study conducted in non-cardiac vascular surgery patients (Poldermans *et al.*, 2003) and a smaller retrospective analysis of coronary artery bypass graft surgery patients (Dotani *et al.*, 2000) this was the first larger retrospective study to show a benefit of statins on early overall mortality following cardiac surgery.

Weaknesses

Apart from the limitations inherent in a retrospective study, this study also suffered from limited statistical power. A previous study by Dotani *et al.* (2000) (323 patients operated on over a course of 6 months) was noted to be underpowered. This study was designed to address the independent association between statin therapy and reduction of acute adverse outcomes. Although 1663 patients were included in the analysis, multivariate regression analysis and propensity matching did not demonstrate an independent effect of statins to decrease MI, stroke or renal dysfunction. Reduction of mortality alone also fell out of the analysis as an independent predictor after propensity matching (p <0.08). Duration of pre- or postoperative statin therapy was not evaluated.

Relevance

Although the study had some important limitations, this was also one of the first investigations that suggested that preoperative therapy with statins might have a beneficial effect to decrease early mortality in a high-risk population of patients with coronary artery disease.

Paper 10: Effects of extended-release metoprolol succinate in patients undergoing non-cardiac surgery (POISE trial): a randomised controlled trial

Author details

POISE Study Group, PJ Devereaux, H Yang, S Yusuf, G Guyatt, K Leslie, JC Villar, D Xavier, S Chrolavicius, L Greenspan, J Pogue, P Pais, L Liu, S Xu, G Málaga, A Avezum, M Chan, VM Montori, M Jacka, P Choi

Reference

Lancet 2008; **371**(9627): 1839–47.

Abstract

Background: Trials of beta blockers in patients undergoing non-cardiac surgery have reported conflicting results. This randomised controlled trial, done in 190 hospitals in 23 countries, was designed to investigate the effects of perioperative beta blockers.

Methods: We randomly assigned 8351 patients with, or at risk of, atherosclerotic disease who were undergoing non-cardiac surgery to receive extended-release metoprolol succinate (n=4174) or placebo (n=4177), by a computerised randomisation phone service. Study treatment was started 2–4 h before surgery and continued for 30 days. Patients, health-care providers, data collectors, and outcome adjudicators were masked to treatment allocation. The primary endpoint was a composite of cardiovascular death, non-fatal myocardial infarction, and non-fatal cardiac arrest. Analyses were by intention to treat. This trial is registered with ClinicalTrials. gov, number NCT00182039.

Findings: All 8351 patients were included in analyses; 8331 (99.8%) patients completed the 30-day follow-up. Fewer patients in the metoprolol group than in the placebo group reached the primary endpoint (244 [5.8%] patients in the metoprolol group vs 290 [6.9%] in the placebo group; hazard ratio 0.84, 95% CI 0.70–0.99; p=0.0399). Fewer patients in the metoprolol group than in the placebo group had a myocardial infarction (176 [4.2%] vs 239 [5.7%] patients; 0.73, 0.60–0.89; p=0.0017). However, there were more deaths in the metoprolol group than in the placebo group (129 [3.1%] vs 97 [2.3%] patients; 1.33, 1.03–1.74; p=0.0317). More patients in the metoprolol group than in the placebo group had a stroke (41 [1.0%] vs 19 [0.5%] patients; 2.17, 1.26–3.74; p=0.0053).

Interpretation: Our results highlight the risk in assuming a perioperative beta-blocker regimen has benefit without substantial harm, and the importance and need for large randomised trials in the perioperative setting. Patients are unlikely to accept the risks associated with perioperative extended-release metoprolol.

Summary

This was the largest multicentre and multinational trial conducted to date in over 8000 patients (history of coronary artery disease, peripheral vascular disease, stroke, congestive heart failure, etc.) to evaluate the beneficial effects of 100 mg extended-release oral metoprolol vs placebo administered 2–4 h before non-cardiac surgery. This dose of beta blocker was repeated 6 h after surgery and followed by metoprolol 200 mg daily for 30 days. The primary endpoint of the study was a composite of cardiovascular death, non-fatal myocardial infarction, and non-fatal cardiac arrest. Although a decreased incidence of adverse cardiac events was observed in the metoprolol group, these patients demonstrated an increased incidence of stroke and this occurred concomitantly with significant hypotension and bradycardia. The latter were the most common reasons for temporary discontinuation of beta blocker. Moreover, there were more deaths in the metoprolol than in the placebo group, highlighting the potential risk of initiating high dose beta-blocker therapy in the immediate perioperative period.

Citation count

518.

Related references

1 Mangano DT, Layug EL, Wallace A, *et al.* Effect of atenolol on mortality and cardiovascular morbidity after noncardiac surgery. Multicenter Study of Perioperative Ischemia Research Group. *N Engl J Med* 1996; **335**: 1713–20.

2 Poldermans D, Boersma E, Bax JJ, *et al.* The effect of bisoprolol on perioperative mortality and myocardial infarction in high-risk patients undergoing vascular surgery. Dutch Echocardiographic Cardiac Risk Evaluation Applying Stress Echocardiography Study Group. *N Engl J Med* 1999; **341**: 1789–94.

3 Raby KE, Brull SJ, Timimi F, *et al.* The effect of heart rate control on myocardial ischemia among high-risk patients after vascular surgery. *Anesth Analg* 1999; **88**: 477–82.

4 Fleisher LA, Poldermans D. Perioperative beta blockade: where do we go from here? *Lancet* 2008; **371**: 1813–4.

5 Fleischmann KE, Beckman JA, Buller CE, *et al.* 2009 ACCF/AHA focused update on perioperative beta blockade: a report of the American college of cardiology foundation/ American heart association task force on practice guidelines. *Circulation* 2009; **120**: 2123–51.

Key message

High-dose beta-blockade initiated within hours of surgery decreased the incidence of postoperative cardiac complications, but at cost of increased stroke and death.

Strengths

The POISE (PeriOperative ISchemic Evaluation) trial was by far the largest prospective, randomized, placebo-controlled trial investigating the benefits and risks of perioperative beta-blockade. The results supported the old adage that 'more is not necessarily better', analogously to similar concerns of hypoglycaemia and worse outcome in patients with hyperglycaemia treated aggressively with insulin. Other strengths of the study included careful monitoring of adverse events throughout the trial and similar patient clinical profiles in the placebo and treatment groups. The study clearly highlights the possible risks associated with cardioprotection using acute beta-blocker administration protocols.

Weaknesses

Despite the size and importance of the trial, the study design had some important shortcomings. A fixed limit rather than a relative lower limit for systolic blood pressure (100 mmHg) was used as an exclusion criterion for receiving metoprolol. This study design feature could have predisposed some patients to develop perioperative organ hypoperfusion. The latter might have occurred because individual variations in baseline blood pressure were not considered. There was no adjustment for a maximum heart rate to trigger an increased dose of beta blocker despite recent findings that incidence of myocardial ischaemia was decreased in patients when heart rate was tightly controlled (Raby *et al.*, 1999). The starting dose of metoprolol was two to eight times higher than that recommended for NYHA Class II heart failure patients (Fleisher and Poldermans, 2008) and in contrast to POISE, another study demonstrated that the incidence of stroke was no greater than placebo when beta-blockade was initiated at least 7 days prior to surgery and at lower doses (Poldermans *et al.*, 1999).

Relevance

This was one of the most controversial, yet important, studies in the area of perioperative cardioprotection in recent years. Despite its undisputed shortcomings, the results clearly indicated that the potential benefit of perioperative beta-blockade (Mangano *et al.*, 1996) must be counterbalanced by a consideration of the risks of initiating such therapy. Perioperative beta-blockade should be individualized and started early enough so that the drug dose can be titrated to the desired clinical effect controlling heart rate *and* avoiding untoward hypotension. These considerations have been clearly addressed in the recent recommendations of the ACC/AHA Guidelines on Perioperative Cardiovascular Evaluation and Care for Noncardiac Surgery (Fleischmann *et al.*, 2009).

Chapter 11

Neuroanaesthesia

K Ferguson and J Dinsmore

Introduction

The central nervous system (CNS) and its pathophysiology differ from other vital systems in several ways. Nowhere is this more apparent or the understanding of the clinical implications of these idiosyncrasies more relevant than when neurosurgical intervention is required to manage natural or unnatural pathology. Advances in the understanding of neuroscience stride on apace yet the functional anatomy and physiological responses of the whole brain and spinal cord under pathological conditions remain less well understood. Further, the unique properties of human CNS function add a dimension of difficulty to the study of mechanisms in available models. Advances in neurosurgical technique are aimed at minimally invasive approaches to diminish resulting neurological deficit and salvage or restitution of function after damage. The role of the neuroanaesthetist includes vital support and monitoring as in all surgical and intensive care procedures but also includes the added dimension of functional monitoring of the brain and cord in the context of the specialized reflexes and responses of the system.

The development of a robust system for the classification of the clinical manifestation of altered brain function has contributed enormously to the advancement in treatment protocols and research strategies in neurosurgery, trauma, anaesthesia, and intensive care. The Glasgow Coma Scale has had minor adjustment in the last 47 years and remains the gold standard in clinical assessment of brain function and the paper describing it is our first Landmark Paper. At the far end of the spectrum of brain function, i.e. brain death, a similar robust classification is required. The Medical Colleges' consensus guidelines go some way to delivering this but controversy still exists. Since a diagnosis of brain death facilitates both the withdrawal of medical support and the procurement of organs for transplantation from heart beating donors, it remains an area of medicine which will continue to develop in line with societies' demands.

Trephination was performed by many ancient civilizations including the Egyptians and Peruvians. Penfold and Pasquet's paper, (Paper 3) reintroduced awake craniotomy to the modern era of neurosurgery. With increased patient safety, improved functional outcome and the opportunity for day case activity, it verges on becoming the norm for supratentorial tumour surgery. For similar reasons the results of the GALA trial were long awaited by vascular and neuroanaesthetists and surgeons alike. Although large numbers were recruited to the trial, insufficient study control led to excessive variability in practice. The trial delivered an inconclusive result. This study demonstrates many of the constraining influences affecting our ability to answer obvious questions in our clinical practice. These include, recruiting sufficient sample numbers to reach statistically significant results and ensuring strict protocol adherence with respect to randomization, blinding, and completion of treatment protocols, whilst avoiding bias.

Primary brain injury, its causes, and prevention are matters of public health and legislative control. Secondary injury accounts for significant morbidity and mortality on a global scale. The Traumatic Coma Data Bank (TCDB) has provided a wealth of information which has permitted the evaluation of hypotension and hypoxia as key factors in outcome from severe head injury, as detailed in Chesnut's paper, Paper 5. Hypotension in association with a severe head injury confers an increase in mortality risk of 150%. This paper set the scene for the publication of the Brain Trauma Foundation guidelines for management of traumatic brain injury. Treatment strategies have been developed to mitigate the effects of secondary brain injury and are described in Papers 6, 7 and 8. Rosner *et al.* and Asgeirsson *et al.* tackled the issue of raised ICP and cerebral oedema from two contrasting physiological standpoints. The debate continues today. Meanwhile triple-H therapy found favour in the treatment of vasopasm secondary to aneurysmal subarachnoid bleeding. Recognition that supranormal physiology produces its own side effects has limited this therapy's universal acceptance.

Many studies of secondary brain injury had suggested that pharmacological manipulation of the cellular mechanisms involved in cerebral oedema and ischaemia might provide a valuable addition to the treatment armamentarium. The Medical Research Council (MRC) CRASH trial was designed to confirm or refute the benefit of corticosteroids in severe head injury. It remains an excellent example of what can be achieved through multicentre collaboration and cooperation. Similarly the ISAT trial, published 2 years earlier, reported on the benefits of clipping versus coiling in ruptured intracranial aneurysms. A definitive answer was found although methodological flaws limit the study findings' application to certain clinical groups. These issues accepted, the way forward in developing neuroanaesthesia and intensive care will rely heavily where possible on large randomized control trials robustly delivered. We await the outcome of the Eurotherm trial. It is also important, however, to support the continued collection of large databases, such as the TCDB, to permit the study of specific questions when ethics will not allow denial of treatment inherent in RCT design. The benefits of such a 'mixed economy' of strategies are apparent in the papers described in this chapter and that mixture of approaches serves as a useful model for the future.

Paper 1: Assessment of coma and impaired consciousness. A practical scale

Author details

G Teasdale, B Jennet

Reference

Lancet 1974; **2**: 81–4.

Summary

The Glasgow Coma Scale (GCS) was developed as a standardized way to evaluate and describe the depth and duration of altered consciousness or coma in patients with head injuries. The fundamental concept was to separately assess the various attributes considered important in the concept of 'conscious level'. The original description in 1974 consisted of a 14-point scale, comprised of three components, and based on the patient's best response in terms of eye opening, motor response, and verbal response. This was then modified in 1976 to a 15-point scale with the addition of numerical values (see Table 11.1). Scores may be expressed as totals or separated into the three categories.

Further details of individual responses were described in the text:

- Eye opening in response to pain should be assessed from stimulus to the limbs so as to avoid triggering the grimacing reflex.

Table 11.1 Glasgow Coma Scale

Eye opening	Score
Spontaneous	4
To speech	3
To pain	2
None	1
Best verbal response	
Orientated	5
Confused	4
Inappropriate	3
Incomprehensible	2
None	1
Best motor response	
Obeying	6
Localizing	5
Withdrawing	5
Flexing	3
Extending	2
None	1

Reprinted from Teasdale G, Jennett B. Assessment of coma and impaired consciousness. A practical scale. *The Lancet*, **304**, 1974; 81–84, with permission from Elsevier.

- Verbal responses were described as: orientated in time, place and person, confused conversation, inappropriate words, or incomprehensible with moans or groans only.
- Motor responses were described in most detail. Localizing was defined as the movement of a limb to avoid a noxious stimulus at more than one site, withdrawing as normal flexion of the elbow or knee to local noxious stimulus, flexing as slow withdrawal with pronation of the wrist, and adduction of the shoulder, extending as adduction and internal rotation of the shoulder with pronation of the forearm. Noxious stimuli were to be applied using pressure on the nail bed with a pencil to test for flexion and the head, neck, or trunk to test for localization.

Citation count

6331.

Related references

1 Teasdale G, Jennet B. Assessment and prognosis of coma after head injury. *Acta Neurochir* 1976; **34**: 45–55.

2 Jennet B, Teasdale G. Aspects of coma after severe head injury. *Lancet* 1977; **309**: 878–81.

3 Teasdale GM, Murray L. Revisiting the Glasgow Coma Scale and Coma Score. *Intensive Care Med* 2000; **26**: 153–4.

Key message

The GCS is a scoring system for describing neurological status in patients with acute brain injury from trauma, stroke, or other causes.

Strengths

At the time of its introduction there was no other standardized method for measuring level of consciousness. The GCS not only provided a quick and simple way to evaluate the severity of a head injury but also to effectively communicate this information. It could be used by all members of the healthcare team and be repeated at different time periods to assess changes in the patient's neurological status. It has become the most widely used scoring system for the measurement of consciousness throughout the world.

Weaknesses

The GCS was developed primarily as a research tool for simple bedside assessment and it has never been subjected to careful statistical evaluation. Yet it is commonly used in guidelines as a trigger for clinical intervention and also to predict outcome with all the associated implications for patients and family. A major criticism in these situations is the use of GCS as single numerical score. Jennet and Teasdale themselves used a summed score for GCS in their assessment of head injured patients and concluded that all combinations resulting in a GCS <8 were definitive of coma. However Teasdale also emphasized that the conscious level of the patient should always be described in terms of the three separate responses. Every GCS score except 3 and 15 consists of a collection of different possible groupings of subscores for motor, verbal, and eye response and, although these different combinations may have a single GCS score, they may also have very different mortalities. Consequently the summed score will not always provide an accurate assessment of the patient's condition. Despite this it is frequently used to aid in management decisions. In addition it is not possible to assess verbal scores if a patient is sedated, intubated, or intoxicated and the GCS does not incorporate any assessment of brainstem reflexes. Some authors have suggested the replacement of the GCS score with the motor score alone as it has been shown to yield similar outcome prediction rates in head injured patients.

Relevance

Despite numerous technological advances and the development of new monitors of cerebral function, clinical assessment of the neurological system remains the gold standard. The GCS has now been in use for over 36 years. It has been incorporated into various other scoring systems such as the Acute Physiology and Chronic Health Evaluation (APACHE) score, Revised trauma score and Trauma and Injury Severity Score (TRISS). Although not perfect it is a difficult to improve on its simplicity and practical usefulness. The description of the GCS was a true landmark paper and it is likely to remain part of our clinical decision-making process in patients with brain injury for many years to come.

Paper 2: Diagnosis of brain death

Author details

Statement issued by the honorary secretary of the Conference of Medical Royal Colleges and their Faculties in the United Kingdom

Reference

British Medical Journal 1976; **2**: 1187–88.

Summary

The Conference of Medical Royal Colleges proposed the concept of brain death in this consensus statement stating, 'permanent functional death of the brainstem constitutes brain death and once this has occurred further artificial support is fruitless and should be withdrawn'. They also issued criteria for its diagnosis. Before a diagnosis of brain death could be made the patient was required to be deeply comatose and apnoeic due to irreversible structural brain damage. There were three diagnostic steps. Essential preconditions must be met, the patient should be in an apnoeic coma and there should be no doubt that the condition is due to irreversible brain damage of known cause. Next any reversible causes of apnoeic coma such as hypothermia, metabolic, endocrine or pharmacological intoxication should be excluded. Finally, clinical examination must confirm the absence of brain stem reflexes and persistent apnoea. These tests should be repeated but additional investigations such as electroencephalography were not required provided that a well-established aetiology for brain death was established.

So in summary, brain death has been defined as complete irreversible loss of brainstem function and the diagnostic criteria for brain death have been agreed.

Citation count

19.

Related references

1 Review by a working group convened by the Royal College of Physicians and endorsed by the Medical Royal Colleges and their Faculties in the United Kingdom Conference. Criteria for the diagnosis of brain stem death. *J R Coll Physicians Lond* 1995; **29**: 381–2.

2 Department of Health. *A code of practice for the diagnosis of brain stem death*. London: HMSO, 1998.

3 Academy of Medical Royal Colleges. *A code of practice for the diagnosis and confirmation of brain death (United Kingdom)*. London: Academy of Medical Royal Colleges, 2008.

Key message

The concept of death has always been difficult to define. Historically the cessation of vital functions, giving rise to apnoea and asystole, were sufficient to confirm the diagnosis. However, with advances in intensive care medicine we are now able to maintain cardiovascular and respiratory function even in the presence of catastrophic and irreversible brain injury. Inevitably this has lead to further diagnostic difficulties. Death can now be defined as the irreversible loss of the capacity for consciousness, combined with the capacity to breathe.

Strengths

In view of the implications of diagnosis of brain death a consensus view is essential and this consensus must be maintained despite changes in medical opinion and practice. A diagnosis of brainstem death serves two purposes; it provides grounds for withdrawal of medical support and facilitates the procurement of organs for transplantation from heart beating donors. A revised UK code of practice in 1998 included guidelines for the identification and management of potential organ and tissue donors. Variations in the interpretations of these guidelines led to calls for more guidance and clarity and in response the latest code of practice were produced in 2008 by a working party on behalf of the Academy of the Royal Medical Colleges. This takes a different approach addressing the diagnosis and confirmation of death in all situations and in isolation from issues surrounding organ donation. These revised guidelines also produced clearer guidance in some areas, such as the apnoea test and the repetition of tests.

Weaknesses

There is no statutory definition of brain death in English law and its diagnosis differs from country to country. Philosophical, cultural, and religious notions of death further complicate the matter. Within existing guidelines there remain several areas of controversy. The major focus of debate is the lack of consensus in diagnostic criteria between different countries. In the UK and many European countries there has been refinement of the original brain death to one of brainstem death. This is based on the premise that cognitive processing is impossible with death of the brainstem and that asystole will inevitably follow. Diagnosis is clinical and is not dependent on confirmatory tests, which are reserved for cases where comprehensive neurological examination is not possible (e.g. extensive maxillofacial injuries, residual sedation, high cervical cord injury) or when diagnosis may be complicated. In contrast in other countries such as the USA, Sweden, and the Netherlands the definition of death requires whole brain death characterized by loss of function of both cerebral hemispheres as well as the brainstem. Here confirmatory testing is recommended or required. Typically guidelines recommend assessment of whole brain blood flow and currently validated diagnostic tests capable of identifying complete cerebral circulatory arrest, include cerebral angiography, ^{99}Tc-HMPAO radionucleotide angiography and positron emission tomography (PET) with $H_2^{15}O$. Other tests used include cerebral electrical activity (electroencephalogram or EEG), transcranial Doppler, or cerebral evoked potentials. Whereas the actual clinical criteria used to determine brainstem death are remarkably similar in most guidelines, there are differences in who performs the tests and time intervals involved. In the UK two medical practitioners, each registered for more than 5 years and competent in the conduct and interpretation of brain stem tests are required for diagnosis. One must be a consultant and there must be no conflicts of interest or involvement with the transplant team. A complete set of tests must be performed on two separate occasions. If the first set of tests confirms death the second set may be performed as soon as the end-tidal carbon dioxide has returned to baseline following the apnoea test. In other countries the number of physicians varies between one to three and the minimum interval between each set of tests between 2–48 h. In addition these are all guidelines, which, in common with all guidelines, accommodate clinical judgement rather than rigidly prescribe process. Consequently there are some areas where interpretation may differ and this has raised concerns. A further criticism has been the lack of scientific rationale for the differences in practice. There have been many publications addressing the issues of the neurological determination of death but there is little evidence-base to support many of our current practices relating to brain and brainstem death determination.

Relevance

There are now over 50 years of patient data and clinical experience and no scientific data to discount the clinical criteria of brain death. Although now almost universally accepted by the medical profession, a diagnosis of brainstem death may still be very difficult for families to accept. In addition some cultures and religions do not equate brainstem death with death of the individual. Dealing with these issues always requires sensitivity, and understanding. However, variability and inconsistency in diagnosis within the medical profession itself will only add to doubts. In view of the implications of a diagnosis of brainstem death the profession must work together, to explore areas where uncertainty still exists. This is essential in order to maintain public trust and protect patients and practitioners.

Paper 3: Combined regional and general anaesthesia for craniotomy and cortical exploration

Author details

W Penfield, A Pasquet

Reference

Anesthesia and Analgesia 1954; **33**: 145–6.

Summary

This paper describes the surgical and anaesthetic aspects of craniotomy under local anaesthesia, intermittent sedation, and analgesia, and consists of two parts. In the first part Penfield discusses the neurosurgical considerations and in the second Pasquet describes the anaesthetic considerations. Each author describes his own personal experience of the procedures, his techniques, and 'tricks of the trade'. However, they both highlight the importance of an informed, cooperative patient and the need for perfect teamwork. Penfield focuses mainly on awake craniotomy for the radical treatment of focal epilepsy, but also describes its use for the excision of brain tumours in the dominant hemisphere. A conscious and alert patient was essential to facilitate electrocorticography and cortical mapping, which would then guide surgical decision-making 'making possible more complete removal without the risk of sacrifice of function'. He went on to describe the anatomy of intracranial pain and methods of analgesia using infiltration of local anaesthesia and nerve block. In the second part of the paper Pasquet reviews the three anaesthetic techniques, which they developed for this type of surgery. The first technique was only suitable for a cooperative patient and entailed being awake for most of the procedure but general anaesthesia for closure. The second technique was suitable for an uncooperative patient or child less than 10 years and consisted of general anaesthesia with awakening for testing and then general anaesthesia for closure. Finally a completely uncooperative patient or child under 4 years of age would require general anaesthesia 'at the lightest possible plane' throughout the procedure. General anaesthesia was induced with pentothal, the nose and respiratory tract anaesthetized with cocaine and the airway secured by blind nasal intubation. Anaesthesia was then maintained with intermittent injection of pentothal and an oxygen, nitrous oxide mixture with or without trilene. Pasquet highlighted the difficulties in these types of cases of providing optimal surgical conditions without compromising patient safety. He concluded that although the techniques described were not perfect and were in a continuous state of transformation, they served their purpose.

Citation count

27.

Related references

1 Taylor MD, Bernstein M. Awake craniotomy with brain mapping as the routine surgical approach to treating patients with supratentorial intraaxial tumor: a prospective trial of 200 cases. *J Neurosurg* 1999; **90**: 35–41.

2 Meyer FB, Bates LM, Goerss SJ, *et al*. Awake craniotomy for aggressive resection of primary gliomas located in eloquent cortex. *Mayo Clin Proc* 2001; **76**: 677–87.

3 McGirt MJ, Chaichana KL, Attenello FJ, *et al*. Extent of surgical resection is independently associated with survival in patients with hemispheric low-grade glioma. *Neurosurgery* 2008; **63**: 700–8.

Key message

Awake craniotomy guides surgical decision-making. Anaesthetic techniques need to evolve to cope with changing surgical requirements. The authors highlight the importance of an informed, cooperative patient, attention to detail, good communication, and the need for perfect teamwork.

Strengths

Awake craniotomies have been performed for many years in one form or other however the modern era of awake craniotomy was heralded by the publication of this landmark paper in 1954. Penfield was undoubtedly one of the most influential surgeons of his time and published extensively his neurosurgical studies of the brain mechanisms of epilepsy and speech. Many of the discussion points from this paper remain just as relevant today.

Weaknesses

This manuscript is a documentation of the authors' personal experience in anaesthesia and surgery for awake craniotomy. In medical practice today where randomized clinical trials and citation indexes count, such case reports rank poorly in the hierarchy of evidence.

Relevance

Wilder Penfield and André Pasquet's early experiences laid the groundwork for the awake craniotomy today. Although anaesthetic drugs and adjuncts have radically changed there are many similarities in practice. Certainly many of the difficulties and management dilemmas highlighted by Pasquet and Penfield are just as relevant today. Whereas in their practice awake craniotomy was mainly for epilepsy surgery it is now increasingly used in the surgical treatment of Parkinson's disease, dystonias, and intractable movement disorders. It is also frequently used for the resection of intracranial tumours in or adjacent to eloquent cortex. The management of low-grade gliomas in these areas presents neurosurgeons with a difficult dilemma. Although the extent of resection may affect survival, this must be balanced against the risk of causing neurological damage. With improved neuronavigation methods and intraoperative MRI radical resection may be achieved more safely but the ability to perform this surgical resection in an awake patient with continuous neurological assessment greatly enhances safety. There is still no consensus regarding best technique, hardly surprising considering the different operative procedures, surgical requirements and patient groups involved. Numerous techniques have been described but, as in Pasquet's paper, they fall into three main categories: local anaesthesia, conscious sedation and asleep–awake–asleep (AAA) technique with or without airway instrumentation. Effective local anaesthesia is essential for all techniques either by field infiltration of the incision area and pins sites, or by individual nerve blockade. The introduction of propofol revolutionized practice. It is now the most popular agent used for awake craniotomy and is often combined with remifentanil using target-controlled infusions. Dexmedetomidine has also been used successfully especially for implantation of deep brain stimulators. It provides rapidly titratable sedative, analgesic and sympatholytic effects without respiratory depression and can be used as a sole agent, an adjunct or as a rescue agent. The AAA technique with or without airway intervention is increasingly popular. It is not so dissimilar to Pasquet's second technique as the patient need only be awake for intraoperative testing minimizing patient discomfort. However it is made much easier today with propofol and remifentanil, titrated against patient response, haemodynamic parameters and possibly bispectral index (BIS) monitoring. Remifentanil can also be used to provide analgesia during awake testing. To minimize the risk of hypoventilation or airway obstruction a variety of airway adjuncts are available, ranging from a nasopharyngeal airway to a modified endotracheal tube. However the laryngeal mask airway is very popular as it is easy to insert and remove, well tolerated at lighter planes of anaesthesia and it allows ventilation to be controlled, providing optimal operative conditions. Non-invasive positive pressure ventilation (biphasic positive airway pressure and proportional assist ventilation) has been used successfully for awake craniotomy, as has pressure support ventilation for patients with obstructive sleep apnoea. These are far removed from Pasquet's blind nasal intubation.

We too find that our techniques are in a 'continuous state of transformation'. However the enthusiasm for awake craniotomy is such now that it has even been suggested that it could become routine for supratentorial tumours irrespective of functional cortex. Awake craniotomy is associated with a lower requirement for high-dependency care, shorter hospital stay and reduced costs.

Paper 4: General anaesthesia versus local anaesthesia for carotid surgery (GALA): a multicentre randomized controlled trial

Author details

GALA Trial Collaborative group, SC Lewis, CP Warlow, AR Bodenham, B Colam, PM Rothwell, D Torgerson, D Dellagrammaticas, M Horrocks, C Liapis, AP Banning, M Gough, MJ Gough

Reference

Lancet 2008; **372**: 2132–42.

Abstract

Background: The effect of carotid endarterectomy in lowering the risk of stroke ipsilateral to severe atherosclerotic carotid-artery stenosis is offset by complications during or soon after surgery. We compared surgery under general anaesthesia with that under local anaesthesia because prediction and avoidance of perioperative strokes might be easier under local anaesthesia than under general anaesthesia.

Methods: We undertook a parallel group, multicentre, randomised controlled trial of 3526 patients with symptomatic or asymptomatic carotid stenosis from 95 centres in 24 countries. Participants were randomly assigned to surgery under general (n=1753) or local (n=1773) anaesthesia between June, 1999 and October, 2007. The primary outcome was the proportion of patients with stroke (including retinal infarction), myocardial infarction, or death between randomisation and 30 days after surgery. Analysis was by intention to treat. The trial is registered with Current Control Trials number ISRCTN00525237.

Findings: A primary outcome occurred in 84 (4.8%) patients assigned to surgery under general anaesthesia and 80 (4.5%) of those assigned to surgery under local anaesthesia; three events per 1000 treated were prevented with local anaesthesia (95% CI -11 to 17; risk ratio [RR] 0.94 [95% CI 0.70 to 1.27]). The two groups did not significantly differ for quality of life, length of hospital stay, or the primary outcome in the prespecified subgroups of age, contralateral carotid occlusion, and baseline surgical risk.

Interpretation: We have not shown a definite difference in outcomes between general and local anaesthesia for carotid surgery. The anaesthetist and surgeon, in consultation with the patient, should decide which anaesthetic technique to use on an individual basis.

Summary

There was no definite difference in outcome between general and local anaesthesia for carotid surgery.

Citation count

50.

Related references

1 Rerkasem K, Rothwell PM. Local versus general anaesthesia for carotid endarterectomy. *Cochrane Database Syst Rev* 2008; **4**: CD000126.

2 Gomes M, Soares MO, Dumville JC, *et al.*; GALA Trial Collaborative group. Cost effectiveness analysis of general anaesthesia versus local anaesthesia for carotid surgery (GALA trial). *Br J Surg* 2010; **97**: 1218–25.

Key message

Carotid endarterectomy improves long-term outcome in patients with recently symptomatic, severe carotid stenosis but there is a significant risk of perioperative complications such as stroke. It was suggested that performing the operation under local anaesthesia rather than general anaesthesia might minimize these risks. This was a parallel group multicentre randomized controlled trial of 3,526 patients conducted in 24 countries between 1999–2007. Patients were randomized to local or general anaesthesia by a central trial office. Analysis was by intention to treat. All patients with symptomatic or asymptomatic carotid stenosis for whom surgery was indicated were eligible. Exclusion criteria included: a definite preference for general or local anaesthesia by clinician or patient, inability to cooperate with awake testing during local anaesthesia, patients requiring bilateral carotid endarterectomy or carotid endarterectomy combined with another procedure such as cardiac bypass, no informed consent. Primary endpoints were the proportion of patients alive, stroke free (including retinal infarction) and without myocardial infarction 30 days post surgery. Secondary endpoints were the proportion of patients alive and stroke-free at 1 year, a comparison of health related quality of life at 30 days, surgical adverse events, re-operation and readmission rates, the relative costs of the two methods of anaesthesia, length of stay, and intensive and high-dependency bed occupancy. There were 1,753 procedures in the general anaesthesia group and 1,773 in the local anaesthesia group. Patient demographics and vascular risk factors were similar for both groups. A primary outcome occurred in 84 (4.8%) patients in the general anaesthesia group and 80 (4.5%) in the local anaesthesia group. Three events per 1,000 treated were prevented with local anaesthesia (95% CI −11 to 17; risk ratio 0.94 [95% CI 0.70–1.27]). The two groups did not differ significantly for quality of life, length of hospital stay, or primary outcome in the pre-specified groups of age, contralateral carotid occlusion and baseline surgical risk.

This study failed to show any statistical difference in the risk of stroke or death between general and local anaesthesia for carotid endarterectomy. The anaesthetist and surgeon should decide on an individual basis, in discussion with the patient, which anaesthetic technique to use.

Strengths

The GALA trial was a good, well-designed study. It was the largest study of its kind to date.

Weaknesses

Neither surgery nor anaesthesia were standardized. Analysis was by intention to treat. However there were 167 crossovers between the study groups before initiation of anaesthesia (75 crossed from local to general anaesthesia and 92 switched from general anaesthesia to local) and 69 patients (3.9%) in the local anaesthesia group were converted to general after initiation of anaesthesia. There was the possibility of selection bias where some high-risk patients were excluded. Other criticisms of the study included the use of intraoperative shunts in each group

(43% of patients in the general anaesthesia group had an intraoperative shunt compared with only 14% in the local group). There was no information given on the type of shunts used and it is possible that some shunts such as atraumatic shunts may be associated with a lower incidence of perioperative strokes. Neither was the use of preoperative statins recorded. Finally the 30-day incidence of stroke and death in the GALA trial was only 4.5% and with this low event rate a substantial difference between local and general anaesthesia would be required to reach statistical significance.

Relevance

Before the GALA trial many centres performing carotid endarterectomy already believed that local anaesthesia was inherently safer than general anaesthesia. However this is not supported by these results. Inevitably this has raised questions and lead to some criticisms of the trial. There are potential advantages to performing a carotid endarterectomy in an awake patient. It enables an accurate and continuous assessment of clinical state and the prompt detection of any neurological deterioration allowing more appropriate use of selective shunting. Cerebral and systemic autoregulation should be preserved minimizing the risk of cerebral hypoperfusion. Regional anaesthetic techniques also provide high quality analgesia and any cardiopulmonary morbidity related to the effects of general anaesthesia is reduced. Finally there may be economic advantages to local anaesthesia, which tends to be cheaper than general anaesthesia and is associated with a reduced length of hospital stay. Indeed an economic analysis of the GALA trial showed that patients undergoing carotid endarterectomy under local anaesthesia incurred fewer costs (mean difference £178) compared to patients having general anaesthesia. However, local anaesthesia may itself present problems. Some surgeons are reluctant to perform surgery under local anaesthesia and surgery may be technically more difficult in an awake patient, increasing the risk of a poor result. Local anaesthetic techniques such as superficial or deep cervical plexus blocks and epidural and spinal blocks carry their own risks. Some patients may find being awake during surgery stressful or painful, potentially increasing the risk of myocardial ischaemia. Local anaesthetic techniques are often combined with sedation or even general anaesthesia as adjuncts or rescue regimes for failed local anaesthetic techniques. This can make it difficult to distinguish the effects of one from the other. Finally, it is possible that general anaesthetics themselves may confer some advantages in terms of neuroprotection.

The optimal anaesthetic technique in the current healthcare environment depends on numerous factors. With so many confounding variables it may be that there is no simple answer to this question. However no trial to date has been powered to detect an effect on mortality reliably and the numbers required to detect an effect (about 20,000 patients) are such that it is unlikely that a sufficiently large randomized trial study will do so in the foreseeable future.

Paper 5: The role of secondary brain injury in determining outcome from severe head injury

Author details

RM Chesnut, LF Marshall, MR Klauber, BA Blunt, N Baldwin, HM Eisenberg, JA Jane, A Marmarou, MA Foulkes

Reference

Journal of Trauma 1993; **34**: 216–22.

Summary

The investigators used data from the TCDB to elaborate on their previous publication detailing the prevalence and significance of secondary systemic insults in severely head-injured patients. In the current paper, the group analysed the data as four mutually exclusive categories: neither hypoxia nor hypotension, hypoxia only, hypotension only, and hypoxia and hypotension combined. Additional controls were applied for age and severe multiple trauma. The investigators confirmed the earlier study findings that secondary insults of hypoxia and hypotension significantly worsen outcome in severe head injury patients. Further analysis separated hypoxia and hypotension into mutually exclusive categories. Hypotension was revealed as the major determinant of overall increased morbidity and mortality. The detrimental effect of hypoxia was significant and the combination of both was significantly greater than hypotension alone. Hypoxia may have less impact in patients >40 years old but remains an independent predictor of outcome. There was a significant trend towards poorer outcome in head injured patients with severe multiple trauma but correction for hypotension and hypoxia removed this significance.

Citation count

1289.

Related references

1 Miller JD, Becker DP. Secondary insults to the injured brain. *J R Coll Surg Edin* 1982; **27**; 292.
2 Bullock MR, Povlishock JT (eds) Brain Trauma Foundation Guidelines for the management of severe traumatic brain injury *J Neurotrauma* 2007; 24(suppl 1): 1–106.

Key message

The authors introduce the concept that the severely head injured patient is, first and foremost, sensitive to the adverse effects of hypotension when associated with multiple injuries. Hypoxia plays a secondary but still significant role. The potentially devastating effect of secondary hypotensive insult in the head injured patient is noted. The authors make a clear case for the prioritization of prevention and immediate corrective treatment of hypotension in traumatic head injury.

Strengths

Noting the significant previous publications on secondary insults, the authors used the large TCDB cohort to substantiate further the frequency and clinical importance of hypotension and hypoxia in the outcome from severe head injury. The methodology is clearly outlined and can be easily followed. They were able to identify the scale of the impact of hypotension and hypoxia on the outcome from severe head injury.

Weaknesses

This study was a retrospective review of previously prospectively collected data on patients with head injury. The methodology identifies inclusion and exclusion criteria; however the sample population is derived from four trauma centres in the USA. Thirty-eight per cent of patients were transferred from other institutions to the TCDB hospitals. The adverse effects of transfer are not commented upon.

Relevance

Hypotension in relation to injury is easily recognized clinically and assessed objectively. The initial treatment strategies of haemorrhage control and volume replacement are vital steps in ensuring that patients with severe head injury have the best possible chance of a good outcome. This paper very simply demonstrates the pivotal role of hypotension and, to a lesser extent, that of hypoxia in the pathogenesis of secondary brain injury. The differences between hypotension and hypoxia are eloquently described by way of the differential sensitivity of the brain to oxygenation and perfusion. Additional treatment strategies are suggested and remain topics for further research today, for example hypertonic saline, colloid versus crystalloid and inotropic or vasopressor drugs. In their closing remarks the authors state that some secondary injuries may not be treatable or preventable and require further research. The visionary aspect of this paper is its proposal, based on the observations made, that outcome in severe head injury with secondary brain injury can be improved by a comprehensive approach to the whole injury including highly directed triage protocols and pharmacological neuronal protection.

Paper 6: Cerebral perfusion pressure: management protocol and clinical results

Author details

MJ Rosner, SD Rosner, AH Johnson

Reference

Journal of Neurosurgery 1995; **83**: 949–62.

Summary

This paper tests the effectiveness of a management protocol designed to prevent cerebral ischaemia after traumatic brain injury (TBI). The protocol describes how CPP is kept at levels adequate to maintain cerebral blood flow and thus prevent ischaemic damage. The study recruited in 158 patients with TBI and GCS of 7 or less. It outlines admission orders for the management of patients with acute TBI thereby entraining the prospective collection of over 100 patient variables. Morbidity and mortality in all GCS categories were compared to Traumatic Coma Data Bank (TCDB) data. The work demonstrates that morbidity and mortality were directly related to admission GCS, the lower the GCS, the worse the outcome. The study highlights the relevance in preventing cerebral ischaemia after TBI by demonstrating that, in all GCS categories, morbidity and mortality improved with CPP management when compared to ICP-based techniques. Similar improvement is seen in favourable outcome rates.

Citation count

699.

Related references

1 Rosner MJ, Daughton S. Cerebral perfusion pressure management in head injury. *J Trauma* 1990; **30**: 933–40.

2 Howells T, Elf K, Jones PA, *et al.* Pressure reactivity as a guide in the treatment of cerebral perfusion pressure in patients with brain trauma. *J Neurosurg* 2005; **102**: 311–17.

Key message

CPP management as the primary treatment target leads to better patient outcome (morbidity and mortality) compared to management strategies using ICP-directed techniques in patients with severe TBI.

Strengths

The paper is an observational study of a CPP management strategy in 158 patients with severe TBI. The two hypotheses being tested are clearly stated. Over 100 variables are measured and relevant criteria are synthesized. Inclusion and exclusion criteria are well defined. Much of the raw data are displayed. The beneficial results of CPP treatment forced previously accepted ICP-targeted strategies to be questioned. This CPP concept remains the mainstay of TBI management strategies today.

Weaknesses

The study uses historical comparisons from the TCDB although this limitation is noted in the study discussion. The timescale during which the study was undertaken is not described thus limiting the reproducibility of the study.

Relevance

Outcome from severe TBI is affected by the severity of cerebral ischaemia produced following injury (secondary brain injury). The primary goal of an adequate CPP is to maintain cerebral blood flow and thus brain tissue oxygenation, metabolism, and function. The CPP is the most amenable variable to clinical manipulation. Prior to the introduction of a CPP-directed management protocol, treatment strategies used ICP as a primary treatment goal. The ICP-goal-directed studies demonstrated little impact on outcome from TBI and this lead some to conclude that ICP monitoring was not useful. It is now recognized that CPP, ICP, and mean arterial pressure are all intimately linked and that CPP has the greatest effect on cerebral haemodynamics. Active management of CPP has afforded significant improvement in the expected outcomes from TBI. The protocol has been refined subsequently based on up-to-date best evidence. Incorporation of the CPP concept into computer-based technologies has lead to the development of new diagnostic and treatment parameters (pressure reactivity index).

Paper 7: A new therapy of post-trauma brain oedema based on haemodynamic principles for brain volume regulation

Author details

B Asgeirsson, PO Grände, CH Nordström

Reference

Intensive Care Medicine 1994; **20**: 260–7.

Abstract

Objective: To evaluate a new therapy of posttraumatic brain oedema, with the main concept that opening of the blood-brain barrier upsets the normal brain volume regulation, inducing oedema formation. This means that transcapillary fluid fluxes will be controlled by hydrostatic capillary and colloid osmotic pressures, rather than by crystalloid osmotic pressure. If so, brain oedema therapy should include reduction of hydrostatic capillary pressure and preservation of normal colloid osmotic pressure.

Patients: 11 severely head injured comatose patients with brain swelling, raised intracranial pressure (ICP), and impaired cerebrovascular response to hyperventilation.

Interventions: To reduce capillary hydrostatic pressure the patients were given hypotensive therapy (beta 1-antagonist, metoprolol and alpha 2-agonist, clonidine) and a potential precapillary vasoconstrictor (dihydroergotamine). The latter may also decrease cerebral blood volume through venous capacitance constriction. Colloid osmotic pressure was maintained by albumin infusions. The concept implies the need of a negative fluid balance with preserved normovolaemia.

Results: ICP decreased significantly within a few hours of treatment with unaltered perfusion pressure in spite of lowered blood pressure. Of 11 patients 9 survived with good recovery/moderate disability, 2 died. This was compared to outcome in a historical control group with identical entry criteria, given conventional brain oedema therapy, where mortality/vegetativity/severe disability was 100%.

Conclusion: The results indicate that the therapy should focus on extracellular rather than intracellular oedema and that ischemia is not the main triggering mechanism behind oedema formation. We suggest that our therapy is superior to conventional therapy by preventing herniation during the healing period of the blood-brain barrier.

Summary

The authors evaluated a new therapy to manage post-traumatic brain oedema. The theory proposes that traumatic brain injury (TBI) damages the blood–brain barrier (BBB) and this disturbs the normal brain volume regulation leading to oedema formation. This extracellular oedema is a major cause of raised intracranial pressure (ICP). The therapeutic intervention aims to reduce raised capillary hydrostatic pressure whilst boosting the colloid osmotic pressure and ensuring the patient is in overall negative fluid balance. Eleven patients were recruited and following therapeutic intervention all patients demonstrated a significant fall in ICP and mean arterial pressure but cerebral perfusion pressure (CPP) was maintained. Nine patients survived with good recovery/moderate disability and two patients died. These outcomes were favourable in comparison to matched historical controls receiving conventional therapy where outcomes of mortality/ vegetative state/severe disability were 100%.

This was a small cohort study consisting of 11 patients. All 11 fulfilled the inclusion criteria: Glasgow Coma Score (GCS) <8 for 12 h or more, CT findings of diffuse brain swelling with absence of space occupying lesion and impaired cerebral vasoreactivity to hyperventilation ($\Delta CBF/\Delta PCO_2$ ≤1 or no reduction in ICP). All patients had ICP monitoring and CBF measurement and six had jugular venous bulb catheters permitting calculation of a-v DO_2. Hyperventilation was not employed. Thiopentone was infused to depress the EEG moderately. Capillary hydrostatic pressure was reduced using dihydroergotamine as a precapillary vasoconstrictor. Mild hypotension was achieved using metoprolol with or without clonidine. Glucose control was tight. The therapeutic concept required simultaneous negative fluid balance with preserved normovolaemia. This was achieved using infusion of albumin, blood and diuretics as required. MAP and ICP were charted from the commencement of therapy for the following 36 h. MAP and ICP decreased in the first 6 h of treatment and thereafter MAP remained stable whilst ICP continued to drop over the next 6 h to reach the desired level of 20 mmHg. According to the Glasgow Outcome Scale nine patients survived, six with good recovery, three with moderate disability, and two died. One of the survivors underwent bilateral frontal craniotomies to prevent impending brainstem herniation.

Citation count

179.

Related references

1 Rosner MJ, Daughton S. Cerebral perfusion pressure management in head injury. *J Trauma* 1990; **30**: 933–41.

2 Miller JD, Dearden MM, Piper IR, *et al.* Control of intracranial pressure in patients with severe head injury. *J Neurotrauma* 1992; **9**(Suppl 1): 317–26.

3 Grände P, Asgeirsson B, Nordström CH. A new potential therapy for treatment of posttraumatic brain oedema based on haemodynamic principles for brain volume regulation. In: Nakamura N, Hashimoto T, Yasue M (eds) *Recent Advances in Neurotraumatology*, pp. 319–22. Tokyo: Springer, 1993.

Key message

In patients with severe head injury, this new therapy based on basic physiological principles effectively reduces ICP and improves outcome.

Strengths

The physiological basis of the new therapeutic regime is logical and well outlined. Physiological variables for the actively treated patients are presented for review. The outcomes of treatment appear to be very favourable compared to the historical controls.

Weaknesses

This is a cohort study of 11 patients. There are several treatment variables included but there is no detail in the text that describes how much of any of the stated drugs were required (metoprolol, clonidine, thiopentone, for example). There is no detail relating to the historical controls—although it is stated that they underwent conventional therapy, it is not clear what this entailed. No detail is given of the two deaths other than that patient 8 was considered beyond treatment at the time of recruitment. It is not clear whether the two deaths were included in the data analysis. Thiopentone was infused to depress the EEG moderately but there is no information of how often burst suppression was induced. Hyperthermia received brief mention simply to say it was restricted.

Relevance

The paper identifies the significance of brain oedema, raised ICP, and altered brain volume regulation in traumatic brain injury. High ICP with low CPP and impaired vasoreactivity to hyperventilation all correlate with poor outcome. Conventional CPP based management is based on the premise that ischaemia is a major factor in secondary brain injury. Current conventional therapies (hyperventilation, barbiturate infusion, osmotic agents, cerebrospinal fluid drainage) all have their downsides. The concept described in this paper relies on hydrostatic capillary pressure and colloid osmotic pressure controlling transcapillary fluid transfer and the development of interstitial oedema and thus advances understanding. The paper concludes that brain oedema following TBI is of two kinds: intracellular and extracellular, the former due to ischaemic damage and the latter due to disturbed haemodynamics. By attending to the latter, permitting BBB to repair in the meantime, the former will be minimized. The paper makes a plea for further research in this area.

Paper 8: Treatment of ischemic deficits from vasospasm with intravascular volume expansion and induced arterial hypertension

Author details

NF Kassel, SJ Peerless, QJ Durward, DW Beck, CG Drake, HP Adams

Reference

Neurosurgery 1982; **11**(3): 337–43.

Summary

Fifty-eight consecutive patients treated with induced hypertension to reverse vasospasm induced neurological deficit were reviewed retrospectively. Vasospasm was confirmed angiographically. The treatment protocol evolved over the course of the case series. Deficits due to raised intracranial pressure (ICP) were managed using mannitol or cerebrospinal fluid (CSF) drainage before addressing blood pressure. Volume expansion was implemented first with either whole blood, packed cells (haematocrit of 40) and supplemented with plasma fractionate or albumin. Crystalloids were used to maintain normal plasma electrolytes. Mineralocorticoids were occasionally used to aid maintenance of the hypervolaemic state. CVP and pulmonary capillary wedge pressure (PCWP) were maintained at 10 mmHg and 18–20 mmHg respectively. Vagal depressor responses were blocked with atropine and vasopressin was given intramuscularly to keep urine output <200 ml h^{-1}. The preferred vasopressors were dopamine and dobutamine and their use if required followed volume expansion. Target blood pressure (BP) was that required to produce reversal of the deficit and thereafter the BP was allowed to drift down to a level required to sustain acceptable neurological function. Complete or partial resolution of deficits occurred in 81% of patients within 1 h of commencement of hypervolaemic/hypertensive therapy. In 7% the improvement was only temporary. Permanent improvement occurred in 74% whilst 6% experienced neurological deterioration during treatment, usually as cerebral infarction had already occurred. Nineteen serious complications were associated with the treatment protocol (aneurysmal rebleed 19%, pulmonary oedema 17%).

Citation count

491.

Related references

1 Denny-Brown D. The treatment of recurrent cerebrovascular symptoms and the question of vasospspam, *Med Clin North Am* 1951; **35**:1457–74.

2 Hunt WE, Kosnik EJ. Timing and peri-operative care in intracranial arterial aneurysm surgery. *Clin Neurosurgery* 1974; **21**: 79–98.

3 Kosnik EJ, Hunt WE. Post-operative hypertension in the management of patients with intracranial aneurysms. *J Neurosurg* 1976; **45**: 148–53.

Key message

Vasospasm accounts for the majority of morbidity and mortality after aneurysmal subarachnoid haemorrhage. Volume expansion and induced arterial hypertension are effective in reversing the ischaemic neurological deficits caused by vasospasm.

Strengths

This paper addresses the hypothesis that induced hypertension and hypervolaemia reverse or remove ischaemic neurological deficits following aneurysmal subarachnoid haemorrhage. Although similar case series were published in the 1980s this was the largest series to date and showed clear neurological functional benefit as a result of intravascular volume expansion and induced arterial hypertension. The study included description of complications and explanation of treatment failures. A major benefit was the publication of an outline for the rationale for treatment of vasospasm after ruptured berry aneurysm.

Weaknesses

The study design is a retrospective case note review of a relatively small number of patients (n=58). The authors noted this and also suggested that a randomized controlled trial was required. There are limited raw data for review in the published paper. The published results of this and other studies of its kind have meant that, ethically, it is difficult to deny treatment in order to undertake an appropriately designed trial.

Relevance

The deleterious effects of vasospasm on cerebral blood flow had been clarified by work during the 1970s. Interest had grown around showing that induced hypertension and hypervolaemia might improve the ischaemic neurological deficit following aneurysmal subarachnoid haemorrhage. Despite advances in the management of vasospasm following subarachnoid haemorrhage, morbidity and mortality remained high. This paper was a landmark in providing evidence of benefit from hypervolaemia and induced hypertension but the study also demonstrated the significant risks involved in increasing blood volume and blood pressure in association with unclipped/uncoiled aneurysms and in the presence of multiple aneurysms. Many of the adverse events were related to overhydration and the inability to predict optimal fluid loading accurately. In addition, 16% of the study group showed no improvement and 10% deteriorated with treatment, highlighting the complex pathophysiology of vasospasm. It remains true today that optimal treatment requires prevention and reversal of post subarachnoid haemorrhage arterial narrowing.

Paper 9: Effect of intravenous corticosteroids on death within 14 days in 10 008 adults with clinically significant head injury (MRC CRASH trial): randomised placebo-controlled trial

Author details

I Roberts, D Yates, P Sandercock, B Farrell, J Wasserberg, G Lomas, R Cottingham, P Svoboda, N Brayley, G Mazairac, V Laloe, A Munoz-Sanchez, B Arango M, Hartzenberg, H Khamis, S Yutthakasemsunt, E Komolafe, F Olldashi, Y Yadav, F Murillo-Cabezas, H Shakur, P Edwards

Reference

Lancet 2004; **364**: 1321–8.

Abstract

Background: Corticosteroids have been used to treat head injuries for more than 30 years. In 1997, findings of a systematic review suggested that these drugs reduce risk of death by 1–2%. The CRASH trial—a multicentre international collaboration—aimed to confirm or refute such an effect by recruiting 20000 patients. In May, 2004, the data monitoring committee disclosed the unmasked results to the steering committee, which stopped recruitment.

Methods: 10008 adults with head injury and a Glasgow coma score (GCS) of 14 or less within 8 h of injury were randomly allocated 48 h infusion of corticosteroids (methylprednisolone) or placebo. Primary outcomes were death within 2 weeks of injury and death or disability at 6 months. Prespecified subgroup analyses were based on injury severity (GCS) at randomisation and on time from injury to randomisation. Analysis was by intention to treat. Effects on out-comes within 2 weeks of randomisation are presented in this report. This study is registered as an International Standard Randomised Controlled Trial, number ISRCTN74459797.

Findings: Compared with placebo, the risk of death from all causes within 2 weeks was higher in the group allocated corticosteroids (1052 [21.1%] vs 893 [17.9%] deaths; relative risk 1.18 [95% CI 1.09–1.27]; p=0.0001). The relative increase in deaths due to corticosteroids did not differ by injury severity (p=0.22) or time since injury (p=0.05).

Interpretation: Our results show there is no reduction in mortality with methylprednisolone in the 2 weeks after head injury. The cause of the rise in risk of death within 2 weeks is unclear.

Summary

In 1997 a systematic review of the use of steroids in head injury was published suggesting a 1–2% decrease in risk of death as compared controls. However the 95% confidence intervals ranged from 6% fewer to 2% more deaths. The CRASH collaborators enrolled 239 hospitals from 49 countries into the study into the randomized trial. The aim was simple: to confirm or refute the effectiveness of steroids in head injury. Patient inclusion criteria were: adults (≥16 years) with head injury, within 8 h of injury and Glasgow Coma Score (GCS) of ≤14. Eligibility was based on the uncertainty principle: if steroid therapy was actively indicated or contraindicated the patient was not recruited. A total of 10,008 patients were recruited. The methodology includes reference to power calculation, randomization and allocation, blinding, 'intention to treat' and analysis. Twenty-one per cent were allocated treatment via a central telephone randomization and 79% were randomized using local packs. Ninety-nine per cent of patients completed the full loading dose ($100\,\mathrm{ml\,h^{-1}}$ infusion of steroid or placebo). Eighty-three per cent completed the full treatment protocol ($20\,\mathrm{ml\,h^{-1}}$ infusion of steroid or placebo for 48 h). Pre-specified subgroup analysis based on injury severity (GCS) at time of randomization and time from injury to randomization did not affect the relative risk of death at 2 weeks post injury.

Citation count

282.

Related references

1 Brachen MB, Shephard MJ, Collins WF, *et al*. A randomised controlled trial of methylprednsiolone or naloxone in the treatment of acute spinal cord injury. *N Engl J Med* 1990; **322**: 1405–11.

2 Alderson P, Roberts I. Corticosteroids in acute traumatic brain injury: a systematic review of randomised trials. *BMJ* 1997; **314**: 1855–9.

3 Bracken MB. Pharmacological interventions for acute spinal cord injury. *Cochrane Database Syst Rev* 2000; **2**: CD001046.

Key message

Methylprednisolone is not useful in the management of patients following traumatic brain injury.

Strengths

This is a remarkable piece of work. It is an excellent example of a large multicentre randomized controlled trial reporting a 98% adherence to treatment protocol. The authors rightly identify their attention to detail in methodology as a strength; the detail taken in randomizing and blinding and the application of intention to treat analysis deserves special mention.

Weaknesses

The group failed to recruit from centres in North America. Only 21% of patients were centrally allocated. The majority were allocated by local pack arrangements there for introducing the possibility of bias. The authors identify that they did not ask participating clinicians for their views on the cause of death. There is no information on the causation of increased mortality in the steroid treatment group. There was no mention of glucose control being considered, hyperglycaemia being a known consequence of steroid therapy. Steroids have been shown to be of benefit in acute spinal cord injury. No data was collected regarding spinal injury. Guidance for treatment in situations of dual injury (brain and spinal cord) cannot be given.

Relevance

For many years, steroids have been used to treat head injuries with the aim of reducing ICP and brain swelling and minimizing post-traumatic inflammatory changes. The healthcare burden of traumatic brain injury is huge with many patients dying or suffering permanent disability. Small changes in overall survival numbers and quality of outcome would have significant global effects. Prior to the CRASH trial publication only small trials amounting to 2000 patients in total had been studied. The sheer size of the sample in the CRASH trial reliably refutes any previous assertions of a benefit with steroid therapy. Previous reports state that 14% of UK intensive care units and 64% of US trauma units used steroids in traumatic head-injured patients. This exemplary study has changed practice globally with clear implications for improving outcome in the management of traumatic brain injury.

Paper 10: International subarachnoid aneurysm trial (ISAT) of neurosurgical clipping versus endovascular coiling in 2143 patients with ruptured intracranial aneurysms: a randomized trial

Author details

AJ Molyneux, RSC Kerr, I Stratton, P Sandercock, M Clarke, J Shrimpton, R Holman; International subarachnoid aneurysm trial (ISAT) Collaborative group

Reference

Lancet 2002; **360**: 1267–74.

Abstract

Background: Endovascular detachable coil treatment is being increasingly used as an alternative to craniotomy and clipping for some ruptured intracranial aneurysms, although the relative benefits of these two approaches have yet to be established. We undertook a randomised, multicentre trial to compare the safety and efficacy of endovascular coiling with standard neurosurgical clipping for such aneurysms judged to be suitable for both treatments.

Methods: We enrolled 2143 patients with ruptured intracranial aneurysms and randomly assigned them to neurosurgical clipping (n=1070) or endovascular treatment by detachable platinum coils (n=1073). Clinical outcomes were assessed at 2 months and at 1 year with interim ascertainment of rebleeds and death. The primary outcome was the proportion of patients with a modified Rankin scale score of 3–6 (dependency or death) at 1 year. Trial recruitment was stopped by the steering committee after a planned interim analysis. Analysis was per protocol.

Findings: 190 of 801 (23.7%) patients allocated endovascular treatment were dependent or dead at 1 year compared with 243 of 793 (30.6%) allocated neurosurgical treatment (p=0.0019). The relative and absolute risk reductions in dependency or death after allocation to an endovascular versus neurosurgical treatment were 22.6% (95% CI 8.9–34.2) and 6.9% (2.5–11.3), respectively. The risk of rebleeding from the ruptured aneurysm after 1 year was two per 1276 and zero per 1081 patient-years for patients allocated endovascular and neurosurgical treatment, respectively.

Interpretation: In patients with a ruptured intracranial aneurysm, for which endovascular coiling and neurosurgical clipping are therapeutic options, the outcome in terms of survival free of disability at 1 year is significantly better with endovascular coiling. The data available to date suggest that the long-term risks of further bleeding from the treated aneurysm are low with either therapy, although somewhat more frequent with endovascular coiling.

Summary

Endovascular coiling was introduced into clinical practice in 1990 and prior to this the standard treatment was surgical clipping of the neck of the aneurysm. However the relative efficacy and safety of the two treatments had not been established. For patients in good clinical condition with ruptured aneurysms, for which endovascular coiling and neurosurgical clipping are both therapeutic options, coiling is associated with a better outcome. Long-term risks of rebleeding from treated aneurysms are low for both interventions but more frequent with coiling.

Citation count

674.

Related references

1 Molyneux AJ, Kerr RSC, Yu L, *et al.* for the International subarachnoid aneurysm trial (ISAT) Collaborative Group. International subarachnoid aneurysm trial (ISAT) of neurosurgical clipping versus endovascular coiling in 2143 patients with ruptured intracranial aneurysms: a randomized comparison of effects on survival, dependency, seizures, re-bleeding, subgroups, and aneurysm occlusion. *Lancet* 2005; **366**: 809–17.

2 Molyneux AJ, Kerr RSC, Birks J, *et al.* for the ISAT collaborators. Risk of recurrent subarachnoid haemorrhage, death, or dependence and standardized mortality ratios after clipping or coiling of an intracranial aneurysm in the International subarachnoid aneurysm trial (ISAT): long term follow up. *Lancet Neurol* 2009; **8**: 427–33.

Key message

In patients with ruptured intracranial aneurysms suitable for both treatments, endovascular coiling is more likely to result in independent survival at 1 year than neurosurgical clipping.

Strengths

ISAT was a statistically powerful study, which has had a greater impact on the management of ruptured intracranial aneurysms than any other study to date and has resulted in significant changes to treatment policy in most countries.

Weaknesses

The most widely aired criticism of the trial has centred on the randomization process. Of the 9,559 patients assessed for eligibility only 2,143 were randomized (22%). Although this may be an indication that only a minority of aneurysms are truly suitable for either coiling or clipping an alternative explanation is that pre-existing bias in participating surgeons prevented referral. In addition there was an increased time from randomization to surgery in the neurosurgical group, which may have led to poorer outcome in this group as a result of re-bleeds. As the majority of aneurysms were small (90%) and in the anterior circulation (95%) the results of the ISAT trial cannot be extrapolated to all aneurysms. Most patients were recruited from centres with enthusiastic interventional neuroradiology services and, although specialist neurovascular surgical experience was not a requirement, the interventional neuroradiologists were all specialists. Consequently it has been suggested that the better outcome in the coiled patients might be explained by differences in practitioner expertise and experience. However at the time of the ISAT trial, interventional radiology was a relatively new specialty with some interventionalists only having begun coiling aneurysms in the previous few years. The third major criticism of the trial has been of the outcome measures. The primary endpoints were measured at one year but not subsequently. Although assessment of secondary endpoints is ongoing this is mostly in the UK. The ability to adequately assess clinical status using a postal questionnaire has also been questioned and, as time passes, it becomes difficult to distinguish any specific effect of the intervention on outcome of morbidity and mortality as patient's age and comorbidities increase. Finally there is the issue of long-term recurrence and late rebleeds. About 20% of patients who have had a subarachnoid haemorrhage from a ruptured aneurysm will have more than one aneurysm at presentation and they remain at continuing risk of developing new aneurysms. Female gender and smoking are known risk factors (unfortunately smoking history was not collected). Although rebleeding rates in both groups were low retreatment was 6.9 times more likely in patients who had endovascular treatment. Younger age, larger lumen size and incomplete occlusion are all risk factors for recurrence. This is of particular importance as many patients who present with subarachnoid haemorrhage are young (mean age at entry into trial was 52 years).

Relevance

ISAT demonstrated that those patients who have rupture of small anterior circulation aneurysms and good World Federation of Neurosurgeons (WFNS) grade have better clinical outcome after endovascular coiling than clipping. It has undoubtedly radically altered the management of patients with ruptured cerebral aneurysms. However concerns about the long-term risks of recurrence and re-bleeding in patients who have been coiled remain.

Chapter 12

Thoracic anaesthesia

J Macdonald and A Macfie

Chapter 12

Thoracic anaesthesia

Fredrik Olsen & A Marshe

Introduction

A thoracic anaesthetist from the first part of the 20th century would have difficulty comprehending the advances made over the past 80 years in the anaesthetic management and perioperative care of the thoracic surgical patient. Up until the early 1930s, thoracic surgeons operated in a 'smash and grab' manner due to the deleterious effects quickly encountered on the creation of a pneumothorax when the operative hemithorax was opened. Resultant lung collapse, mediastinal shift, disruption of respiratory mechanics, and hypoxaemia afforded little time for surgical deliberation. In the ensuing years advances in anaesthetic equipment and practice have allowed safe and successful complex surgeries in patients with more comorbidities and in poorer preoperative condition.

The introduction of reliable equipment and methods for lung isolation and differential ventilation heralded a major advance. This afforded a safe (isolated) environment for the dependent lung, together with a suitable surgical environment. The Carlens tube provided the substrate for Robertshaw's modifications producing a double-lumen tube with an improved airway resistance profile; today, several manufacturers produce disposable double-lumen tubes still based upon Robertshaw's original design, and hence this is our first Landmark Paper. Malposition of double-lumen tubes (and indeed bronchial blockers) is an important cause of hypoxaemia and potential morbidity during one-lung anaesthesia. Benumof's paper, based upon anatomical airway measurements coupled with a series of double-lumen tube lengths and diameters, highlights the margin of safety in double-lumen tube positioning. This paper details a number of important clinical recommendations, and is our second Landmark Paper. To complete this theme, Smith's paper on the use of fibreoptic bronchoscopy to delineate tube position is Paper 3; it heralded much debate as to the requirement for the routine use of fibreoptic bronchoscopy in ascertaining double-lumen tube position.

Appropriate patient selection for thoracic surgery is paramount. Without surgery, survival from lung cancer is very poor. Balanced against this is the major surgical insult imposed upon the patient, especially if the patient's physical reserve is questionable. Evidence exists that traditional patient selection criteria as to suitability for lung resection may be too stringent and that high-risk patients can do well, implying that we may be denying patients surgery. The Brunelli paper influenced the new British Thoracic Society Guidelines on the radical management of patients with lung cancer, and is our fourth Landmark Paper.

There is accumulating evidence that lung inflammation plays a pivotal role in lung injury associated with one-lung ventilation, as well as in post lung resection acute lung injury. This was recognized in the early 1980s by Zeldin and termed 'post pneumonectomy edema'. However, this was mistakenly attributed to excess fluid administration, rather than being attributed to inflammation per se. Zeldin's paper is thus our fifth Landmark Paper. Further evidence suggests that mechanical ventilation per se triggers a dysregulated inflammatory response even in the normal lung (ventilator induced lung injury), and this response is further exaggerated during one-lung ventilation. Ventilator induced Inflammatory injury appears related to high tidal volume and high peak inspiratory pressure ventilation, and thus may be modified by a protective ventilatory strategy akin to that employed in the critical care setting in acute lung injury (ALI) and acute respiratory distress syndrome (ARDS). Schilling's paper is our sixth Landmark Paper, documenting a significantly enhanced inflammatory response to higher tidal volume ventilation, suggesting that a protective ventilator strategy should be employed during one-lung ventilation. Paper 7 by Yang moves this hypothesis a step forward in a prospective randomized trial, finding that a protective ventilation strategy would appear to reduce the risk of pulmonary complications after lung cancer surgery. Fortunately, it would also appear that this inflammatory response can be reduced by inhalational anaesthetic agents.

Attention has turned toward the potential for the choice of post-thoracotomy analgesia regimen to modulate outcomes from thoracic surgery. Richardson, the main author of our Paper 8, generated much debate with his findings that paravertebral analgesia appeared to be superior to epidural blockade on a number of fronts, including analgesia and postoperative respiratory morbidity. A well-conducted systematic review by Davies and colleagues (Paper 9) found no difference in analgesia with paravertebral block techniques when compared to epidural regimens. Paravertebral blockade was, however, associated with improvements in respiratory function and a reduction in complications, findings complemented by the recently published UKPOS study of analgesia and outcome after pneumonectomy.

So what does the future hold? We have already seen advances in ventilation strategy translated from the critical care arena to the thoracic surgery setting. The new technologies of pumpless interventional lung assist (iLA) devices have a developing role in critical care. Our final Landmark Paper from Wiebe breaks new ground by taking these techniques into the operating room. This offers new challenges to anaesthetists and surgeons, but may improve outcomes in some of the highest risk cases.

Paper 1: Low resistance double-lumen endobronchial tubes

Author details

FL Robertshaw

Reference

British Journal of Anaesthesia 1962; **34**: 576–9.

Abstract

A new double-lumen endobronchial tube, suitable for thoracic anaesthesia is described. Both left-and right-sided versions have been developed, in three sizes, suitable for adults and adolescents. It has been designed to have the maximum possible size of lumen. This ensures low resistance to gas flows, and facilitates the use of suction catheters. The resistance has been compared with that of Carlens tubes under conditions simulating those of actual use. The tubes have been in constant use for more than a year, and have been found clinically satisfactory. They are durable and comparatively inexpensive.

Robertshaw FL, 'Low resistance double-lumen endobronchial tubes', *British Journal of Anaesthesia,* 1962, 34, 8, pp. 576–579, by permission of Oxford University Press and British Journal of Anaesthesia.

Summary

Robertshaw describes the development and clinical introduction of a double-lumen endotracheal tube with an improved airway resistance profile (Fig. 12.1).

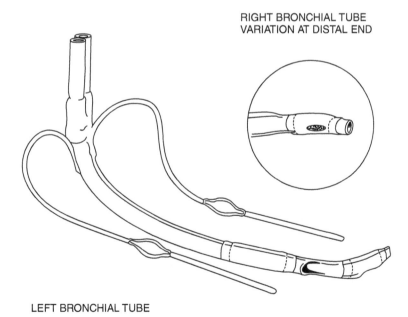

RIGHT BRONCHIAL TUBE
VARIATION AT DISTAL END

LEFT BRONCHIAL TUBE

Fig. 12.1 Robertshaw's double-lumen tube. Reproduced from F.L. Robertshaw, Low resistance double-lumen endobronchial tubes, *British Journal of Anaesthesia*, 1962, **34**, pp. 576–579, Oxford University Press, by permission of British Journal of Anaesthesia.

Citation count

72.

Related references

1 Carlens E. A new flexible double-lumen catheter for bronchospirometry. *J Thorac Surg* 1949; **18**: 742–6.

2 Bjork VO, Carlens E. The prevention of spread during pulmonary resection by use of a double-lumen catheter. *J Thorac Surg* 1950; **20**: 151–7.

3 Narayanaswamy M, McRae K, Slinger P, *et al*. Choosing a lung isolation device for thoracic surgery: a randomized trial of three bronchial blockers versus double-lumen tubes. *Anesth Analg* 2009; **108**: 1097–101.

Key message

Robertshaw's design for a low resistance double-lumen endobronchial tube provides an effective and improved conduit for lung isolation and one-lung ventilation.

Strengths

The paper describes the introduction of a piece of anaesthetic equipment in the early 1960s which remains pivotal to the safe conduct of thoracic anaesthesia and surgery today, as well as being of great historical significance. It is the 'gold standard'.

Weaknesses

The paper is mainly a narrative, describing the author's own clinical experience over a year, without any rigorous comparison with other double-lumen tubes, or representation from other clinical users. There is also no indication of numbers of tubes inserted.

Relevance

Differential lung isolation and ventilation is pivotal to the safe and effective conduct of thoracic surgery. As well as allowing an optimal surgical field with the collapse of the operated lung, cuffed double-lumen endobronchial tubes afford protection from soiling to the non-operated lung. Double-lumen tubes developed by Carlens (initially for differential broncho-spirometry) paved the way for selective one-lung ventilation. However, the clinical use of double-lumen tubes was initially hampered by issues with accurate endobronchial placement and high airway resistance characteristics. The introduction of Robertshaw's rubber double-lumen tube went a long way to addressing the latter. In Robertshaw's words 'After some years of experience with Carlens catheters, an effort has been made to develop a similar double lumen tube with the largest possible lumina'. Indeed, Robertshaw invented a curved rubber double-lumen tube which could be placed in a relatively straightforward manner, had wider lumina, and was less susceptible to kinking, thereby improving gas flow during one-lung ventilation. Importantly, this was produced in both right- and left-sided versions. Nowadays, a number of manufacturers produce disposable plastic double-lumen tubes based upon this original design by Robertshaw. Whether or not the design will be superseded or alternative methods of lung isolation will prove superior, only time will tell. However, Robertshaw's design has passed the test of time thus far.

Paper 2: Margin of safety in positioning modern double-lumen endotracheal tubes

Author details

JL Benumof, BL Partridge, C Salvatierra, J Keating

Reference

Anesthesiology 1987; **67**: 729–38.

Summary

The authors have defined the 'margin of safety in positioning modern double-lumen endotracheal tubes', as being the 'length of tracheobronchial tree over which it may be moved or positioned without obstructing a conducting airway'. Using three independent methods to obtain average mainstem bronchial length measurement, in combination with right upper lobe and left lower bronchial diameter, and coupled with a series of lengths and diameters of double-lumen tube segments, the authors calculate the margin of safety in positioning of three manufacturers' double-lumen tubes.

Citation count

220.

Related references

1 Ehrenfeld JM, Walsh JL, Sandberg WS. Right- and left-sided mallinckrodt double-lumen tubes have identical clinical performance. *Anesth Analg* 2008; **106**: 1847–52.

2 Ehrenfeld JM, Mulvoy W, Sandberg WS. Performance comparison of right- and left-sided double-lumen tubes among infrequent users. *J Cardiothorac Vasc Anesth* 2010; **24**: 598–601.

Key message

Left-sided double-lumen tubes should be used preferentially, where possible, due to a much greater positioning margin of safety.

The position of all double-lumen tubes should be confirmed with the aid of fibreoptic bronchoscopy.

Larger, rather than smaller, sized double-lumen tubes should be used in practice as the margin of safety either remains constant or increases with increasing tube size (with the attendant reduction in airway resistance and improved secretion removal). A positive correlation between patient height and mainstem bronchial length suggests the use of 39- and 41-French tubes in patients 5 foot 8 inches (174 cm) or taller, and 35–39-French tubes in patients who are shorter.

In view of the small margin of safety in positioning double-lumen tubes, head movement and changes in patient position can displace a previously well-positioned tube. Hence, the position of the tube should be rechecked with the fibreoptic bronchoscope once the patient has been turned into a lateral decubitus position.

Strengths

This is a well thought-out, pragmatic study. Consideration is given to validity of definitions and accuracy of measurements, with anatomical findings in agreement with previous studies.

Weaknesses

Double-lumen tube manufacture, population characteristics, and the normal distribution of anatomical measurements have changed since the paper was published.

Relevance

Issues with airway, ventilation, and perfusion lead to hypoxaemia during one-lung anaesthesia. Malposition of the device used to secure lung isolation remains an important cause of hypoxaemia. This paper details a number of recommendations which were, and continue to be, important in the provision of safe anaesthesia for thoracic surgery when using double-lumen tubes. The preferential use of left-sided double-lumen tubes will be contested by many. Indeed, evidence from a large retrospective study does not support the hypothesis that left-sided double-lumen tubes are safer than right-sided when placed by a thoracic anaesthetist under bronchoscopic control. Interestingly, this finding is replicated in a similar retrospective study amongst infrequent double-lumen tube users. Nevertheless, this paper gives sound evidence-based clinical advice pertaining to the safe conduct of thoracic anaesthesia, which is as pertinent today as it was at the time of publication.

Paper 3: Placement of double-lumen endobronchial tubes. Correlation between clinical impressions and bronchoscopic findings

Author details

GB Smith, NP Hirsch, J Ehrenwerth

Reference

British Journal of Anaesthesia 1986; **58**: 1317–20.

Abstract

Double-lumen endobronchial tubes were placed 'blindly' in 23 patients undergoing thoracotomy. Clinical criteria suggested satisfactory positioning in all cases; however, subsequent fibreoptic bronchoscopy revealed malposition in 48%. Bronchoscopic findings included the inability to view the bronchial cuff, narrowing of the bronchial lumen of the tube at the level of the cuff and herniation of the cuff over the carina. The potential hazards associated with these findings are discussed.

Smith GB, Hirsch NP, Ehrenwerth J, 'Placement of double-lumen endobronchial tubes. Correlation between clinical impressions and bronchoscopic findings', *British Journal of Anaesthesia*, 1986, 58, 11, pp. 1317–1320, by permission of Oxford University Press and British Journal of Anaesthesia.

Summary

Twenty-three consecutive patients undergoing elective thoracotomy requiring the use of a double-lumen tube were studied prospectively. Double-lumen tube (Bronchcath™) insertion was followed by clinical assessment of tube position both before and after positioning each patient for surgery. Fibreoptic bronchoscopy was then undertaken in the lateral position to determine whether bronchoscopic findings confirmed the clinical impression (accurate placement necessitated achieving a number of bronchoscopic criteria). Despite positioning being deemed clinically satisfactory in all 23 patients, fibreoptic bronchoscopy revealed that in only 52% was the position optimal.

Citation count

112.

Related references

1 Klein U, Karzai W, Bloos F, *et al.* Role of fibreoptic bronchoscopy in conjunction with the use of double-lumen tubes for thoracic anaesthesia: a prospective study. *Anesthesiology* 1998; **88**: 346–50.

2 Pennefather SH, Russell GN. Placement of double lumen tubes – time to shed light on an old problem. *Br J Anaesth* 2000; **84**: 308–10.

Key message

Fibreoptic bronchoscopy should be used routinely during double-lumen tube placement to allow accurate confirmation of position and facilitate repositioning.

Strengths

This was the first well-publicized study to prospectively examine the correlation between clinical assessment of double-lumen tube position and the subsequent fibreoptic bronchoscopy findings.

Weaknesses

The study group was small (n=23). There was a lack of standardization in cuff inflation technique and no comment as to the standardization of anaesthetist, or fibreoptic bronchoscopist. The clinical significance of malpositioned tubes in this study is debateable in view of the lack of documented clinical sequelae in the patients studied.

Relevance

Satisfactory placement of a double-lumen tube (or other device such as a bronchial-blocker) is fundamental to the practice of thoracic anaesthesia where lung isolation is necessary. Although Smith's paper describes a small number of subjects, it heralded much debate as to the necessity of fibreoptic bronchoscopy as a routine. 'Minor' malpositions may not lead to any significant clinical sequelae, but 'critical' malpositions and their frequency, as described by Klein and colleagues, cannot and must not be ignored. Hence it would appear difficult to argue against the routine use of fibreoptic bronchoscopy to check tube placement. Pennefather and Russell's (2000) editorial 'Placement of double lumen tubes—time to shed light on an old problem' further references compelling support for its routine use.

Paper 4: Predicted versus observed FEV$_1$ and DLCO after major lung resection: a prospective evaluation at different postoperative periods

Author details

A Brunelli, M Refai, M Salati, F Xiumé, A Sabbatini

Reference

Annals of Thoracic Surgery 2007; **83**: 1134–9.

Abstract

Background: The objective of this study was to prospectively assess the agreement between predicted and observed postoperative values of forced expiratory volume in 1 second (FEV$_1$) and carbon monoxide lung diffusion capacity (DLCO) after major lung resection.

Methods: Two hundred consecutive patients undergoing lobectomy or pneumonectomy for lung cancer in a single center were prospectively evaluated with complete preoperative and repeated postoperative measurements of FEV$_1$ and DLCO. Predicted postoperative (ppo) values were compared with the observed postoperative values. The precision of ppoFEV$_1$ and ppoDLCO at 3 months was subsequently evaluated by plotting the cumulative predicted postoperative values against the observed ones.

Results: After lobectomy, observed values were 11% lower at discharge (p <0.0001), and 6% higher at 3 months (p <0.0001), compared with ppoFEV$_1$. No differences were noted at 1 month. Observed DLCO values were 12% lower than predicted at discharge (p <0.0001) and 10% higher than predicted at 3 months (p <0.0001), without differences noted at 1 month. After pneumonectomy, no differences were noted between predicted and observed values of FEV$_1$ at every evaluation time, and of DLCO at discharge and 1 month. However, the observed DLCO value was 17% higher than predicted at 3 months (p = 0.002). Plots of predicted and observed postoperative values at 3 months showed that ppoFEV$_1$ predicted worse at lower levels of ppoFEV$_1$, and ppoDLCO was constantly lower than the observed values at every ppoDLCO levels.

Summary

In 200 thoracic surgical patients, postoperative FEV$_1$ was lower at discharge and higher at 3 months than that calculated by the postoperative predicted FEV$_1$. This has significant implications for guidelines on the fitness of patients for lung resection.

In this study, the criteria used for inoperability or lesser resections were predicted postoperative FEV$_1$ and predicted postoperative DLCO <30% of predicted in association with insufficient exercise tolerance (height at preoperative stair climbing test less than 12 m or maximum volume oxygen consumption (VO$_{2max}$) measured at cycle ergometry less than 10 ml kg^{-1}min^{-1}). The early postoperative mortality was still only 4% despite this low cut-off.

Citation count

26.

Related references

1 Lim E, Baldwin D, Beckles M, *et al*. Guidelines on the radical management of patients with lung cancer. *Thorax* 2010; **65**: iii1–iii27.

Key message

Given the imprecision of the prediction of postoperative function, particularly of gas exchange determinants after pneumonectomy, and at low ppoFEV$_1$ levels, the use of ppoFEV$_1$ and ppoDLCO for risk stratification needs to be reconsidered.

Strengths

This was a large (n=200) prospective study in a single centre. The patient group was homogenous (all lung cancer patients).

Weaknesses

This study has several potential limitations

* The first limitation is one common to most of the follow-up analyses and concerns the dropped-out patients. As these patients could have been those with the worst functional status, their inclusion in the analysis could have perhaps changed the results, and that should be taken into account when interpreting the results.

* Secondly, a certain proportion of the patients had adjuvant chemotherapy; because chemotherapy has been proved to impair the gas exchange, the inclusion of these patients could have influenced the results. As most of the patients started chemotherapy 4–6 weeks after operation, the problem refers mainly to the last evaluation time (3 months). However, only 20 of the 200 patients studied at 3 months underwent adjuvant chemotherapy. Another 21 patients, who performed the 1-month evaluation test, dropped out for concomitant chemotherapy at 3 months. The authors decided to include the 20 patients under chemotherapy after a preliminary analysis did not show differences in PFTs at 3 months compared with the other patients.

* Finally, the calculation the authors used to estimate ppoFEV$_1$ and ppoDLCO was the one recommended by the British Thoracic Society (BTS) guidelines, which takes into account the degree of obstruction and function of the segments removed during operation. Furthermore, all pneumonectomy candidates and all those lobectomy patients with a FEV$_1$ <70% underwent a quantitative lung perfusion scan, the results of which were used to estimate the percentage of functioning tissue removed. Although these methods are not universally used in clinical practice, recent studies have shown the substantial equivalency of different methods of prediction of residual postoperative function.

Relevance

Recent data show that there is a poor correlation between TLCO and FEV$_1$ (r=0.35) reflecting the fact that they measure very different aspects of lung function. The findings of this study influenced the new joint BTS/SCTS guidelines on the radical management of patients with lung cancer which recommend the measurement of TLCO in all patients undergoing lung resection. This study showed that particularly after pneumonectomy, the postoperative predicted DLCO underestimated the TLCO at 3 months. These data could help the risk stratification of patients undergoing lung resection. An acceptable mortality was achieved using a cut off for post operative predicted FEV$_1$ and TLCO of 30% with careful assessment of functional capacity.

Paper 5: Postpneumonectomy pulmonary edema

Author details

RA Zeldin, D Normandin, D Landtwing

Reference

Journal of Thoracic and Cardiovascular Surgery 1984; **87**: 359–65.

Abstract

Postpneumonectomy pulmonary edema has become a worldwide problem. Study of data available from some of these patients implicates the excessive perioperative volumes of intravenous fluid. A study done on dogs supports the clinical conclusion. The risk factors for this complication are right pneumonectomy, large perioperative fluid load, and high intraoperative and postoperative urine outputs. Patients undergoing pneumonectomy are at greater risk from intravenous fluid than other types of patients.

Summary

This paper investigates the clinical entity of postoperative pulmonary oedema associated with pneumonectomy. The authors have collected a case series of ten patients with postoperative pulmonary oedema from multiple centres and compared the clinical data with 15 patients with uncomplicated pneumonectomy in the author's own hospital. A subset of these patients were then compared (4 pulmonary oedema vs. 6 non-postoperative pulmonary oedema patients). Patients with postoperative pulmonary oedema had higher fluid intakes and higher urinary outputs (67 vs. 46 ml kg^{-1} and 21 vs. 11 ml kg^{-1} respectively). The researchers then went to the animal laboratory and developed an animal model on dogs for postoperative pulmonary oedema. They studied 13 dogs who were subjected to right pneumonectomy and randomized to receiving Ringer's lactate by rapid infusion of 100 ml kg^{-1} before pneumonectomy (Group A n= 8), a slower infusion of 50 ml kg^{-1} at start and an additional 50 ml kg^{-1} during (Group B n= 5). A control group (n=4) received 100ml h^{-1} preoperatively and had no pneumonectomy. The presence of pulmonary oedema was assessed by weighing the removed right lung at pneumonectomy and the weight of the left lung at 48 h when the 'dogs put to death'. A left lung to body weight ratio of >0.68% was used to diagnose pulmonary oedema. L/R lung weight ratio confirmed findings. Six dogs had pulmonary oedema and seven did not. Of these, no controls had pulmonary oedema. There was an overlap in fluid balances between dogs that developed pulmonary oedema and those who did not however all dogs in the fast infusion group (Group A0) developed pulmonary oedema.

Pulmonary oedema occurs when the balance of the factors described by the Starling equation favour the net filtration from capillaries. The Starling equation is as follows:

$$J_f = K_f A \left([P_c - P_t] - \sigma [II_c - II_t] \right),$$

where J_f is quantity of fluid filtered, K_f is filtration constant, A is area of capillary bed perfused, Pc is pulmonary capillary hydrostatic pressure, P_t is pulmonary interstitial hydrostatic pressure, σ is protein reflectance coefficient, II_c is serum colloid osmotic pressure, and II_t is tissue colloidal pressure.

The haemodynamic data revealed that the pulmonary wedge pressure was normal which rules out cardiogenic shock as a contributory feature. However, the high preoperative fluid load resulted in increased cardiac output and pulmonary artery pressure which would elevate the pulmonary capillary hydrostatic pressure if precapillary tone was reduced or unaltered. Serum colloid osmotic pressure was no different between the groups of dog; therefore haemodilution did not appear to be responsible.

It should be noted that the lymphatic system can normally accommodate up to a sevenfold increase in lymphatic flow. However, after right pneumonectomy 55% of the lymphatic system is excised.

The risk factors for postoperative pulmonary oedema were right pneumonectomy, excessive positive perioperative fluid balance and high urine volumes in first 24 h.

Citation count

123.

Related references

1 Wiedemann HP, Wheeler AP, Bernard GR, *et al.* Comparison of two fluid-management strategies in acute lung injury. *N Engl J Med* 2006; **354**: 2564–75.

Key message

Zeldin states controversially that 'Anesthesiologists must not boldly load the patient up with fluids prior to induction'. In summary, PPE appears to result from an infusion of excessive volumes of fluid. This causes an increase in cardiac output and pulmonary artery pressure, which alter the balance of forces in the Starlings equation, increasing net filtration beyond the limited lymphatic pump capacity of the remaining lung. The result is pulmonary oedema in the presence of a normal wedge pressure.

Strengths

This study was well constructed and linked clinical pathophysiology with laboratory investigation. It tackled the life-threatening clinical syndrome of postpneumonectomy pulmonary oedema. Thus was a fantastic piece of work back in 1984.

Weaknesses

There are however, many weaknesses in the scientific design and the subsequent conclusions of this study, including:

- The clinical patient study was a retrospective case note review.
- The patients numbers were small, and the study design was non randomized and multi-institutional.
- The animal study was designed to generate postoperative pulmonary oedema by the infusion of very large volumes of Ringer's Lactate in excess of what would be administered in the clinical context of patients undergoing surgery. They did however show that after pneumonectomy, dogs handled the large fluid load less well and developed pulmonary oedema. Patients in the study who developed pulmonary oedema had a net fluid intake of 37 ml kg^{-1}; in contrast the dogs in the study had a net positive fluid balance of 100 ml kg^{-1} which is three times as much.

The authors have made the assumption that the greater fluid intake of patients with postoperative pulmonary oedema, compared to non randomized controls after pneumonectomy, was causative although evidence to this is absent.

Relevance

This landmark paper from 1984 which has influenced thoracic surgical practice for decades was written by North American thoracic surgeons. In the discussion the author states 'the most important thing that we can do in terms of recognizing this problem is to watch our anesthesiologists as they start loading the patient up with fluid'. The intolerance of excessive administration of crystalloid fluids during and after pneumonectomy is demonstrated by this study and is accepted; however the study and conclusions have been found to be flawed. Later work has shown that excessive fluid administration is not the primary cause of acute lung injury (ALI) associated with pneumonectomy. The pathological findings in postoperative pulmonary oedema are indistinguishable from acute respiratory distress syndrome (ARDS) and ALI. There is an acute lung injury with increased capillary permeability and polymorphoneutrophil sequestration due to inflammatory mediated injury. The exact mechanisms of PPE have still to be defined by future research. The focus on the administration of fluids by anaesthetic and intensive care staff was unhelpful and misleading. There is however a place for conservative fluid management strategies in the care of the lung resection patient as well as the patient with an acute lung injury and or ARDS. Subsequent research published in the *New England Journal of Medicine* in 2006 has shown in ARDS that a conservative strategy of fluid management improved lung function and shortened the duration of mechanical ventilation and intensive care without increasing non-pulmonary organ failures. These results support the use of a conservative strategy of fluid management in patients with acute lung injury. This is however rather different from suggesting that the fluid therapy is the primary cause of the pulmonary oedema.

Paper 6: The pulmonary immune effects of mechanical ventilation in patients undergoing thoracic surgery

Author details

T Schilling, A Kozian, C Huth, F Bühling, M Kretzschmar, T Welte, T Hachenberg

Reference

Anesthesia and Analgesia 2005; **101**: 957–65.

Summary

The data suggest that OLV initiates a proinflammatory response in the alveolar compartment of the dependent lung. Intra-alveolar concentrations of IL-8, TNF-α, PMN elastase, protein, and albumin, as well as cell numbers in the BAL fluids, increased during and after OLV, and anti-inflammatory IL-10 decreased.

Ventilation with Vt $5\,ml\,kg^{-1}$ in comparison with Vt $10\,ml\,kg^{-1}$ significantly decreased alveolar TNF-α and sICAM-1 and increased IL-10 after OLV. However, 2 h postoperatively there were no differences between groups; only sICAM-1 showed a consistent trend to decrease after mechanical ventilation with Vt $5\,ml\,kg^{-1}$.

Citation count

78.

Related references

1 Wrigge H, Zinserling J, Stuber F, *et al.* Effects of mechanical ventilation on release of cytokines into systemic circulation in patients with normal pulmonary function. *Anesthesiology* 2000; **93**: 1413–17.

2 Licker M, de Perrot M, Spiliopoulos A, *et al.* Risk factors for acute lung injury after thoracic surgery for lung cancer. *Anesth Analg* 2003; **97**: 1558–65.

3 Schilling T, Kozian A, Kretzschmar M, et al. Effect of propofol and desflurane anaesthesia on the alveolar inflammatory response to one-lung ventilation. *Br J Anaesth* 2007; **99**: 368–75.

Key message

OLV provokes an inflammatory response in the dependant lung. Small tidal volumes (Vt = $5\,ml\,kg^{-1}$) and a protective ventilator strategy may diminish this response. This study and others suggest that a protective ventilator strategy should be adopted as this may reduce the ventilation induced inflammatory injury to the dependant lung.

Strengths

This comprehensive study, in contrast to Wrigge's paper, used sampling of bronchoalveolar lavage (BAL) fluid to assess the release of inflammatory mediators.

Weaknesses

The main weaknesses of this paper are as follows:

- No attempt is made to link inflammatory response to clinical outcomes; therefore the clinical significance of the findings is unknown.
- The number of study patients is low (n=32).
- One concern is that the very procedure of performing a BAL with bronchoscopic manipulation may itself be responsible for inducing an inflammatory reaction.
- Blinding of investigators was not possible.
- Neither the high nor low Vt group received any PEEP (positive end-expiratory pressure) to correct for loss of lung volume and prevent mechanical injury secondary to repeated opening and closing of alveoli.

Relevance

This paper provides evidence that OLV may contribute to lung injury after thoracic surgery, and also that this injury may be modified by a protective ventilation strategy. Respiratory complications after lung resection are unpredictable and have a multifactorial aetiology. Susceptibility to lung injury due to the effects of lung cancer and/or chemotherapy on oxidative stress, respiratory disease processes, surgical factors (such as trauma), lymphatic drainage loss, respiratory infection, intraoperative ventilator induced injury, blood product transfusion (transfusion-related acute lung injury or TRALI), subclinical aspiration, and inappropriate fluid administration all may contribute to the risk of postoperative ALI and respiratory complications.

This paper adds to the scientific knowledge of the causes of respiratory complications in patients after lung resection, which occurs in up to 30% of patients with the attendant morbidity and mortality, and financial implications of intensive care unit admission and prolonged hospital stay. A subsequent study by Schilling in 2007 using a similar OLV model interestingly indicated that pro-inflammatory reactions during OLV were influenced by the type of general anaesthesia. Different patterns of alveolar cytokines may be a result of increased granulocyte recruitment during propofol anaesthesia.

Paper 7: Does a protective ventilation strategy reduce the risk of pulmonary complications after lung cancer surgery? A randomized controlled trial

Author details

M Yang, HJ Ahn, K Kim, JA Kim, CA Yi, MJ Kim, HJ Kim

Reference

Chest 2011; **139**: 530–7.

Summary

To test their hypothesis, the authors conducted a prospective randomized trial to assess the impact of a standardized protective ventilatory regime as compared to a conventional ventilatory regime on safety during, and on the occurrence of lung complications following, elective lobectomy. They found that the primary endpoint of pulmonary dysfunction was significantly lower in the protective ventilation group than in the conventional ventilation group, with a satisfactory intra-operative safety profile.

Citation count

3.

Related references

1 Michelet P, D'Journo XB, Roch A, *et al.* Protective ventilation influences systemic inflammation after esophagectomy: a randomized controlled study. *Anesthesiology* 2006; **105**: 911–19.

2 De Conno E, Steurer MP, Wittlinger M, *et al.* Anesthetic-induced improvement of the inflammatory response to one-lung ventilation. *Anesthesiology* 2009; **110**: 1316–26.

3 Licker M, Diaper J, Villiger Y, *et al.* Impact of intraoperative lung-protective interventions in patients undergoing lung cancer surgery. *Crit Care* 2009; **13**: R41.

Key message

A protective ventilation strategy, when employed during one-lung ventilation, would appear to reduce the risk of pulmonary complications after lung cancer surgery.

Strengths

This represents the first prospective randomized trial assessing the impact of a standardized protective ventilatory regime on intraoperative safety during, and on the occurrence of lung complications following, lung cancer surgery. Anaesthesia was standardized and although the anaesthetists were not blinded to the strategy used, they were not involved in data collection; the operating surgeon, ITU physicians and radiologists involved, however, were blinded to the strategy used. The sample size appears reasonable and the study is appropriately powered on the basis of best available evidence.

Weaknesses

The generalizability of the study findings appears questionable when considering, for example, the patient population (ASA physical status 1 to 2), and patient admission to ICU for at least 24 h following surgery (although the level of care in the ICU is not defined). Other weaknesses include:

- 30% of patients in the CV group needed to change ventilation modes from volume- to pressure-controlled because of high peak inspiratory pressures, but were still analysed as 'conventional ventilation.

- The PaO_2/FIO_2 ratio was apparently only measured at two time points (2 h after ICU admission and at 0300 during ICU stay); the second time point was not standardized with respect to time of operation/ICU admission.

- Results and statistical analysis should be interpreted with caution.

- The follow-up was of short duration.

- The PV strategy was only used during the period of one-lung anaesthesia, rather than throughout surgery.

Relevance

This paper illustrates the concept of translating advances in critical care and science into the operating theatre environment. Accumulating evidence suggests an inflammatory response is triggered by mechanical ventilation, especially during one-lung ventilation. It would appear that this inflammatory response can be attenuated by employing protective lung ventilation strategies and utilizing inhalational anaesthetic agents. In critical care, a protective ventilatory strategy has been shown to reduce ventilator-induced lung injury in patients with ARDS and is considered standard practice. Licker and colleagues' observational study (2009), implementing an intraoperative protective lung ventilation strategy protocol in patients undergoing lung cancer resection, demonstrated an association with improved postoperative respiratory outcomes (significantly reduced incidences of acute lung injury and atelectasis), along with reduced utilization of intensive care resources. Despite its shortcomings, Yang *et al.*'s paper moves the evidence in the right direction by undertaking a prospective randomized 'partially-blinded' study. Their conclusion that a protective ventilation strategy leads to a reduced risk of pulmonary complications after lung cancer surgery requires further clarification by more robust investigation.

Paper 8: A prospective, randomized comparison of preoperative and continuous balanced epidural or paravertebral bupivacaine on post-thoracotomy pain, pulmonary function and stress responses

Author details

J Richardson, S Sabanathan, J Jones, RD Shah, S Cheema, AJ Mearns

Reference

British Journal of Anaesthesia 1999; **83**: 387–92.

Abstract

Both epidural and paravertebral blocks are effective in controlling post-thoracotomy pain, but comparison of preoperative and balanced techniques, measuring pulmonary function and stress responses, has not been undertaken previously. We studied 100 adult patients, premedicated with morphine and diclofenac, allocated randomly to receive thoracic epidural bupivacaine or thoracic paravertebral bupivacaine as preoperative bolus doses followed by continuous infusions. All patients also received diclofenac and patient-controlled morphine. Significantly lower visual analogue pain scores at rest and on coughing were found in the paravertebral group and patient-controlled morphine requirements were less. Pulmonary function was significantly better preserved in the paravertebral group who had higher oxygen saturations and less postoperative respiratory morbidity. There was a significant increase in plasma concentrations of cortisol from baseline in both the epidural and paravertebral groups and in plasma glucose concentrations in the epidural group, but no significant change from baseline in plasma glucose in the paravertebral group. Areas under the plasma concentration vs. time curves for cortisol and glucose were significantly lower in the paravertebral groups. Side effects, especially nausea, vomiting and hypotension, were troublesome only in the epidural group. We conclude that with these regimens, paravertebral block was superior to epidural bupivacaine.

Summary

This prospective randomized study sought to compare two common regional analgesia techniques employed for thoracic surgery as part of a standardized multimodal analgesia regime, investigating their relative contributions to postoperative analgesia and pulmonary function (using peak expiratory flow rate or PEFR as the main outcome measure in the study), and their effects on the stress response to thoracic surgery. Data collection took place in the immediate 48-h postoperative period,with serious complications at any point, length of hospital stay, and pain at 6-month follow-up also recorded. The authors found that paravertebral block provided significantly better pain scores, both at rest and on coughing, which was accompanied by lower PCA morphine requirements and fewer opioid-related side effects. The patients in the paravertebral group as compared to the epidural group also had:

- Superior pulmonary function and oxygenation, with lower postoperative respiratory morbidity.
- A lower neuroendocrine stress response (as assessed by blood glucose and cortisol).
- Less hypotension.

Citation count

177.

Related references

1 Davies RG, Myles PS, Graham JM. A comparison of the analgesic efficacy and side-effects of paravertebral vs. epidural blockade for thoracotomy – a systematic review and meta-analysis of randomized trials. *Br J Anaesth* 2006; **96**: 418–26.

2 Joshi GP, Bonnet F, Shah R, *et al*. A systematic review of randomized trials evaluating regional techniques for postthoracotomy analgesia. *Anesth Analg* 2008; **107**: 1026–40.

3 Powell ES, Cook D, Pearce AC, *et al*. A prospective, multicentre, observational cohort study of analgesia and outcome after pneumonectomy. *Br J Anaesth* 2011; **106**: 364–70.

Key message

Continuous paravertebral and epidural blocks, instituted prior to the surgical incision as part of a multimodal approach to analgesia, are highly effective for post-thoracotomy pain. Paravertebral analgesia was found to be superior in terms of analgesia, pulmonary function, neuroendocrine stress response, side effect profile, and postoperative respiratory morbidity.

Strengths

This was a well-constructed prospective, randomized study, with strong methodology under-pinning the data collection and findings, and clear and valid representation of results and statistical analysis.

Weaknesses

The use of plain bupivacaine solution in the epidural group, i.e. the lack of a local anaesthetic–opioid combination, is often quoted as a weakness, and also brings into question the generalizability of the findings of the study when opioid–local anaesthetic epidural solutions are widely used. In response, the authors have argued that most patients in the epidural group in their study had pain scores and postoperative pulmonary function comparable to other published prospective rand-omized studies, including those where combinations of epidural local anaesthetics with opioids were used. Also, the use of PEFR as the sole tool for spirometry and thereby the main outcome measure for the study could be questioned, as well as the generalization of neuroendocrine stress response based upon just two end markers (cortisol and glucose). In addition, mortality is not considered outside the hospital admission period. There are also some potential confounding factors in the study, for example:

♦ Approximate dosage of bupivacaine local anaesthetic in the paravertebral group was twice that recorded in the epidural group.

♦ Differences in PEFR *per se* between the two groups could have been skewed by both the increased opioid requirement in the epidural group, with attendant effects on respiratory function and opioid-related side effects, and the bilateral nature of thoracic epidural blockade with attendant intercostal muscle weakness and resultant direct effects on PEFR.

Relevance

Despite increasing evidence for (1) paravertebral blockade being at least as efficacious as epidural blockade for post-thoracotomy analgesia, and (2) paravertebral blockade having a better side effect profile, with a concomitant reduction in pulmonary complications, when compared with epidural blockade for thoracic surgery, the anaesthetic community seem reluctant to acknowledge that paravertebral blockade may be the superior choice. Undoubtedly, high-quality studies are required to address this further. The recently-reported UKPOS study examined associations between analgesic technique and major complications in pneumonectomy patients. This large, multicentred, prospective, observational cohort study concluded that epidural analgesia was associated with an increased incidence of clinically important major post-pneumonectomy complications when compared with paravertebral blockade, but highlighted a need for a large, multicentre randomized controlled trial to provide robust evidence for a change in practice. Time will tell whether or not the scepticism is founded.

Paper 9: A comparison of the analgesic efficacy and side-effects of paravertebral vs. epidural blockade for thoracotomy—a systematic review and meta-analysis of randomized trials

Author details

RG Davies, PS Myles, JM Graham

Reference

British Journal of Anaesthesia 2006; **96**: 418–26.

Abstract

Epidural analgesia is considered by many to be the best method of pain relief after major surgery. It is used routinely in many thoracic surgery centres. Although effective, side-effects include hypotension, urinary retention, incomplete (or failed) block, and, in rare cases, paraplegia. Paravertebral block (PVB) is an alternative technique that may offer comparable analgesic effectiveness and a better side-effect profile. The authors undertook a systematic review and meta-analysis of all relevant randomized trials comparing PVB with epidural analgesia in thoracic surgery. Data were abstracted and verified by both authors. Studies were tested for heterogeneity, and meta-analyses were done with random effects or fixed effects models. Weighted mean difference (WMD) was used for numerical outcomes and odds ratio (OR) for dichotomous outcomes, both with 95% CI. Ten trials were identified that enrolled 520 thoracic surgery patients. All of the trials were small (n<130) and none were blinded. There was no significant difference between PVB and epidural groups for pain scores at 4–8, 24 or 48 h, WMD 0.37 (95% CI: −0.5, 121), 0.05 (−0.6, 0.7), -0.04 (−0.4, 0.3), respectively. Pulmonary complications occurred less often with PVB, OR 0.36 (0.14, 0.92). Urinary retention, OR 0.23 (0.10, 0.51), nausea and vomiting, OR 0.47 (0.24, 0.53), and hypotension, OR 0.23 (0.11, 0.48), were less common with PVB. Rates of failed block were lower in the PVB group, OR 0.28 (0.2, 0.6). PVB and epidural analgesia provide comparable pain relief after thoracic surgery, but PVB has a better side-effect profile and is associated with a reduction in pulmonary complications. PVB can be recommended for major thoracic surgery.

Summary

This systematic review found no difference in analgesia with PVB techniques when compared with epidural regimens. PVB was associated with improvements in respiratory function and a reduction in complications. It appears that PVB is advantageous and can be recommended for major thoracic and upper abdominal surgery.

Citation count

183.

Related references

1 Joshi GP, Bonnet F, Shah R, *et al.* A systematic review of randomized trials evaluating regional techniques for postthoracotomy analgesia. *Anesth Analg* 2008; **107**: 1026–40.

Key message

PVB and epidural analgesia provide comparable pain relief after thoracic surgery, but PVB has a better side effect profile and is associated with a reduction in pulmonary complications. PVB can be recommended for major thoracic surgery.

Strengths

This is a well conducted meta-analysis. All included studies were randomized. The statistical approach is correct and the data are well presented.

Weaknesses

Despite trawling all the world's literature, only ten studies of adequate quality were identified which enrolled a total of 520 thoracic surgical patients. This is a low number to find significant differences in outcomes. The techniques used were very heterogeneous, both in terms of PVB and thoracic epidural analgesia (TEA) procedure, but also drug concentration, administration, and additional analgesic agents. In short the techniques were not standardized. Individual studies were all small (n <130).

Surprisingly the use of morphine in the PVB group was comparable to the TEA group which raises questions about the epidural insertion technique and how their position and function was confirmed. As most centres give patients with a PVB PCA morphine for additional analgesia it is surprising that the TEA group have the same morphine use. The study demonstrated a lower rate of failed technique in the PVB group. As the endpoint of PVB is less well defined when compared with the loss of resistance used for TEA and no systematic measurement of dermatomal block in the awake patients was included, this finding may be unreliable.

None of the studies were blinded to technique which may have introduced some bias.

Relevance

This meta-analysis has challenged the belief that TEA provides superior analgesia after thoracotomy. In 2010, in the Association of Cardiothoracic Anaesthetists (ACTA) UK survey of thoracic practice, 60% of anaesthetists used TEA and 32% PVB for major thoracic surgery. Further research is needed to resolve this clinical question. Any randomized controlled study would need high patient numbers and should address efficacy, complications and cost effectiveness.

Paper 10: Thoracic surgical procedures supported by a pumpless interventional lung assist

Author details

K Wiebe, J Poeling, M Arlt, A Philipp, D Camboni, S Hofmann, C Schmid

Reference

Annals of Thoracic Surgery 2010; **89**: 1782–8.

Abstract

Background: For support of pulmonary function during complex thoracic surgical procedures, especially in respiratory compromised patients, a pumpless interventional lung assist (iLA) was applied. Feasibility and effectiveness for this novel indication were evaluated.

Methods: Ten patients underwent thoracic surgery with respiratory support by iLA. Indication for iLA application was the need for intraoperative prolonged discontinuation of ventilation (tracheal surgery and lung resections after pneumonectomy [n = 6], and emergency procedures in patients with acute respiratory failure [n = 4]). The pumpless extracorporeal system was inserted percutaneously into the femoral blood vessels before surgery. Blood flow through the iLA, cardiac output, and gas exchange were monitored.

Results: In all patients, the surgical procedure was successfully performed because of the support by the pumpless iLA. Mean blood flow across the iLA was $1.58 \pm 0.31 \, \mathrm{l\,min^{-1}}$ ($1.2 \, \mathrm{l\,min^{-1}}$ to $2.2 \, \mathrm{l\,min^{-1}}$). Low-dose norepinephrine was required to maintain sufficient systemic blood pressure. There was a moderate improvement in oxygenation ($49 \, \mathrm{ml\,min^{-1}}$ transfer of O2) and a very efficient elimination of carbon dioxide ($121 \, \mathrm{ml\,min^{-1}}$ transfer of CO_2). Thus, extended periods of apnoeic oxygenation were possible during surgery. The device was removed immediately after surgery in 6 patients. In 4 patients with severe respiratory insufficiency, the iLA was continued for a mean of 6.8 days to allow for protective postoperative ventilation.

Summary

The Novalung iLA represents a valuable alternative to conventional extracorporeal membrane oxygenation (ECMO) systems and certainly has potential in lung surgery. Its major advantage is the low incidence of adverse effects and uncomplicated handling, while allowing protective ventilatory strategies. The heparin coated system allows operation without anticoagulation which makes its use feasible during major non cardiac surgery. In this study, before cannula insertion, a single bolus of heparin (500 or 1000 IU) was given prophylactically. Only in those patients where the iLA was used for prolonged postoperative period then an activated clotting time (ACT) of 130–150 s or an activated partial thromboplastin time (aPTT) of 40–50 s was targeted by the infusion of unfractionated heparin. In this study, the Novalung iLA was used in the management of a heterogeneous group of both elective and emergency thoracic patients. All had severe respiratory compromise and the Novalung iLA corrected hypercapnia and acidosis very effectively. Oxygenation was also improved in the five patients with respiratory failure. In four patients apnoeic ventilation was utilized in theatre to facilitate surgery, and a subgroup had early closure of bronchopleural fistula after pneumonectomy. Four patients had the Novalung iLA continued for several days for postoperative respiratory failure. The use of the Novalung iLA also allowed the use of a protective lung ventilation strategy.

Citation count

2.

Related references

1 Bein T, Weber F, Philipp A, *et al.* A new pumpless extracorporeal interventional lung assist in critical hypoxemia/hypercapnia. *Crit Care Med* 2006; **34**: 1372–7.

2 Iglesias M, Jungebluth P, Petit C, *et al.* Extracorporeal lung membrane provides better lung protection than conventional treatment for severe postpneumonectomy noncardiogenic acute respiratory distress syndrome. *J Thorac Cardiovasc Surg* 2008; **135**: 1362–71.

Key message

The application of pumpless iLA was haemodynamically well tolerated, and allowed for safe procedures in respiratory compromised patients, avoiding the application and consequences of cardiopulmonary bypass or pump-driven ECMO.

Strengths

This is a well-conducted, detailed observational case series of ten patients which adds to the literature on the use of the Novalung iLA in the treatment of thoracic surgical patients with severe respiratory compromise.

Weaknesses

This is an observational case series and is not a randomized trial so it is impossible to say whether the Novalung iLA improved outcomes of these patients. The group of patients were clearly very high risk and the death of two of the six emergency patients with the survival of all four elective patients is suggestive that the treatment was effective, but is not conclusive.

Relevance

The new technologies of pumpless interventional lung assist have a developing role in critical care; however, this paper breaks new ground by taking these techniques into the operating room. There is a potential in this area due to the lesser requirement for anticoagulation and diminished inflammatory responses when compared to pump assisted ECMO. This offers new challenges to anaesthetists and surgeons but may improve outcomes in some of the highest risk patients. Further work is needed to refine the indications for the use of pumpless interventional lung assist and confirm that outcomes are indeed improved by this intervention.

In critical care, pumpless interventional lung support may well have a role in respiratory failure after thoracic surgery, particularly in acute lung injury after pneumonectomy where protective ventilation is critical. The use of pumpless interventional lung support may be limited by the presence of cardiovascular failure, however, which can commonly coexist. An adequate driving pressure is essential and all patients in this study received norepinephrine to support the mean arterial pressure to range of 70–90 mmHg. These potential benefits must be tempered against the risk of limb ischaemia.

Chapter 13

Anaesthesia for vascular surgery

A Lumb and L Jobling

Introduction

Operative surgery for vascular disease is a relatively new surgical speciality, having effectively been born in the mid 20th century when the first synthetic grafts were introduced for bypassing occluded arteries or replacing aneurysmal ones. As surgical techniques and graft materials improved, the range of possible procedures expanded, and vascular surgeons became subspecialists in their own right. In the last two decades, the expansion of vascular radiology, again driven mostly by advances in technology, has begun to replace some of the operations traditionally done by vascular surgeons.

Patients who require vascular surgery invariably have multisystem pathology, with their requirement for an operation acting as an indicator of advanced vascular disease. This advanced vascular pathology is commonly asymptomatic, with the classic example of intermittent claudication from femoral arterial disease preventing the patient from walking fast enough to get angina. Data on comorbidity in patients presenting for vascular surgery in our unit are typical with 32.6% smokers, 64.2% with hypertension, 19.4% with angina, 17.4% with diabetes, and 25.2% with impaired renal function. It is therefore not surprising that vascular surgery is one of the most high-risk specialities for perioperative mortality with around 7% of patients dying within 30 days of surgery, a figure that has changed little in recent decades.

Most of the papers chosen for this chapter therefore relate to how mortality and morbidity associated with vascular surgery can be reduced. Avoiding such high-risk surgical procedures completely would be the patient's best approach to survival but for the fact that the stakes are so high in taking a non-operative approach. With an abdominal aortic aneurysm, for example, rupture risks almost certain death, and high-risk prophylactic surgery has been a reasoned approach to take. Thus endovascular aneurysm repair offered a way out of this dreadful dilemma, and Paper 1 considers the first evidence that the technique was truly helpful in some groups. Paper 2 considers ways of identifying those patients most at risk of mortality following aneurysm surgery, and offers a glimmer of hope that stratification will eventually be suitably robust to advise patients in whom aneurysm surgery really is best avoided.

As therapeutic advances have occurred in cardiovascular medicine, the same interventions have been transferred to perioperative use in vascular patients. Vascular anaesthesia has led the way in this respect, with perioperative use of beta-blockers, statins, and better control of blood glucose metabolism featuring in our next Papers 3–6. These interventions are now routine practice in vascular units, and probably should be adopted in other specialities for similarly high-risk patients.

Our remaining four papers consider the part played by the choice and management of anaesthesia on vascular surgical patient outcomes. Regional anaesthesia for carotid endarterectomy has followed the usual story of enthusiastic proponents of a new technique publishing impressive case-series and small randomized trials before a suitably powered multicentre randomized control trial fails to find any benefit. Two other vascular procedures are at different stages of this process, with debate about an effect of anaesthetic technique on surgical outcomes for lower limb revascularization and arteriovenous fistula formation both being unresolved.

Paper 1: The EVAR Trial Participants: Comparison of endovascular aneurysm repair with open repair in patients with abdominal aortic aneurysm (EVAR trial 1), 30-day operative mortality results: randomised controlled trial

Author details

The EVAR trial participants

Reference

Lancet 2004; **364**: 843–8.

Abstract

Background: Endovascular aneurysm repair (EVAR) is a new technology to treat patients with abdominal aortic aneurysm (AAA) when the anatomy is suitable. Uncertainty exists about how endovascular repair compares with conventional open surgery. EVAR trial 1 was instigated to compare these treatments in patients judged fit for open AAA repair.

Methods: Between 1999 and 2003, 1082 elective (non-emergency) patients were randomised to receive either EVAR (n=543) or open AAA repair (n=539). Patients aged at least 60 years with aneurysms of diameter 5.5 cm or more, who were fit enough for open surgical repair (anaesthetically and medically well enough for the procedure), were recruited for the study at 41 British hospitals proficient in the EVAR technique. The primary outcome measure is all-cause mortality and these results will be released in 2005. The primary analysis presented here is operative mortality by intention to treat and a secondary analysis was done in per-protocol patients.

Findings: Patients (983 men, 99 women) had a mean age of 74 years (SD 6) and mean AAA diameter of 6.5 cm (SD 1). 1047 (97%) patients underwent AAA repair and 1008 (93%) received their allocated treatment. 30-day mortality in the EVAR group was 1.7% (9/531) versus 4.7% (24/516) in the open repair group (odds ratio 0.35 [95% CI 0.16–0.77], p=0.009). By per-protocol analysis, 30-day mortality for EVAR was 1.6% (8/512) versus 4.6% (23/496) for open repair (0.33 [0.15–0.74], p=0.007). Secondary interventions were more common in patients allocated EVAR (9.8% vs 5.8%, p=0.02).

Interpretation: In patients with large AAAs, treatment by EVAR reduced the 30-day operative mortality by two-thirds compared with open repair. Any change in clinical practice should await durability and longer term results.

Summary

EVAR 1, a multicentre randomized control trial, recruited 1,082 patients from 41 UK hospitals between 1999 and 2003. Patients with AAA >5.5cm in diameter and considered fit for conventional surgical repair were randomized to receive either open or endovascular repair. This first paper from the EVAR study presents operative mortality by intention to treat and reported 30-day mortality as 1.6% amongst patients treated with EVAR versus 4.6% in the group undergoing open repair.

Citation count

743.

Related references

1 EVAR trial participants. Endovascular aneurysm repair versus open repair in patients
   with abdominal aortic aneurysm (EVAR trial 1): Randomised control trial. *Lancet* 2005;
   365: 2179–6.

Key message

EVAR results in significantly reduced 30-day mortality when compared with open AAA repair in
patients considered clinically fit to undergo open repair. The improved survival demonstrated in
this study applied only to the short term, but subsequent reports from the EVAR study confirmed
longer term (4 years) benefit (Evar trial participants, 2005).

Strengths

EVAR 1 recruited a large number of patients into this randomized control trial. This was a substantial achievement considering that EVAR was considered to be an almost 'experimental' procedure at the time, and the devices available still under active development. The participating
hospitals were representative of contemporary UK practice in specialist centres.

Weaknesses

This paper was an early report of selective findings of the EVAR 1 trial and not strictly representative of EVAR's wider findings published later in 2005 (Evar trial participants, 2005). Perhaps
the compelling findings of this early report of EVAR, viewed in isolation, may have bolstered
enthusiasm for the technique when a more measured approach would have been appropriate.

Relevance

In the UK rupture of AAA accounts for around 2% of all deaths in men aged 65 and over, and
mortality from either elective repair (see paper 2) or from AAA rupture has changed little in
recent decades. The arrival of a viable alternative to these two options for patients with an AAA
was momentous.

Subsequent studies showed that in the longer term EVAR reduced aneurysm related mortality
(4% for EVAR versus 7% for open repair) but there was no difference in all cause mortality at
4 years (Evar trial participants, 2005). Also, there was no difference between groups in health
related quality of life and a higher number of complications and re-interventions in the EVAR
group, requiring constant surveillance and extra cost. Thus the decision patients currently face is
whether to have a procedure associated with a reduced early mortality but with an unknown
chance of long-term 'cure' from the potential disaster of AAA rupture and an equivalent chance
of death from all causes in the mid term, as well as a need for long-term monitoring.

The use of EVAR requires an anatomically suitable aneurysm and for this reason open repair
will not be supplanted by current technologies and open AAA repair will continue to form a proportion of the vascular anaesthetist's workload. Even so, improvements in endovascular technology and increased expertise of the whole vascular team mean that the proportion of AAAs
treatable by EVAR continues to increase. EVAR techniques are also now being employed in the
emergency management of ruptured aneurysms, which offers fantastic potential for improved
outcomes compared to open repair from which currently only 20–30% of patients survive.

Paper 2: Mid-term survival after abdominal aortic aneurysm surgery predicted by cardiopulmonary exercise testing

Author details

J Carlisle, M Swart

Reference

British Journal of Surgery 2007; **94**: 966–9.

Abstract

Background: Cardiopulmonary exercise (CPX) testing measures how efficiently subjects meet increased metabolic demand. This study aimed to determine whether preoperative CPX testing predicted postoperative survival following elective abdominal aortic aneurysm (AAA) repair.

Methods: Some 130 patients had CPX testing before elective open AAA repair. Additional preoperative, operative and postoperative variables were recorded prospectively. Median follow-up was 35 months. The correlation of variables with survival was assessed by single and multiple regression analyses.

Results: CPX testing identified 30 of 130 patients who had been unfit before surgery. Two years after surgery the Kaplan–Meier survival estimate was 55 per cent for the 30 unfit patients, compared with 97 per cent for the 100 fit patients. The absolute difference in survival between these two groups at 2 years was 42 (95 per cent confidence interval 18 to 65) per cent (P <0.001).

Conclusion: Preoperative CPX testing, combined with simple co-morbidity scoring, identified patients unlikely to survive in the mid-term, even after successful AAA repair.

Summary

This observational study recorded a variety of clinical risk factors and performed preoperative CPX testing on 130 patients having elective AAA repair. Patients were then followed-up for almost 3 years. The two single most accurate predictors of survival were the RCRI (revised cardiac risk index, a score of 0–6 clinical predictors) and the ventilatory equivalent for carbon dioxide from the CPX test. These two predictors were retrospectively used to divide the patients into 'fit' (100/130) and 'unfit' (30/130) groups, which were shown to have significantly different postoperative survival curves (Fig. 13.1). Of the patients considered 'fit', 97% were alive at 3 years compared with only 55% of the 'unfit' group.

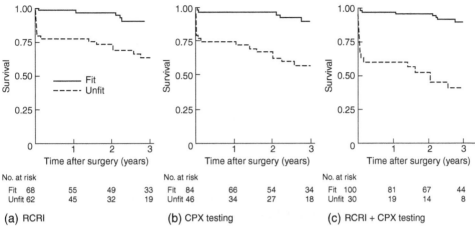

Fig. 13.1 Kaplan–Meier overall survival curves for 130 patients who underwent open abdominal aortic aneurysm repair categorized as 'fit' or 'unfit' respectively by (a) a Revised Cardiac Risk Index (RCRI) of 1 (no co-morbidities) or >1 (at least one comorbidity), (b) ventilatory equivalent for carbon dioxide ($\dot{V}_E/\dot{V}_{CO_2}$) below 43 or above 42 on cardiopulmonary exercise (CPX) testing, and (c) no comorbidity (or comorbidity and a $\dot{V}_E/\dot{V}_{CO_2}$ below 43) or comorbidity with a $\dot{V}_E/\dot{V}_{CO_2}$ above 42 (RCRI + CPX testing). Note that the estimation of risk using a combination of clinical and CPX scoring is more predictive than either alone. Reproduced from J. Carlisle, M. Swart, Mid-term survival after abdominal aortic aneurysm surgery predicted by cardiopulmonary exercise testing, *British Journal of Surgery*, 2007; **94**: 966–9, Wiley, © British Journal of Surgery Society Ltd, DOI: 10.1002/BJS.5734 with permission.

Citation count

45.

Related references

1 Older P, Smith R, Courtney P, *et al.* Preoperative evaluation of cardiac failure and ischemia in elderly patients by cardiopulmonary exercise testing. *Chest* 1993; **104**: 701–4.

2 Older P, Hall A, Hader R. Cardiopulmonary exercise testing as a screening test for perioperative management of major surgery in the elderly. *Chest* 1999; **116**: 355–62.

Key message

A combination of simple clinical risk scoring and the results of CPX testing may be suitably predictive of mortality following AAA surgery to be used in the clinical decision of whether an operation is worthwhile for an individual patient.

Strengths

Use of medium-term follow-up (3 years) rather than the usual in-hospital or 30-day mortality measures. The study compared numerous clinical risk scores and several measures obtained from CPX testing to identify the most predictive combination.

Weaknesses

A small sample size for a study assessing multiple factors. The inhospital mortality of the cohort was high (9.6%) compared with generally accepted outcomes.

Relevance

A preoperative test that is a reliable predictor of postoperative survival has been sought for many years. Many clinical scores exist but for some time focus has been on the anaerobic threshold derived from a CPX test (Older *et al.*, 1993). Increased perioperative mortality rates with an AT of <11 ml min^{-1} kg^{-1} have led to this measure being used to help inform clinical decisions both about whether intervention for AAA is justified at all, or the level of critical care required following surgery (Older *et al.*, 1999). The expectation that a single physiological measure could fulfil this important predictive role was always naïve, and the study by Carlisle and Swart has shown that a combination of clinical history and physiological reserve is a much more useful approach.

Paper 3: Effect of atenolol on mortality and cardiovascular morbidity after noncardiac surgery

Author details

DT Mangano, EL Layug, A Wallace, I Tateo

Reference

New England Journal of Medicine 1996; **335**: 1713–20.

Summary

A randomized controlled trial of atenolol administered from the day of surgery until 7 days post-operatively in patients at risk of cardiovascular complications based on clinical evidence of ischaemic heart disease or a positive stress test. Death or a major cardiovascular event within 2 years of surgery were significantly less frequent in the atenolol treated group.

Citation count

1428.

Related references

1 Sear JW, Giles JW, Howard-Alpe G, *et al.* Perioperative beta-blockade, 2008: What does POISE tell us, and was our earlier caution justified? *Br J Anaesth* 2008; **101**: 135–8.

2 Poldermans D, Boersma E, Bax JJ, *et al.* The effect of bisoprolol on perioperative mortality and myocardial infarction in high-risk patients undergoing vascular surgery. *N Engl J Med* 1999; **341**: 1789–95.

3 Sear JW, Foëx P. Recommendations on perioperative beta-blockers: differing guidelines: so what should the clinician do? *Br J Anaesth* 2010; **104**: 273–5.

Key message

In patients deemed at high risk of cardiovascular complications on simple clinical grounds the short-term use of a beta-blocker in the perioperative period can improve survival and reduce cardiovascular events in the long term.

Strengths

A pragmatic study with a simple intervention (intravenous or oral atenolol) commenced on the day of surgery and discontinued on discharge from hospital. The recommendations of the study were easily adopted by vascular anaesthetists worldwide.

Weaknesses

A small sample size for a study addressing such an important and multifactorial problem. Retrospective criticism of the study (Sear *et al.*, 2008) became intense—in particular regarding the failure to include in the analysis events that occurred during hospitalization, and the acute withdrawal of long-term beta-blocker therapy in patients randomized to the control group.

Relevance

Many anaesthetic techniques were studied to try and reduce the stress response to surgery and so ameliorate its effects on the cardiovascular system in susceptible patients. This study was the first to take the alternative approach of simply blocking the effects of the neurohumoral response, with seemingly impressive results. Other studies soon followed, with more invasive identification of 'high risk' patients by using pre-operative stress echocardiography and more complex beta-blocker therapy using variable doses of beta blocker and target heart rates (Poldermans *et al.*, 1999). In this study only 173 patients met the criteria for being high risk out of 1351 patients screened, but again, beta-blockers produced impressive reductions in cardiovascular events, e.g. 3.4% died of a cardiac cause in the beta-blocker group compared with 17% in the placebo group. Perioperative beta-blocker use was soon adopted in guidelines around the world.

Over the next few years evidence of the dangers of stopping beta-blocker therapy in the periop-erative period began to emerge, the use of beta-blockers for other indications changed, and the requirement to closely monitor perioperative beta-blockade became apparent (Sear *et al.*, 2008; Sear and Foëx, 2010). Enthusiasm for the widespread use of beta blockers began to wane, and a large randomized controlled trial was established (see Paper 4) that undermined Mangano's recommendations almost completely.

Paper 4: Effects of extended-release metoprolol succinate in patients undergoing non-cardiac surgery (POISE trial): a randomized controlled trial

Author details

POISE study group

Reference

Lancet 2008; **371**: 1839–47.

Abstract

Background: Trials of β blockers in patients undergoing non-cardiac surgery have reported conflicting results. This randomised controlled trial, done in 190 hospitals in 23 countries, was designed to investigate the effects of perioperative β blockers.

Methods: We randomly assigned 8351 patients with, or at risk of, atherosclerotic disease who were undergoing non-cardiac surgery to receive extended-release metoprolol succinate (n=4174) or placebo (n=4177), by a computerized randomisation phone service. Study treatment was started 2–4 h before surgery and continued for 30 days. Patients, health-care providers, data collectors, and outcome adjudicators were masked to treatment allocation. The primary endpoint was a composite of cardiovascular death, non-fatal myocardial infarction, and non-fatal cardiac arrest. Analyses were by intention to treat. This trial is registered with ClinicalTrials. gov, number NCT00182039.

Findings: All 8351 patients were included in analyses; 8331 (99.8%) patients completed the 30-day follow-up. Fewer patients in the metoprolol group than in the placebo group reached the primary endpoint (244 [5.8%] patients in the metoprolol group vs 290 [6.9%] in the placebo group; hazard ratio 0.84, 95% CI 0.70–0.99; p=0.0399). Fewer patients in the metoprolol group than in the placebo group had a myocardial infarction (176 [4.2%] vs 239 [5.7%] patients; 0.73, 0.60–0.89; p=0.0017). However, there were more deaths in the metoprolol group than in the placebo group (129 [3.1%] vs 97 [2.3%] patients; 1.33, 1.03–1.74; p=0.0317). More patients in the metoprolol group than in the placebo group had a stroke (41 [1.0%] vs 19 [0.5%] patients; 2.17, 1.26–3.74; p=0.0053).

Interpretation: Our results highlight the risk in assuming a perioperative β-blocker regimen has benefit without substantial harm, and the importance and need for large randomised trials in the perioperative setting. Patients are unlikely to accept the risks associated with perioperative extended-release metoprolol.

Summary

This large trial evaluated the effect of perioperative beta-blockers in patients undergoing non-cardiac surgery. Patients received either placebo or metoprolol, which was commenced 2–4 h preoperatively and continued for the 30 days coincident with the duration of follow-up. While the primary outcome measure (a composite of cardiovascular death, non-fatal myocardial infarction (MI), and non-fatal cardiac arrest) was found to differ between the two groups, favouring the use of metoprolol, clinically significant hypotension and bradycardia, stroke and all cause mortality were significantly higher in the intervention group.

Of the patients in the study who had an MI less than one-third went on to require coronary intervention, develop congestive cardiac failure, or have a non-fatal cardiac arrest; indeed for most of these patients, diagnosis of MI was made on electrocardiogram (ECG) and biochemical findings in the absence of ischaemic pain. In contrast, a majority of patients who had a non-fatal stroke required help to perform everyday activities or were incapacitated, and few were considered to have fully recovered (15% in the metoprolol and 21% in the placebo group), although assessment of recovery was made 7 days following stroke onset or discharge, whichever was earlier.

Citation count

523.

Related references

1 Sear JW, Giles JW, Howard-Alpe G, *et al*. Perioperative beta-blockade, 2008: What does POISE tell us, and was our earlier caution justified? *Br J Anaesth* 2008; **101**: 135–8.

2 Opie LH. Beta-blockade should not be among several choices for initial therapy of hypertension. *J Hypertens* 2008; **26**: 161–3.

3 Chen ZM, Pan HC, Chen YP, *et al*. Early intravenous then oral metoprolol in 45,852 patients with acute myocardial infarction: randomised placebo-controlled trial. *Lancet* 2005; **366**: 1622–32.

4 Sear JW, Foëx P. Recommendations on perioperative beta-blockers: differing guidelines: so what should the clinician do? *Br J Anaesth* 2010; **104**: 273–5.

Key message

This trial confirms the cardiovascular benefits of perioperative beta-blockade previously shown in smaller trials, but also, for the first time, demonstrates that the adverse effects of the chosen beta-blocker regime outweigh the benefits.

Strengths

This is a huge, worldwide, multicentre trial in which patients, healthcare workers, data collectors, and outcome adjudicators (although not data analysts) were blind to treatment allocation. Central monitoring of data was thorough, including on-site audit of hospital charts and all supporting documents, with the result that 947 participants from 17 centres were excluded from the trial due to suspected fraudulent activity. Very few patients were lost to follow-up considering the scale of this trial (99.8% were followed for the required postoperative 30 days).

Weaknesses

The study followed patients for a relatively short time. Whether longer term follow-up will lead to observed findings commensurate with other studies such as that of Mangano *et al*. (see Paper 3) remains to be seen. The study did not look exclusively at vascular patients, though vascular procedures made up a large proportion of operations (approximately 41% in both groups). The study was stopped before the full recruitment goal of 10,000 patients was achieved.

The acute administration of a beta-blocker in this study may not reflect ideal clinical practice and may moreover contribute to the hypotension and bradycardia which has been postulated to have a causal role in the excess morbidity in the metoprolol group. Similar concerns relate to the dose of metoprolol used, which was felt to be high (Sear *et al*., 2008).

Relevance

This study highlighted the need for such large randomized trials in order to balance the benefits and risks of any perioperative intervention at a time when the tide of opinion regarding their use in other contexts was also changing. Beta-blockers are no longer recommended as a first-line drug in the management of hypertension in light of the findings of large trials and meta-analyses demonstrating that other drugs are superior in preventing the risk of stroke (Opie, 2008). A randomized controlled trial of >45,000 patients with acute myocardial infarction showed no impact of beta-blockers on 30-day mortality (Chen et al., 2005). And now the POISE trial has also shown that serious consideration needs to be given about whether the use of perioperative beta blockers with the sole indication of managing perioperative risk is warranted in the face of such potentially serious adverse effects. If beta-blockers are used perioperatively their effect needs to be closely monitored (Sear and Foëx, 2010).

A more significant problem with perioperative interventions is raised by the POISE trial. If, as some commentators believe, the POISE study results simply reflect too high a dose of beta-blocker, will a lower dose, that does not cause such significant side effects, still be effective at reducing cardiovascular risk? If each regime tested requires a worldwide study of over 8,000 patients we will wait a long time for definitive advice. In the meantime, clinicians must continue to balance the risks and benefits of interventions in each individual patient they treat.

Paper 5: Reduction in cardiovascular events after vascular surgery with atorvastatin: A randomized trial

Author details

AES Durazzo, FS Machado, DT Ikeoka, C De Bernoche, MC Monachini, P Puech-Leão, B Caramelli

Reference

Journal of Vascular Surgery 2004; **39**: 967–76.

Abstract

Objectives: This prospective, randomized, placebo-controlled, double-blind clinical trial was performed to analyze the effect of atorvastatin compared with placebo on the occurrence of a 6-month composite of cardiovascular events after vascular surgery. Cardiovascular complications are the most important cause of perioperative morbidity and mortality among patients undergoing vascular surgery. Statin therapy may reduce perioperative cardiac events through stabilization of coronary plaques.

Methods: One hundred patients were randomly assigned to receive 20 mg atorvastatin or placebo once a day for 45 days, irrespective of their serum cholesterol concentration. Vascular surgery was performed on average 30 days after randomization, and patients were prospectively followed up over 6 months. The cardiovascular events studied were death from cardiac cause, nonfatal myocardial infarction, unstable angina, and stroke.

Results: Fifty patients received atorvastatin, and 50 received placebo. During the 6-month follow-up primary end points occurred in 17 patients, 4 in the atorvastatin group and 13 in the placebo group. The incidence of cardiac events was more than three times higher with placebo (26.0%) compared with atorvastatin (8.0%; P = 0.031). The risk for an event was compared between the groups with the Kaplan–Meier method, as event-free survival after vascular surgery. Patients given atorvastatin exhibited a significant decrease in the rate of cardiac events, compared with the placebo group, within 6 months after vascular surgery (P = 0.018).

Conclusion: Short-term treatment with atorvastatin significantly reduces the incidence of major adverse cardiovascular events after vascular surgery.

Summary

This randomized control trial evaluated the effect of statins on cardiovascular events in patients having vascular surgery randomly allocating 100 patients to receive either 20 mg of atorvastatin or placebo daily for 45 days. Patients received the drug for an average 31 days before surgery and were followed-up for 6 months postoperatively. A composite endpoint of death due to a cardiac cause, myocardial infarction (MI), unstable angina, or stroke was studied and found to differ significantly between the two groups (P = 0.031).

Citation count

373.

Related references

1 Poldermans D, Bax JJ, Kertai MD, *et al*. Statins are associated with a reduced incidence of perioperative mortality in patients undergoing major noncardiac vascular surgery. *Circulation* 2003; **107**: 1848–51.

2 Schouten O, Boersma E, Hoeks SE, *et al*. Fluvastatin and perioperative events in patients undergoing vascular surgery. *N Engl J Med* 2009; **361**: 980–5.

Key message

The use of perioperative atorvastatin from approximately 1 month preoperatively reduces the incidence of serious cardiovascular complications in the first 6 months after vascular surgery.

Strengths

This was the first randomized controlled clinical trial examining the effect of preoperative introduction of stains. Follow-up was complete, an assessment made of drug compliance, and analysis performed on an intention to treat basis.

Weaknesses

This was a small study using a composite endpoint at 6 months and not powered to assess 30-day postoperative outcomes. The difference observed between the groups only just achieved statistical significance. No reference is made to compliance with the atorvastatin medication in the 6 months following surgery or the potential impact of this on the results.

Relevance

The pathophysiology of perioperative myocardial ischaemia in vascular patients is not fully elucidated, but coronary plaque rupture has a significant role to play in around half of perioperative MIs and the systemic inflammatory response to surgery may also play a role. Statins are accepted to have a long-term cardioprotective role in patients with, or at risk of, coronary heart disease in the non-surgical setting. This effect results not only from their lipid lowering properties but also from effects on endothelial function, plaque stability, immunomodulation and inhibition of thrombogenic responses—all of which help to stabilize the vulnerable atherosclerotic plaques thought to underlie many perioperative cardiac events. Much like perioperative beta blockade (see Papers 3 and 4), the idea that perioperative outcome in vascular surgery might be improved by introducing a drug preoperatively is attractive. Evidence to support such a role for statins is in its infancy relative to the beta blocker debate but is of great interest to the vascular anaesthetist.

   This study should be placed in the context of evidence regarding the use of statins in a medical setting and retrospective studies supporting the use of perioperative statin therapy (Poldermans *et al.*, 2003). Also, there has since been a larger, more robust RCT (Schouten *et al.*, 2009), the findings of which support the view that vascular surgical patients may benefit from initiating statin therapy in the perioperative period. However, questions remain about the use of statins in this setting such as the optimal run in time, dose, and the choice of specific drug. The debate may already be becoming irrelevant as NICE (National Institute for Health and Clinical Excellence) guidelines now recommend that all patients with significant vascular disease should be taking statins long term, and in the authors' unit the only patients not taking the drugs preoperatively are those with a contraindication to statin therapy.

Paper 6: Continuous perioperative insulin infusion decreases major cardiovascular events in patients undergoing vascular surgery

Author details

B Subramaniam, PJ Panzica, V Novack, F Mahmood, R Matyal, JD Mitchell, E Sundar, R Bose, F Pomposelli, JR Kersten. DS Talmor

Reference

Anesthesiology 2009; **110**: 970–7.

Summary

This randomized trial assessed the effects of two different methods for control of perioperative blood glucose on significant cardiac events in patients having vascular surgery. In both groups, the target blood glucose concentration was 5.5–8.3 mmol l^{-1}. When compared to patients managed with 4-hourly intravenous boluses of insulin, a continuous insulin 'sliding scale' produced better control of blood glucose levels. In the continuous insulin group the relative risk for a major cardiovascular events was 0.29, and there were twice as many occurrences of moderate hypoglycaemia (glucose <3.3) though no severe or neurologically damaging hypoglycaemia occurred.

Citation count

28.

Related references

1 Van den Berghe G, Wouters P, Weekers F, *et al.* Intensive insulin therapy in critically ill patients. *N Engl J Med* 2001; **345**: 1359–67.

2 Watkinson P, Barber VS, Young JD. Strict glucose control in the critically ill: May not be such a good thing for all critically ill patients. *BMJ* 2006; **332**: 865–6.

3 Houle TT. Reporting the results of a study that did not go according to plan. *Anesthesiology* 2009; **110**: 957–8.

Key message

Tight perioperative control of blood glucose in both diabetic and non-diabetic patients by continuous insulin infusion is associated with a lower incidence of major cardiovascular events.

Strengths

This is a pragmatic study of vascular patients having a variety of procedures which uses a minimally invasive intervention to produce significant outcome benefits.

Weaknesses

With only 236 patients randomized this is a small study. The authors admit to having intended to recruit 993 patients, but slow recruitment and changing practices in the routine management of blood glucose in their hospital led to early termination of the study: the authors' honesty in describing this was commended in an accompanying Editorial (Houle, 2009).

Relevance

Tight control of blood glucose by insulin infusion in critical care patients had been shown to have improve mortality since 2001 (Van den Berghe *et al.*, 2001), and was widely adopted in clinical practice. It was therefore not a surprise that a similar benefit was observed perioperatively in vascular surgery patients. Enthusiasm for tight glucose control in critical care has, however, now declined as more recent studies have found little benefit in some patient groups, and more evidence of harmful episodes of hypoglycaemia has emerged (Watkinson *et al.*, 2006). The study of vascular patients reported here used a modest target level for glucose (5.5–8.3 mmol l^{-1} compared with 4.4–6.1 in the critical care studies) so reducing the likelihood of hypoglycaemia and making the target levels more easily achievable. The study also provides some evidence that reduced variability in glucose concentration may be more protective than the mean level, as the standard deviation of readings in the continuous insulin group was lower than in the bolus group. Finally, this study provides some early evidence that, irrespective of whether the patient has diabetes or not, blood glucose should be monitored and carefully controlled in the perioperative period in vascular patients.

Paper 7: General anaesthesia versus local anaesthesia for carotid surgery (GALA): a multicentre, randomised controlled trial

Author details

GALA Trial Collaborative group: SC Lewis, CP Warlow, AR Bodenham, B Colam, PM Rothwell, D Torgerson, D Dellagrammaticas, M Horrocks, C Liapis, AP Banning, M Gough, MJ Gough

Reference

Lancet 2008; **372**: 2132–42.

Abstract

Background: The effect of carotid endarterectomy in lowering the risk of stroke ipsilateral to severe atherosclerotic carotid-artery stenosis is offset by complications during or soon after surgery. We compared surgery under general anaesthesia with that under local anaesthesia because prediction and avoidance of perioperative strokes might be easier under local anaesthesia than under general anaesthesia.

Methods: We undertook a parallel group, multicentre, randomised controlled trial of 3526 patients with symptomatic or asymptomatic carotid stenosis from 95 centres in 24 countries. Participants were randomly assigned to surgery under general (n=1753) or local (n=1773) anaesthesia between June, 1999 and October, 2007. The primary outcome was the proportion of patients with stroke (including retinal infarction), myocardial infarction, or death between randomisation and 30 days after surgery. Analysis was by intention to treat. The trial is registered with Current Control Trials number ISRCTN00525237.

Findings: A primary outcome occurred in 84 (4.8%) patients assigned to surgery under general anaesthesia and 80 (4.5%) of those assigned to surgery under local anaesthesia; three events per 1000 treated were prevented with local anaesthesia (95% CI –11 to 17; risk ratio [RR] 0.94 [95% CI 0.70 to 1.27]). The two groups did not significantly differ for quality of life, length of hospital stay, or the primary outcome in the prespecified subgroups of age, contralateral carotid occlusion, and baseline surgical risk.

Interpretation: We have not shown a definite difference in outcomes between general and local anaesthesia for carotid surgery. The anaesthetist and surgeon, in consultation with the patient, should decide which anaesthetic technique to use on an individual basis.

Summary

This was a large randomized controlled trial comparing general anaesthesia (GA) and local anaesthesia (LA) for carotid endarterectomy (CEA) surgery, using stroke, myocardial infarction or death within 30 days of surgery as the primary outcome measures. No differences were found between the anaesthetic techniques studied. The study was not large enough for a formal subgroup analysis, but there was a non-statistically significant trend in favour of using regional anaesthesia in patients whose contralateral carotid artery was occluded. A summary of the results is shown in Table 13.1.

Citation count

50.

Table 13.1 Summary of the GALA trial results

	General anaesthesia	Local anaesthesia
Preoperative data:		
n	1753	1773
Age	70 (8.8)	69 (8.8)
Male	1232 (70%)	1256 (71%)
Hypertension	1334 (76%)	1382 (78%)
Coronary heart disease	647 (37%)	627 (35%)
Cardiac failure	90 (5%)	93 (5%)
Diabetes	435 (25%)	437 (25%)
Contralateral carotid occlusion	150 (9%)	160 (9%)
Procedural data:		
n	1720	1730
Conversion to GA during LA	0	69
Shunt usage:		
Total	738 (43%)	248 (14%)
Reason for using shunt:		
Used routinely	369	35
Neurological deterioration	N/A	150
Drop in velocity on TCD	45	3
Low stump pressure	108	15
Blood pressure manipulation		
Manipulated up	667 (43%)	267 (17%)
Manipulated down	208 (13%)	433 (28%)
Manipulated up and down	259 (17%)	153 (10%)
Not manipulated	435 (28%)	717 (46%)
Outcome data:		
Stroke	70 (4.0%)	66 (3.7%)
Myocardial infarction	4 (0.2%)	9 (0.5%)
Other vascular death	9	5
Death (any cause)	26 (1.5%)	19 (1.1%)
Stroke (including retinal infarction), myocardial infarction, or death	84 (4.8%)	80 (4.5%)
Events prevented per 1000 patients with local anaesthesia		3 (95% CI –11 to 17)

Data are mean (SD) or number (%).

Data from GALA Trial Collaborative group (2008) General anaesthesia versus local anaesthesia for carotid surgery (GALA): a multicentre, randomised controlled trial. *The Lancet* 2008; **372**: 2132–42.

Related references

1 Rothwell PM, Eliasziw M, Gutnikov SA, *et al.*, for the Carotid Endarterectomy Trialists Collaboration. Endarterectomy for symptomatic carotid stenosis in relation to clinical subgroups and timing of surgery. *Lancet* 2004; **363**: 915–24.

2 Rothwell PM, Giles MF, Chandratheva A, *et al.* Effect of urgent treatment of transient ischaemic attack and minor stroke on early recurrent stroke (EXPRESS study): a prospective population-based sequential comparison. *Lancet* 2007; **370**: 1432–42.

Key message

The incidence of major cardiovascular complications or death in patients having CEA is not significantly influenced by the choice of anaesthetic technique.

Strengths

This was a large, randomized study using clinically relevant outcome measures that occur in almost 5% of patients following CEA. Achieving a sample size of 3,526 for such a specialized procedure was impressive. This study is a rare example of a direct comparison of GA and LA techniques.

Weaknesses

To achieve the required number of patients, the study took place in 95 centres in 24 countries, with inevitable variation in both anaesthetic and surgical techniques between centres.

Relevance

After many years of LA versus GA debate, this study showed that any benefit in terms of avoiding major adverse outcomes was too small to be proven by a study of this size, and therefore unlikely to be clinically relevant. However, between commencing and reporting the study, practice in managing patients who require CEA had changed, with greater emphasis now placed on performing the surgery as soon as possible after a neurological event (Rothwell *et al.*, 2004, 2007). This recent move towards performing acute surgery on neurologically unstable patients has changed the patient population away from that studied in the GALA trial.

Paper 8: Superficial or deep cervical plexus block for carotid endarterectomy: a systematic review of complications

Author details

JJ Pandit, R Satya-Krishna, P Gration

Reference

British Journal of Anaesthesia 2007; **99**: 159–69.

Abstract

Carotid endarterectomy is commonly conducted under regional (deep, superficial, intermediate, or combined) cervical plexus block, but it is not known if complication rates differ. We conducted a systematic review of published papers to assess the complication rate associated with superficial (or intermediate) and deep (or combined deep plus superficial/intermediate). The null hypothesis was that complication rates were equal. Complications of interest were: (1) serious complications related to the placement of block, (2) incidence of conversion to general anaesthesia, and (3) serious systemic complications of the surgical-anaesthetic process. We retrieved 69 papers describing a total of 7558 deep/combined blocks and 2533 superficial/intermediate blocks. Deep/combined block was associated with a higher serious complication rate related to the injecting needle when compared with the superficial/intermediate block (odds ratio 2.13, P<0.006). The conversion rate to general anaesthesia was also higher with deep/combined block (odds ratio 5.15, P<0.0001), but there was an equivalent incidence of other systemic serious complications (odds ratio 1.13, P=0.273; NS). We conclude that superficial/intermediate block is safer than any method that employs a deep injection. The higher rate of conversion to general anaesthesia with the deep/combined block may have been influenced by the higher incidence of direct complications, but may also suggest that the superficial/ combined block provides better analgesia during surgery.

Summary

Complications as a result of >10,000 cervical plexus blocks derived from 69 different papers were analysed in this meta-analysis. Serious complications were more than twice as common in patients who received a deep cervical plexus block compared with superficial or intermediate blocks. This observation was true irrespective of whether deep blocks were performed alone or in combination with a superficial block. Conversion to general anaesthesia was more common in patients receiving a deep block, though the authors were unable to determine if these cases required a general anaesthetic due to complications of, or inadequate anaesthesia from, the block.

Citation count

42.

Related references

1 Stroup DF, Berlin JA, Morton SC, *et al.* Meta-analysis of observational studies in epidemiology: a proposal for reporting. Meta-analysis of observational studies in Epidemiology (MOOSE) group. *J Am Med Assoc* 2000; **283**: 2008–12.

Key message

When providing regional anaesthesia for carotid endarterectomy, superficial or intermediate cervical plexus block is a safer technique than any that involves a deep injection in the neck.

Strengths

The large number of procedures that a meta-analysis of this type generates allows assessment of the relative rates at which infrequent complications occur. The authors adhered to the published guidelines for the performance of a meta-analysis of observational studies (Stroup *et al.*, 2000).

Weaknesses

Only two of the 69 papers included reported randomized controlled trials (RCTs), each of which did not find differences in complication rates. An RCT of suitable size to address the question posed would be challenging. Some studies from more than 30 years ago were included, and the authors acknowledge that these studies may affect the results because clinical practice has changed significantly in this time period.

Relevance

The complications included were serious, including life-threatening complications of the local anaesthetic injections, conversion to general anaesthesia, and serious cardiovascular complications in the early postoperative period such as death, stroke, or myocardial infarction. Evidence that any individual approach to regional anaesthesia of the cervical plexus is more effective than another is lacking. Though not directly assessed by this paper, the higher rate of conversion to general anaesthesia in the deep block group leads the authors to conclude that failure to provide adequate operative conditions may be five times more common with this technique. More importantly, the higher rate of such serious complications with deep blocks should make all clinicians who perform these procedures reconsider their choice of regional anaesthetic technique.

Paper 9: Anesthesia type does not influence early graft patency or limb salvage rates of lower extremity arterial bypass

Author details

ET Pierce, FB Pomposelli, GD Stanley, KP Lewis, JL Cass, FW LoGerfo, GW Gibbons, DL Campbell, DV Freeman, EF Halpern, RH Bode

Reference

Journal of Vascular Surgery 1997; **25**: 226–33.

Abstract

Purpose: The effect of anesthesia type on 30-day graft patency and limb salvage rates was evaluated in patients who underwent femoral to distal artery bypass.

Methods: Of 423 patients randomly assigned to receive general, spinal, or epidural anesthetic, 76 did not meet protocol standards and 32 had inadequate anesthesia. A chart review of the remaining 315 patients was undertaken to obtain surgical information not recorded in the original study. All patients were monitored with radial and pulmonary artery catheters. After surgery, patients were in a monitored setting for 48 to 72 hours and had graft function assessments hourly during the first 24 hours and then every 8 hours until discharge.

Results: Fifty-one patients were lost to follow-up (15 general, 22 spinal, 14 epidural). Baseline clinical characteristics were similar for the three groups except prior carotid artery surgery, which was more common in the spinal group. Indications for surgery were also similar except for a higher incidence of nonhealing ulcer in the epidural group. There were no differences among groups for 30-day graft patency with or without reoperation, 30-day graft occlusion, death, amputation, or length of hospital stay.

Conclusion: These results suggest that the type of anesthetic given for femoral to distal artery bypass does not significantly affect 30-day occlusion rate, limb salvage rate, or hospital length of stay.

Summary

A study designed to compare the influence of general (GA) versus epidural or spinal anaesthesia (RA) on perioperative cardiac morbidity and mortality in patients undergoing lower limb revascularization surgery recruited 423 patients. Patients were randomly allocated to one of the three types of anaesthesia, and in the study reported in this paper the records of 315 of these patients were reviewed to compare further outcome measures between the groups. A variety of factors known to influence the success of lower limb revascularization surgery were recorded, along with postoperative graft patency rates. The type of anaesthetic had no influence on 30-day graft patency rates (with or without re-operation), amputation rates or deaths.

Citation count

32.

Related references

1 Cook PT, Davies MJ, Cronin KD, *et al*. A prospective randomized trial comparing spinal anaesthesia using hyperbaric cinchocaine with general anaesthesia for lower limb vascular surgery. *Anaesth Intensive Care* 1986; **14**: 373–80.

2 Tuman KI, McCarthy RJ, March RJ, *et al*. Effects of epidural anesthesia and analgesia on coagulation and outcome after major vascular surgery. *Anesth Analg* 1991; **73**: 696–704.

3 Christopherson R, Beattie C, Frank SM, *et al*. Perioperative morbidity in patients randomized to epidural or general anesthesia for lower extremity vascular surgery. *Anesthesiology* 1993; **79**: 422–34.

Key message

The choice of general, epidural, or spinal anaesthesia does not influence the early patency rates of lower limb arterial reconstructions.

Strengths

Previous studies of anaesthetic type and graft patency had not included the numerous surgical factors which may have affected surgical success such that differences in outcome previously reported may have resulted from an uneven distribution of these variables rather than an effect of anaesthesia. The paper provides a detailed description of what constituted graft failure. It also involved a larger number of subjects than had been included in all of the three previous reports together which examined the effect of anaesthesia on graft patency (Cook *et al.*, 1986; Tuman *et al.*, 1991; Christopherson *et al.*, 1993).

Weaknesses

The original study considered cardiovascular complications and was not designed to evaluate the effect of anaesthesia type on early graft patency. Despite its size relative to earlier studies, this study still fell short of the 2,300 recruits which the authors estimated would be needed to detect a difference between anaesthetic technique given the low graft failure rates seen in this study.

Other management strategies used in the study may have influenced the results such as the universal avoidance of protamine and the use of aspirin and anticoagulants postoperatively. Similarly, intraoperative haemodynamic monitoring was intensive and continued into the post-operative period. Without this aggressive approach to maintaining graft patency, a benefit of regional anaesthesia may still exist, possibly explaining the difference between the results of this study and the earlier, smaller trials.

Relevance

The findings of the earlier studies provided some evidence that graft patency might be influenced by choice of anaesthetic. With a graft failure rate variously quoted as between 5–10%, the idea that regional anaesthesia might alter surgical outcome will understandably influence the risk benefit analysis performed by the anaesthetist when choosing an anaesthetic technique for an individual patient. Based on their findings, the authors of this study refute the view that RA should be the anaesthetic of choice, and that a patient preference for GA should not be discouraged.

This paper adds significantly to the GA versus RA debate, but does not provide a definitive answer to the question 'does regional anaesthesia reduce the risk of graft failure?' In a discussion accompanying the paper, the commentators agree that 'a good anaesthetic is not going to salvage a bad operation; and a less-than-optimal anaesthetic is not likely to compromise a well-performed bypass grafting procedure' which still remains a reasonable summary of the situation.

Paper 10: Regional anesthesia for vascular access surgery

Author details

E Malinzak, TJ Gan

Reference

Anesthesia and Analgesia 2009; **109**: 976–80.

Summary

This review outlines contemporary evidence regarding the effects of anaesthesia on the success of vascular access surgery based on seven papers. A number of factors which might impact on the successful creation of vascular access for dialysis are discussed, including patient characteristics and comorbidities, and the type of fistula. The authors conclude that the sympathetic block produced by the use of regional anaesthesia may increase arm blood flow and reduce vasospasm during the procedure, leading to reduced maturation time and improved fistula patency rates in the long term.

Citation count

3.

Related references

1 Department of Health. *National Service Framework for Renal Services—part two: Chronic kidney disease, acute renal failure and end of life care.* London: Crown Copyright, 2005.

Key message

The use of regional block may improve the success of renal dialysis vascular access procedures.

Strengths

The review brings together the scant evidence in this field, and the authors acknowledge that a large-scale, prospective clinical trial is necessary before conclusions can be drawn.

Weaknesses

There are only a small number of papers included, each reporting small numbers of patients and employing a range of outcome measures. Little comment is made regarding the relative validity of the various measures of graft failure and the clinical heterogeneity of the studies.

Relevance

The formation of vascular access for dialysis is already a common procedure, and will become more common as the incidence of end stage renal disease increases by 6–8% per annum in the UK (Department of Health, 2005). Radiocephalic arteriovenous fistulas have a primary failure rate of 24–35% secondary to thrombosis or inadequate blood flow. The emergence of evidence in favour of regional anaesthesia compared with general anaesthesia with regard to graft patency would lead to substantial changes in anaesthetic practice. This change will be aided by the wider adoption of ultrasound-guided regional anaesthesia which improves the safety and efficacy of upper limb regional blocks.

Evidence that an anaesthetic technique lasting just a few hours can have a significant effect on the success of a procedure measured in months or years is novel and requires explanation. In the case of arteriovenous fistula there is at least a feasible reason: sympathetic blockade with regional anaesthesia normally produces obvious vasodilatation in the limb and this increase in size of both arteries and veins may well make the anastomosis performed by the surgeon more functional.

Chapter 14

Anaesthesia for major abdominal surgery

MC Bellamy and S Flood

Introduction

Major abdominal surgery is an important component of elective and emergency anaesthesia. In addition to the common challenges of all major surgery it involves managing patients at risk of aspiration, large intraoperative fluid shifts, painful incisions, and postoperative gut functional impairment. In selecting only ten landmark papers in anaesthesia for major abdominal surgery, we were in many ways spoilt for choice. We aimed to include a spectrum of papers from those that have changed clinical practice on the grounds of very little evidence to those well-conducted studies, with large patient numbers, which have so far failed to influence modern anaesthesia. The papers we have chosen cover the important topics of preoperative assessment and optimization, intraoperative fluid administration, and several aspects of postoperative management. We hope this chapter will allow the experienced anaesthetist and seasoned journal reader to re-examine the evidence for their own practice whilst helping the trainee anaesthetist to appreciate the historical context for many aspects of modern anaesthetic practice.

Paper 1: Cricoid pressure to control regurgitation of stomach contents during induction of anaesthesia

Author details

BA Sellick

Reference

Lancet 1961; **19**: 404–6.

Summary

Pulmonary aspiration of gastric contents during anaesthesia has been recognized as a cause of significant morbidity and mortality since the classic publication by Mendelson in 1946. Prior to the adoption of the Sellick technique into mainstream UK anaesthetic practice, options for protecting the airway during induction included performing an inhalation technique, positioning the patient in a head-down, left lateral position or giving an intravenous induction in the sitting position. The latter predisposed the seriously ill patient to cardiovascular collapse and if active vomiting occurred, soiling of the airway was common. Sellick identified a simple manoeuvre that could prevent passive regurgitation of gastric contents until a cuffed tube in the trachea could be secured. He demonstrated first with cadaveric studies and then with real patients that posterior pressure on the cricoid cartilage against the bodies of the cervical vertebrae caused temporary occlusion of the upper oesophagus. This occlusion prevented passive regurgitation of stomach contents even with steep Trendelenburg positioning. He went on to show with lateral radiographs and a contrast containing latex tube in the oesophagus that the manoeuvre was effective in an anaesthetized and paralysed patient. Finally he used the technique in 26 patients at risk of regurgitation and aspiration during induction. The cohort consisted of two obstetric patients, two patients with achalasia, three with pyloric stenosis, a patient with a lower oesophageal tumour, and 18 patients with acute bowel obstruction. No patient suffered an aspiration event during induction. In three patients, release of the cricoid pressure post intubation was followed by immediate reflux of gastric content into the pharynx. Sellick also suggested the manoeuvre might be effective in preventing gastric distension during positive pressure ventilation by facemask.

Citation count

605.

Related references

1 Salem MR, Sellick BA, Elam JO. The historical background of cricoid pressure in anesthesia and resuscitation. *Anesth Analg* 1974; **53**: 230–2.

2 Rice MJ, Mancuso AA, Gibbs C, *et al.* Cricoid pressure results in compression of the postcricoid hypopharynx: the esophageal position is irrelevant. *Anesth Analg* 2009; **109**: 1546–52.

Key message

Posterior pressure of the cricoid cartilage against the cervical vertebrae can be used to occlude the oesophagus and prevent passive regurgitation of stomach contents during induction of anaesthesia.

Strengths

Sellick demonstrated the effectiveness of the technique with both cadaveric and patient studies. His article included line diagrams, photographs, and radiographs.

Weaknesses

There was only a small sample size and no mention by the author of the expected incidence of regurgitation in a similar cohort of patients using either the upright sitting position or left lateral, head-down position. Sellick failed to describe how he confirmed the presence or absence of regurgitation during induction of anaesthesia.

Relevance

The increasing use of muscle relaxants to assist rapid, intravenous induction of anaesthesia in this period placed patients at risk of aspiration from gastric regurgitation. Sellick identified a novel, effective method of protecting the unconscious, paralysed patient from passive regurgitation of stomach contents that required no specialist equipment and only minimal training to perform. This study had an exaggerated influence on UK anaesthetic practice considering the lack of evidence presented in this paper. No comparison between Sellick's manoeuvre and the alternative options for prevention of aspiration was performed. Cricoid pressure is a common technique in UK-based anaesthetic practice, but its importance is not accepted internationally.

Paper 2: Multifactorial index of cardiac risk in non-cardiac surgical procedures

Author details

L Goldman, DL Caldera, SR Nussbaum, FS Southwick, D Krogstad, B Murray, DS Burke, TA O'Malley, AH Goroll, CH Caplan, J Nolan, B Carabello, EE Slater

Reference

New England Journal of Medicine 1977; **297**: 845–50.

Summary

The authors sought to find a more specific tool than the American Surgical Association (ASA) score to predict cardiac risk in patients undergoing non-cardiac surgery. They identified every patient over the age of 40 years undergoing general, urological, or orthopaedic surgery in Massachusetts General Hospital in a 6-month period. Each patient had a preoperative cardiac history and examination by one of the authors, or as soon as possible postoperatively in cases of emergency surgery. Clinically 'important' aortic stenosis was defined as a mid systolic murmur Grade 2 out of 6. Premature ventricular contractions were assessed by reviewing the medical notes, palpation of the pulses and performing an electrocardiogram (ECG) preoperatively. The patient was given an ASA score by their anaesthetist. Apart from a planned ECG on day 5, post-operative cardiac complications were identified by reported symptoms and clinical signs, with the use of ECGs and measurement of cardiac enzymes as necessary. A cardiac death was defined as that occurring directly from an arrhythmia or from refractory low cardiac output that was not part of an inexorable downhill course primarily caused by a non-cardiac condition. From a total of 1,001 patients that participated, 19 had a cardiac death and 39 suffered a potentially life threatening cardiac complication (myocardial infarction, pulmonary oedema, or ventricular tachycardia). Analysis identified nine factors that correlated significantly with cardiac outcome: third heart sound or raised jugular venous pressure (JVP), myocardial infarction in preceding 6 months, rhythm other than sinus, >5 premature ventricular contractions/min, intraperitoneal or thoracic surgery, age >70 years, aortic stenosis, emergency surgery, and poor general medical condition. The authors computed a cardiac risk index by converting the multivariate discriminant-function coefficients to 'points'. They identified four risk groups, with a stepwise progression (group 1 to group 4) in the risk of patients developing a life-threatening cardiac complication or suffering a cardiac death.

Citation count

2006.

Related references

1 Noblett SE, Snowden CP, Shenton BK, *et al*. Randomized clinical trial assessing the effect of Doppler-optimized fluid management on outcome after elective colorectal resection. *Br J Surg* 2006; **93**: 1069–76.

2 Abbas SM, Hill AG. Systematic review of the literature for the use of oesophageal Doppler monitor for fluid replacement in major abdominal surgery. *Anaesthesia* 2008; **3**: 44–51.

3 Lahner D, Kabon B, Marschalek C, *et al*. Evaluation of stroke volume variation obtained by arterial pulse contour analysis to predict fluid responsiveness intraoperatively. *Br J Anaesth* 2009; **103**: 346–51.

Key message

The risk of postoperative cardiac complications in patients undergoing non-cardiac surgery may be estimated by preoperative history taking and clinical examination. Patients with a third heart sound, raised JVP or who have suffered a myocardial infarction in the preceding 6 months are at the greatest risk.

Strengths

The study had large patient numbers and wide inclusion criteria, so to that these findings were applicable to all patients undergoing non-cardiac surgery.

Weaknesses

The reliance on ward doctors identifying cardiac complications from patients' signs and reported symptoms is likely to have underestimated the number of postoperative events. A more systematic approach to postoperative ECGs and cardiac enzymes may have captured more cardiac complications. The authors acknowledge the interobserver variability in assessment of preoperative symptoms, signs and even in the interpretation of ECGs. However they state that no patient was classified into a different risk group by a duplicate observer.

Relevance

This paper gives a historical snapshot of the real concerns anaesthetists at the time had in avoiding intraoperative cardiac complications. The ASA classification is of limited value in predicting post-operative cardiac complications following non-cardiac surgery. This paper gave anaesthetists a practical, easily applied index, based on preoperative clinical findings, to assess cardiac risk for the individual patient. The study's emphasis on the ability of history taking and good clinical examination to accurately assess risk has ensured its high profile in modern anaesthetic training. The study was a milestone in the development of a philosophy regarding patients' overall fitness for general anaesthesia. Concerns for preventing intraoperative myocardial infarction have widened into a desire to prevent cardiac, respiratory, renal, and surgical complications. Preoperative history taking and examination are now supplemented by stress echocardiography, shuttle run tests, and cardiopulmonary exercise testing. The Goldman risk index was the first step towards providing the patient with individualized risk assessments of morbidity and mortality that is the goal of modern preoperative assessment.

Paper 3: A randomized clinical trial of the effect of deliberate perioperative increase of oxygen delivery on mortality in high-risk surgical patients

Author details

O Boyd, RM Grounds, ED Bennett

Reference

Journal of the American Medical Association 1993; **70**: 2699–707.

Summary

This study was the first modern perioperative optimization study. The authors noted that Clowes and Del Guercio observed in the 1960s that high-risk patients, surviving operations tended to have higher postoperative cardiac output and oxygen delivery. Shoemaker demonstrated on a small number of patients in 1988 that mortality and morbidity could be reduced by optimizing perioperative cardiac output and oxygen delivery. In this paper Boyd, Grounds, and Bennett from St George's Hospital, London performed a randomized control trial with well-matched, large patient groups, examining the benefits of preoperative optimization of oxygen delivery.

One hundred and seven high-risk patients undergoing major surgery were randomized to either 'best conventional care' in the control arm or preoperative optimization of oxygen delivery in the protocol arm. All patients were admitted to the intensive care unit (ICU) preoperatively and underwent insertion of a peripheral arterial line and central pulmonary artery occlusion catheter. Modified fluid gelatin was given to all patients either until the pulmonary capillary wedge pressure was 12–14 mmHg, urine output >100 ml h^{-1} or there was no further increase in cardiac output. Packed red cells were administered to ensure the patient's haemoglobin reached a minimum of 12 g dl^{-1} and oxygen was delivered by facemask if the SpO$_2$ was <94%. A set of baseline observations were then recorded: heart rate, systemic blood pressure, pulmonary pressure, cardiac output, mixed venous and arterial oxygen saturations and serum lactate. In the protocol group patients, dopexamine was started at 0.5 mg kg^{-1} min^{-1} and the infusion rate doubled every 30 min until a target oxygen delivery index (DO$_2$I) of 600 ml min^{-1} m^{-2} was achieved. Escalation of the dopexamine dose was halted in the event of chest pain, ST depression, an increase in heart rate of >20% from baseline or the maximum dose of 8 mg/kg^{-1} min^{-1} was reached. Once patients left the ICU and proceeded to theatre, intraoperative management was directed by the theatre anaesthetist. The only difference between control and protocol patients was that the latter continued on their dopexamine infusion during surgery. Postoperatively all patients were readmitted to the ICU with treatment targets being the same as preoperatively: pulmonary wedge pressure 12–14 mmHg, haemoglobin 12 g dl^{-1} and SpO$_2$ >94%. Protocol patients had their dopexamine infusions titrated to DO$_2$I as previously. Dopexamine was discontinued once serum lactate normalized. Discharge from ICU was directed by the ICU team, not the authors and final discharge from hospital was instigated by the surgical team. Patient notes were reviewed 28 days following discharge and all postoperative complications noted. Protocol patients received a mean infusion rate of 1.18 µg kg^{-1} min^{-1} of dopexamine pre operatively and 1.32 µg kg^{-1} min^{-1} postoperatively. The infusion was continued for a median of 6.5 h postoperatively. There were no significant differences in mean arterial pressure, central venous pressure, or pulmonary wedge pressure between the two groups either pre- or postoperatively, confirming the poor predictive value of these indices. As expected, there was a significantly higher CI and DO$_2$I in the protocol patients pre- and postoperatively (P <0.01). Protocol patients had a significantly lower 28-day mortality rate (5.7%) compared to controls (22.2%) (P=0.015). The greatest difference in mortality was observed in patients who had abdominal surgery; none of 17 patients in the protocol group died and five (25%) of 20 patients in the control group died (P=0.049). Significantly fewer patients suffered complications in the protocol group compared to controls (P=0.008).

Citation count

768.

Related references

1 Wilson J, Woods I, Fawcett J, *et al.* Reducing the risk of major elective surgery: randomised controlled trial of preoperative optimisation of oxygen delivery. *BMJ* 1999; **24**: 1099–103.

Key message

Deliberately increasing cardiac output and oxygen delivery perioperative with an infusion of dopexamine, reduces morbidity and mortality in high-risk surgical patients.

Strengths

This was a randomized control trial with pre-study power calculations.

Weaknesses

The authors state that both the theatre anaesthetist and operating surgeon were blinded to the patient's group allocation, however no details are given as to how the dopexamine infusion was concealed in the protocol group. Nine patients in the treatment group did not receive dopexamine according to protocol (four patients did not have the infusion titrated correctly and five patients failed to receive it at all preoperatively). As the data was analysed on an intention-to-treat basis, the differences in mortality and morbidity between groups may have been even greater than observed. The study included patients who only received dopexamine post operatively after being recruited and randomized intraoperatively. The authors acknowledge that the study lacked the power to adequately compare the effects of pre- and postoperative dopexamine with postoperative infusion alone.

Relevance

This was the first randomized control trial with well-matched patients groups of adequate size to demonstrate the effectiveness of this regimen for increasing perioperative DO_2I in reducing morbidity and mortality in high-risk surgical patients. It is difficult to elucidate from this paper exactly why the protocol patients did so much better. It may have been the vasodilator effects of dopexamine encouraging adequate fluid filling, its inotrope properties on oxygen delivery or its known anti-inflammatory effects. The study protocol would be demanding in both time and financial resources to roll out into standard clinical practice, requiring a significant expansion of critical care beds. The real legacy of this paper may prove to be that it led us to debate the merits of target driven versus goal directed patient pre-optimization and paved the way for future trials.

Paper 4: Central venous pressure and its effect on blood loss during liver resection

Author details

RM Jones, CE Moulon, KJ Hardy

Reference

British Journal of Surgery 1998; **85**: 1058–60.

Summary

Hepatic resection surgery has historically been associated with a significant risk of intraoperative haemorrhage. Bleeding not only impairs the operating conditions for the surgeon but also increases the likelihood of the patient needing a blood transfusion. Any steps taken by the anaesthetist to minimize intraoperative haemorrhage would make surgery easier for the surgeon and safer for the patient. This study prospectively documented the central venous pressure in 100 consecutive patients undergoing liver resection performed between 1986 and 1996. The main outcome measures documented were volume of intraoperative blood loss and blood transfusion requirements. Other details noted were age, gender, intercurrent disease, length of surgery, number of segments resected, and duration of Pringle manoeuvre. The authors divided the total number of patients into two groups: CVP >5 cmH$_2$O and CVP ≤5 cmH$_2$O. The median blood loss in all patients was 450 ml. However for those patients with a CVP >5 cmH$_2$O median blood loss was 1000 ml compared to 200 ml in the group with CVP ≤5 cmH$_2$O (P <0.0001). In the group with a CVP >5 cmH$_2$O 48% patients required blood transfusion compared to only 5% in CVP ≤5 cmH$_2$O group (P=0.0008). These trends were found to be independent of duration of Pringle manoeuvre, duration of surgery, number of segments resected, method of dissection or the presence of cirrhosis.

Citation count

220.

Related references

1 Melendez JA, Arslan V, Fischer ME, *et al*. Perioperative outcomes of major hepatic resections under low central venous pressure anesthesia: blood loss, blood transfusion, and the risk of postoperative renal dysfunction. *J Am Coll Surg* 1998; **187**: 620–5.

2 Chen H, Merchant NB, Didolkar MS. Hepatic resection using intermittent vascular inflow occlusion and low central venous pressure anesthesia improves morbidity and mortality. *J Gastrointest Surg* 2000; **4**: 162–7.

3 Vassiliou I, Arkadopoulos N, Stafyla V, *et al*. The introduction of a simple manoeuvre to reduce the risk of postoperative bleeding after major hepatectomies. *J Hepatobiliary Pancreat Surg* 2009; **16**: 552–6.

Key message

A low CVP during hepatic resection is associated with reduced blood loss and blood transfusion requirements.

Strengths

The study cohort included a wide range of indications for surgery (metastases, hepatomas, hydatid disease) and type of operation (left lobectomy, right hemihepatectomy, left hemihepatectomy, right lobectomy, submentectomy, and subsegmentectomy).

Weaknesses

The authors do not make clear in the method section whether the CVP was merely observed without modification from the theatre anaesthetists or whether any attempts were made to reduce it with a specific target in mind (e.g. <5 cmH$_2$O). If the study involved actively trying to keep the CVP low, then again no details are given as to whether this was achieved through fluid restriction or infusion of vasodilators. In addition no details are provided as to patient positioning. The authors state clearly than CVP was measured from a zero point at the level of the right atrium, but if the patients were head-up then hepatic vein pressure would exceed CVP whereas in a head-down position hepatic vein pressure would be lower than CVP. The authors refer to a possible increased risk of air embolism in patients with a low/negative central venous pressure. Two patients reportedly suffered an air embolism during the study, but it is not clear which group the patients originated.

Relevance

This paper has greatly influenced clinical practice with maintenance of a low CVP being a central tenant of modern liver resection anaesthesia. There is however inadequate evidence in this observational study to allow the authors to conclude that active maintenance of a low CVP reduces intraoperative bleeding during liver resection. The influence of volume status, use of vasodilators and patient positioning were not mentioned. This paper may suggest an association between CVP and bleeding but fell short of proving active intervention reduces intraoperative haemorrhage.

Paper 5: Effects of the combination of blood transfusion and postoperative infectious complications on prognosis after surgery for colorectal cancer

Author details

T Mynster, LJ Christensen, F Moesgaard, HJ Nielsen

Reference

British Journal of Surgery 2000; **87**: 1553–62.

Summary

Perioperative transfusion of allogenic blood is a known risk factor for the development of post-operative infectious complications. It has been suggested that blood transfusion impairs immunity and leaves the patient more vulnerable to pathogenic organisms. The authors wished to examine whether this relative state of immunosuppression following blood products impacted on tumour recurrence rates and/or overall survival in patients with colorectal adenocarcimoma. There were 740 patients listed for elective colorectal cancer surgery recruited to this multicentre study. All patients received antibiotic prophylaxis at induction. Blood transfusion was defined as transfusion of SAGM (saline–adenine–glucose–mannitol) blood or fresh frozen plasma 30 days prior to or 14 days following surgery. Postoperative infection was defined as the presence of pus, either discharging spontaneously or requiring interventional drainage. All patients were reviewed every 3 months in the outpatient clinic. Those patients receiving a perioperative blood transfusion had a significantly greater risk of developing a postoperative infection (p = 0.001). Those patients who developed a postoperative infection following a perioperative transfusion had a lower overall survival than those patients who had a blood transfusion or developed an infection or neither. The hazard ratio for death in patients who received a transfusion and developed postoperative infection was 1.38 (CI 1.05–1.81) compared to non-infected/no transfusion patients. The same patient cohort (transfusion and infection) were found to have a significantly higher rate of disease recurrence (hazard ratio 1.79 CI 1.13–2.82). Rectal site and Duke's stage were other independent risk factors for disease recurrence. The combination of blood transfusion and a post operative infection is likely to be synergistic in increasing the risk of disease recurrence and death. The mechanism for this synergistic interaction may be either immunomodulation or tumour cell stimulation. Stored blood contains angiogenesis stimulating factors such as vascular endothelial growth factor (VEGF) which may promote tumour progression. Delayed wound healing from an infection can activate granulocytes which may stimulate production of angiogenic factors.

Citation count

107.

Related references

1 Miller GV, Ramsden CW, Primrose JN. Autologous transfusion: an alternative to transfusion with banked blood during surgery for cancer. *Br J Surg* 1991; **78**: 713–15.

2 Edna TH, Bjerkeset T. Perioperative blood transfusions reduce long-term survival following surgery for colorectal cancer. *Dis Colon Rectum* 1998; **41**: 451–9.

3 Davis M, Sofer M, Gomez-Marin O, *et al.* The use of cell salvage during radical retropubic prostatectomy: does it influence cancer recurrence? *BJU Int* 2003; **91**: 474–6.

4 Miki C, Hiro J, Ojima E, *et al.* Perioperative allogeneic blood transfusion, the related cytokine response and long-term survival after potentially curative resection of colorectal cancer. *Clin Oncol (R Coll Radiol)* 2006; **18**: 60–6.

Key message

The combination of a perioperative blood transfusion and subsequent postoperative infection is associated with an increased risk of both tumour recurrence and death in colorectal cancer patients.

Strengths

This was a multicentre study, with a large sample size, in which no patients were lost to follow-up— despite the need for up to 8 years of outpatient surveillance.

Relevance

This study confirmed previously published evidence that the need for perioperative blood transfusion is associated with increased morbidity and mortality. The authors suggest that one possible explanation for their findings may be the synergistic effect of transfusion and infection in predisposing to disease recurrence. It is not clear however whether the need for transfusion and development of a postoperative infection may simply be surrogate markers for the size of the surgical insult. The authors also found that rectal location of tumour, advanced stage, extent of blood loss, and duration of surgery were risk factors for recurrence or death.

Paper 6: Effect of thoracic epidural anaesthesia on colonic blood flow

Author details

TH Gould, K Grace, G Thorne, M Thomas

Reference

British Journal of Anaesthesia 2002; **89**: 446–51.

Abstract

Background: The effect of thoracic epidural block on splanchnic blood flow is unclear. It remains to be resolved if sympathetic block, increases or decreases regional splanchnic blood flow and whether regional splanchnic flow becomes dependent on cardiac output or perfusion pressure. A clear understanding of the regional haemodynamic consequences of an epidural block may modify practice with respect to epidural anaesthesia.

Methods: Fifteen patients, who underwent anterior resection for rectal cancer, had invasive intra-operative monitoring of arterial pressure, central venous pressure, cardiac output, inferior mesenteric artery flow (Doppler flow probe), and colonic serosal red cell flux (laser Doppler probe), while an epidural block was established with local anaesthetic. In three consecutive time periods, arterial pressure was first allowed to fall (to a mean arterial pressure of 60 mmHg), then treated with colloid fluid resuscitation and finally by vasopressors until the pre-epidural arterial pressure had been restored.

Results: On induction of epidural block, there was a reduction in mean colonic serosal red cell flux to 65% and inferior mesenteric artery flow to 80% (mean) of pre-epidural levels. There was a strong association between mean arterial pressure and both measured inferior mesenteric artery blood flow (P <0.004) and colonic serosal red cell flux (P <0.0001). Changes in cardiac output were poorly associated with either inferior mesenteric artery blood flow (P = 0.638) or colonic serosal red cell flux (P = 0.265). Inferior mesenteric artery blood flow and colonic serosal red cell flux were restored to pre-epidural levels after arterial pressure had been improved with a vasopressor.

Conclusion: Once intraoperative epidural block has been established, colonic serosal red cell flux and inferior mesenteric artery flow are more closely associated with changes in mean arterial pressure than changes in cardiac output. The measured reduction in colonic flow does not respond to an increase in cardiac output with fluid resuscitation, but requires the use of a vaso-pressor to increase arterial pressure, before colonic blood flow is improved.

Summary

This paper, originally designed as a pilot study, set out to clarify the haemodynamic effects of thoracic epidurals on splanchnic blood flow. Several previous studies examining the relationship between epidural blockade and gut blood flow had conflictingly shown no effect, increase in flow and decreased flow. The Bristol authors consented 15 patients undergoing anterior resection for colonic carcinoma to have intraoperative Doppler measurement of inferior mesenteric artery blood flow and laser Doppler colonic serosal red cell flux measurements taken directly. Following a standardized induction of general anaesthesia, insertion of invasive monitoring, positioning of an oesophageal Doppler probe and insertion of a low (T9–10) thoracic epidural catheter, the abdomen was opened. A laser Doppler probe was attached to the serosal surface of the colon and a Doppler ultrasound probe to the inferior mesenteric artery. After 5 min of baseline measurements, epidural blockade was initiated with 0.5 mg kg^{-1} of 0.5% bupivacaine and the mean arterial pressure (MAP) allowed to fall to 60 mmHg. In phase 2 this fall in MAP was treated with a bolus of colloid, the infusion stopping when cardiac output (CO) and central venous pressure (CVP) had returned to baseline values. Phase 3 saw any remaining hypotension treated with 2-mg boluses of methoxamine. During all 3 phases, data on inferior mesenteric artery blood flow and red cell flux were recorded. Colonic blood flow fell with MAP following epidural bupivacaine (Phase 1). In Phase 2 an increase in CO and CVP with infusion of a colloid bolus failed to restore flow. Colonic blood flow only returned to pre epidural levels after the restoration of MAP with a vasopressor (Phase 3).

The authors demonstrated that both inferior mesenteric artery blood flow and serosal red cell flux correlate closely to MAP and are poorly associated with CO.

Citation count

50.

Related references

1 Lundberg J, Lundberg D, Norgren L, et al. Intestinal hemodynamics during laparotomy: effects of thoracic epidural anesthesia and dopamine in humans. Anesth Analg 1990; 71: 9–15.

Key message

Hypotension following low thoracic epidural blockade decreases splanchnic blood flow. Restoration of pre-epidural cardiac output and/or central venous pressure is inadequate in reversing the reduction in gut perfusion. As colonic blood flow closely follows mean arterial pressure, perfusion may be restored with the appropriate use of vasospressors.

Strengths

The study used two direct methods of measuring colonic blood flow.

Weaknesses

Patients with cardiovascular disease or taking any cardiovascular medication were excluded from the study. The relationships between colonic blood flow, MAP, CO, and CVP may therefore differ in the many patients undergoing surgery who have a history of ischaemic heart disease or those taking antihypertensive medication. Complete data were collected for only 11 of the 15 patients recruited and no power calculation was used to estimate required sample size.

Relevance

This was the first study to directly measure colonic blood flow continuously during the establishment of an epidural block and subsequent management of the associated hypotension. Epidural anaesthesia is a commonly used technique and suboptimal management of the associated hypotension may impact on ileus duration, bacterial translocation and anastomotic failure rates. Despite the publication of this persuasive, well-conducted study, standard management of epidural related hypotension continues to focus on fluid boluses in many centres. Routine use of vasopressors to treat hypotension in colonic surgery is not widespread. It may be that theatre anaesthetists do not observe the postoperative complications of intraoperative gut hypoperfusion or that postoperative ileus and translocation leading to sepsis are attributed to surgical technique. The advent of laparoscopic colonic surgery may mean patients can be managed without thoracic epidurals or the central venous catheters that would be required to adequately manage their complications.

Paper 7: Colonic surgery with accelerated rehabilitation or conventional care

Author details

L Basse, JE Horbol, K Lossol, H Kehlet

Reference

Diseases of the Colon and Rectum 2004; **47**: 271–8.

Summary

Several studies had already shown reduced duration of urinary catheterization and early oral feeding allowed postoperative stay following colonic surgery to be reduced from 6–10 days to 2–3 days and that the routine insertion of nasogastric tubes following surgery was unnecessary. This study set out to compare the complication rates of patients in the first month following 'fast track' surgery to historical controls. One hundred and thirty consecutive patients undergoing fast track rehabilitation following colonic surgery were followed up for 30 days. Outcomes recorded were time to first defecation, readmission rate, and incidence of medical and surgical complications. The fast track patient group was comparable to historical controls for age, gender, underlying disease, and type of surgery. The fast track group had a significantly higher ASA score compared to controls. All patients received a general anaesthetic and thoracic epidural. The main components of the fast track program were: no premedication, intraoperative crystalloids limited to 1,500 ml, intraoperative ondansetron and ketorolac, transverse surgical incision, epidural out after 2 days, multimodal postoperative analgesia, cisapride postoperatively, and urinary catheter removal on the first postoperative day.

The mean hospital stay was 2 days in the fast track group and 8 days in the control group (P <0.05). Median time to first defecation was 2 days in fast track patients versus 4.5 days in controls (P <0.05). There were significantly more postoperative complications in historical controls than the fast track patients. Individual categories of complication reaching statistical significance included cardiovascular, pulmonary and wound complications. There was no significant difference in readmission rates with 20% of patients readmitted in the fast track group compared to 12% of patients in the control group (P >0.05).

Citation count

290.

Related references

1 Hjort Jakobsen D, Sonne E, Basse L, *et al.* Convalescence after colonic resection with fast-track versus conventional care. *Scand J Surg* 2004; **93**: 24–8.

2 Noblett SE, Watson DS, Huong H, *et al.* Pre-operative oral carbohydrate loading in colorectal surgery: a randomised controlled trial. *Colorectal Dis* 2006; **8**: 563–9.

3 Gouvas N, Tan E, Windsor A, *et al.* Fast-track vs. standard care in colorectal surgery: a meta-analysis update. *Int J Colorectal Dis* 2009; **24**: 1119–31.

Key message

A 'fast track' package of rehabilitation following colonic surgery allows a shorter postoperative hospital stay and decreases the incidence of postoperative complications in the first month.

Strengths

The authors demonstrated a significant reduction in cardiovascular, pulmonary and wound related complications despite a higher median ASA score in the fast track group.

Weaknesses

This was not a randomized control trial. One major weakness in this study is that the authors retrospectively analysed patient records in a different hospital to form a control group. By examining the effectiveness of a 'bundle' of interventions, the value of individual components of that bundle cannot be deduced. Patients undergoing acute surgery or having a stoma were excluded and therefore these results may not be applicable to these patient groups.

Relevance

This was one of the first papers to suggest the potential benefits of standardized, protocol-based postoperative care. Any package of interventions that reduces length of stay and incidence of complications is beneficial to both the individual patient and the healthcare provider. Significant improvements to patient care may be obtained from using 'bundles' of interventions. Scientific curiosity may lead us to try to attribute value to individual components of these bundles, but large patient numbers would be required for any such study to have adequate power. In reality this package comprises of several low-cost, high-impact interventions that could easily be adopted into routine National Health Service (NHS) practice without elucidating the importance of individual components. This study reinforces the benefits of multimodal analgesia and early mobilization following surgery.

Paper 8: Intraoperative oesophageal Doppler guided fluid management shortens postoperative hospital stay after major bowel surgery

Author details

HG Wakeling, MR McFall, CS Jenkins, WG Woods, WF Miles, GR Barclay, SC Fleming

Reference

British Journal of Anaesthesia 2005; **95**: 634–42.

Abstract

Background: Occult hypovolaemia is a key factor in the aetiology of postoperative morbidity and may not be detected by routine heart rate and arterial pressure measurements. Intraoperative gut hypoperfusion during major surgery is associated with increased morbidity and postoperative hospital stay. We assessed whether using intraoperative oesophageal Doppler guided fluid management to minimize hypovolaemia would reduce postoperative hospital stay and the time before return of gut function after colorectal surgery.

Methods: This single centre, blinded, prospective controlled trial randomized 128 consecutive consenting patients undergoing colorectal resection to oesophageal Doppler guided or central venous pressure (CVP)-based (conventional) intraoperative fluid management. The intervention group patients followed a dynamic oesophageal Doppler guided fluid protocol whereas control patients were managed using routine cardiovascular monitoring aiming for a CVP between 12 and 15 mmHg.

Results: The median postoperative stay in the Doppler guided fluid group was 10 *vs.* 11.5 days in the control group *P* <0.05. The median time to resuming full diet in the Doppler guided fluid group was 6 *vs.* 7 for controls *P* <0.001. Doppler patients achieved significantly higher cardiac output, stroke volume, and oxygen delivery. Twenty-nine (45.3%) control patients suffered gastrointestinal morbidity compared with nine (14.1%) in the Doppler guided fluid group *P* <0.001, overall morbidity was also significantly higher in the control group *P*=0.05.

Conclusions: Intraoperative oesophageal Doppler guided fluid management was associated with a 1.5-day median reduction in postoperative hospital stay. Patients recovered gut function significantly faster and suffered significantly less gastrointestinal and overall morbidity.

Summary

Intraoperative hypovolaemia leading to poor organ perfusion is a known risk factor for postoperative morbidity after major surgery. Heart rate and even invasive arterial pressure monitoring are insensitive indicators of intraoperative fluid balance and may not prevent occult hypovolaemia. This study was designed to examine whether oesophageal Doppler-guided fluid management reduced postoperative hospital stay and time to return of gut function by avoiding intraoperative hypovolaemia. Patients presenting for elective large bowel resections were randomized to either Doppler or control groups. Following a standard propofol/fentanyl induction and cannulation of a central vein, a CardioQ oesophageal probe was inserted to a length of approx 35–40 cm from

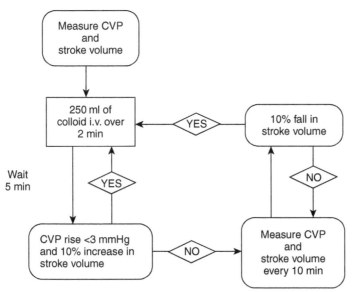

Fig. 14.1 Stroke volume output fluid algorithm. Reproduced from H.G. Wakeling, M.R. McFall, C.S. Jenkins, W.G. Woods, W.F. Miles, G.R. Barclay, S.C. Fleming, Intraoperative oesophageal Doppler guided fluid management shortens postoperative hospital stay after major bowel surgery, *British Journal of Anaesthesia*, 2005, **95**, pp. 634–642, Oxford University Press, by permission of British Journal of Anaesthesia.

the teeth. In the control group cardiac output (CO) and stroke volume (SV) measurements were taken before the operation, immediately after laparotomy and at the end of the operation. The anaesthetist was blinded to these measurements and fluid balance was directed by keeping CVP between 12 and 15 mmHg. In the Doppler group CO and SV measurements were made continuously throughout surgery. Fluid therapy was directed by changes in SV to a 250-ml bolus of colloid (see Fig. 14.1). All patients received standard postoperative care. The authors' primary outcome measure was duration of hospital stay: 10 days in the Doppler group versus 11.5 days in the control group (P <0.05). Their secondary outcome measure was time to return of tolerating a full diet: 6 days in the Doppler group versus 7 days in the control group (P <0.001). Doppler group patients received significantly larger volumes of colloid fluids intraoperatively, achieved a higher SV and CO at end of surgery. There was no significant difference in CVP between the groups at end of surgery. The authors also demonstrated significant reductions in gastrointestinal and overall postoperative morbidity with the use of Doppler-guided fluid management.

Citation count

233.

Related references

1 Sinclair S, James S, Singer M. Intraoperative intravascular volume optimisation and length of hospital stay after repair of proximal femoral fracture: randomised controlled trial. *BMJ* 1997; **315**: 909–12.

2 Noblett SE, Snowden CP, Shenton BK, *et al.* Randomized clinical trial assessing the effect of Doppler-optimized fluid management on outcome after elective colorectal resection. *Br J Surg* 2006; **93**: 1069–76.

3 Abbas SM, Hill AG. Systematic review of the literature for the use of oesophageal Doppler monitor for fluid replacement in major abdominal surgery. *Anaesthesia* 2008; **63**: 44–51.

4 Lahner D, Kabon B, Marschalek C, *et al.* Evaluation of stroke volume variation obtained by arterial pulse contour analysis to predict fluid responsiveness intraoperatively. *Br J Anaesth* 2009; **103**: 346–51.

5 NHS Technology Adoption Centre. *Doppler Guided Intraoperative Fluid Management.* Available at: http://www.technologyadoptioncentre.nhs.uk/doppler-guided-intraoperative-fluid-management/executive-summary.html (accessed 3 February 2010).

Key message

Oesophageal Doppler-guided intraoperative fluid management is associated with shorter postoperative hospital stay and more rapid recovery of gut function compared to titrating fluid therapy to CVP alone in patients undergoing large bowel surgery.

Strengths

This was a randomized controlled trial with pre-study power calculations to estimate minimum sample sizes.

Weaknesses

Although the authors suggest the benefits of higher CO at the end of surgery is in the avoidance of gut hypoperfusion, they found no differences in small bowel permeability, translocation of endotoxin or levels of interleukin-6 between the two groups. The mechanism by which Doppler-guided fluid therapy improves patient outcome remains to be demonstrated.

Relevance

This study clearly demonstrates several benefits of intraoperative cardiac output measurement over 'standard' anaesthetic monitoring. Oesophageal Doppler monitoring is relatively minimally invasive and inexpensive, its use in directing intraoperative fluid administration can improve outcomes for individual patients and allow more efficient use of healthcare resources. Its value has recently been recognized by the NHS Technology Adoption Centre and this should improve access to this important clinical tool across all NHS Trusts.

Paper 9: Liberal or restrictive fluid administration in fast-track colonic surgery: a randomized, double-blind study

Author details

K Holte, NB Foss, J Anderson, L Valentiner, C Lund, P Bie, H Kehlet

Reference

British Journal of Anaesthesia 2007; **99**: 500–8.

Abstract

Background: Evidence-based guidelines on optimal peri-operative fluid management have not been established, and recent randomized trials in major abdominal surgery suggest that large amounts of fluid may increase morbidity and hospital stay. However, no information is available on detailed functional outcomes or with fast-track surgery. Therefore, we investigated the effects of two regimens of intraoperative fluids with physiological recovery as the primary outcome measure after fast-track colonic surgery.

Methods: In a double-blind study, 32 ASA I–III patients undergoing elective colonic surgery were randomized to 'restrictive' (Group 1) or 'liberal' (Group 2) peri-operative fluid administration. Fluid algorithms were based on fixed rates of crystalloid infusions and a standardized volume of colloid. Pulmonary function (spirometry) was the primary outcome measure, with secondary outcomes of exercise capacity (submaximal exercise test), orthostatic tolerance, cardiovascular hormonal responses, postoperative ileus (transit of radio-opaque markers), postoperative nocturnal hypoxaemia, and overall recovery within a well-defined multimodal, fast-track recovery programme. Hospital stay and complications were also noted.

Results: 'Restrictive' (median 1640 ml, range 935–2250 ml) compared with 'liberal' fluid administration (median 5050 ml, range 3563–8050 ml) led to significant improvement in pulmonary function and postoperative hypoxaemia. In contrast, we found significantly reduced concentrations of cardiovascularly active hormones (renin, aldosterone, and angiotensin II) in Group 2. The number of patients with complications was not significantly different between the groups [1 ('liberal' group) [corrected] vs. 6 ('restrictive' group) [corrected] patients, P = 0.08].

Conclusions: A 'restrictive' [corrected] fluid regimen led to a transient improvement in pulmonary function and postoperative hypoxaemia but no other differences in all-over physiological recovery compared with a 'liberal' [corrected] fluid regimen after fast-track colonic surgery. Since morbidity tended to be increased with the 'restrictive' fluid regimen, future studies should focus on the effect of individualized 'goal-directed' fluid administration strategies rather than fixed fluid amounts on postoperative outcome.

Summary

Clinical practice varies widely regarding the administration of perioperative fluids. The 'liberal' compared to 'restrictive' fluid debate is a controversial one with both approaches seeming to have their own evidence base. Several randomized clinical trials preceding this paper indicated a liberal fluid policy increased postoperative morbidity and lengthened hospital stay. The authors wished to pursue whether the same was true in fast track colorectal surgery patients. Fast-track patients are allowed to eat and drink freely immediately after surgery, thereby minimizing the impact of postoperative fluids. Thirty two patients out of 103 undergoing elective colonic surgery met the inclusion criteria and were recruited to the study. All patients received a standard general anaesthetic and thoracic epidural. Patients were randomized by sealed envelope to 'liberal' or 'restrictive' groups. The liberal group patients received $10\,ml\,kg^{-1}$ crystalloid preload, $18\,ml\,kg^{-1}\,h^{-1}$ crystalloid and $7\,ml\,kg^{-1}$ colloid intraoperatively and $10\,m\,kg^{-1}$ in recovery. The restrictive group patients received no preload, $7\,ml\,kg^{-1}$ for the first hour then $5\,ml\,kg^{-1}$ crystalloid and $7\,ml\,kg^{-1}$ colloid intraoperatively and no additional fluid in recovery. Duration of GA and surgery did not differ between the groups. Liberal patients received a median of 5,050 ml versus 1,640 ml in the restrictive group. Intraoperative haemodynamic data did not differ between the two groups although the restrictive group did tend towards lower systolic blood pressure (P = 0.06). A significant decrease in FVC and FEV_1 was found in liberal patients compared to restrictive at 6h post surgery (P <0.05). In addition, liberal patients were found to have significantly lower oxygen saturation and more frequent desaturations to <90% on the second postoperative night (P <0.05). There was however no difference in exercise capacity between the two groups. In contrast, liberal patients had reduced postoperative rises in plasma renin, aldosterone and angiotensin II hormones compared to the restrictive patients. There was a reduced duration of hospital stay (P = 0.03) and fewer post operative complications (P <0.01) in the liberal group.

Citation count

110.

Related references

1 Holte K, Klarskov B, Christensen DS, *et al.* Liberal versus restrictive fluid administration to improve recovery after laparoscopic cholecystectomy: a randomized, double-blind study. *Ann Surg* 2004; **240**: 892–9.

2 Nisanevich V, Felsenstein I, Almogy G, *et al.* Effect of intraoperative fluid management on outcome after intraabdominal surgery. *Anesthesiology* 2005; **103**: 25–32.

3 Bundgaard-Nielsen M, Secher NH, Kehlet H. 'Liberal' vs. 'restrictive' perioperative fluid therapy—a critical assessment of the evidence. *Acta Anaesthesiol Scand* 2009; **53**: 843–51.

Key message

A liberal approach to perioperative fluid administration may be associated in fast-track patients with a shorter hospital stay and fewer total postoperative complications.

Strengths

This was a double blinded, prospective, randomized controlled trial.

Weaknesses

Due to relatively restrictive inclusion criteria (e.g. age <50) only a small sample of 32 patients were selected to participate out of a possible 105 patients undergoing surgery. The two treatment groups are likely to represent the extremes of clinical practice, with $18\,ml\,kg^{-1}\,h^{-1}$ in the liberal group being in excess of most published guidelines. Spirometry is known to be a poor predictor of postoperative pulmonary complications.

Relevance

Similar studies published around the same time came to differing conclusions regarding the relative merits of restrictive vs. liberal administration of fluids. Nisanevich *et al.* (2005) compared $4\,ml\,kg^{-1}\,h^{-1}$ to $12\,ml\,kg^{-1}\,h^{-1}$ in patients undergoing major abdominal surgery. He found that a restrictive protocol reduced time to return of gut function, hospital stay and the incidence of complications. Aside from the sample size (Holte 32 patients, Nisanevich 152 patients) the main difference between the studies was that in Holte's study, patients received no intravenous fluids routinely postoperatively, with patients being allowed to eat and drink following surgery. In the Nisanevich study patients received up to $1.5\,ml\,kg^{-1}\,h^{-1}$ of dextrose saline for 3 days postoperatively. Holte's liberal group therefore received a similar total volume of intravenous fluid (5,050 ml) as Nisanevich's restrictive group (7,585 ml), although the latter was spread across 3 days. Neither paper indicates either the optimum volume or ideal timing of administration of perioperative fluid. Combining the two papers we might conclude that $5\,ml\,kg^{-1}\,h^{-1}$ intraoperatively with no postoperative intravenous fluids is too little and $18\,ml\,kg^{-1}\,h^{-1}$ intraoperatively followed by $1.5\,ml\,kg^{-1}\,h^{-1}$ for 3 days too much. Holte *et al.* concluded that further studies examining optimal fluid management in the perioperative period should abandon the restrictive and liberal comparisons and instead focus on individual 'goal directed' strategies.

Paper 10: The analgesic efficacy of transversus abdominis plane block after abdominal surgery: A prospective randomized controlled trial

Author details

JG McDonnell, B O'Donnell, G Curley, A Heffernan, C Power, JG Laffey

Reference

Anesthesia and Analgesia 2007; **104**: 193–7.

Summary

Reduced postoperative pain scores and decreased incidence of side effects from systemic analgesics are recognized benefits of regional analgesia. Ilioinguinal and hypogastric nerve blocks are commonly used following hernia and scrotal surgery. This randomized controlled trial investigated a novel approach to providing regional analgesia to the whole anterior abdominal wall for patients undergoing a midline laparotomy incision. Patients were randomized to either a standard postoperative analgesia package of morphine PCAS + paracetamol + diclofenac or to TAP block plus standard package. Following induction of general anaesthesia using fentanyl and propofol, patients randomized to TAP + standard analgesia received bilateral injections into the triangle of Petit of 0.375% bupivacaine to a maximum of $1\,mg\,kg^{-1}$ each side. The blocks were performed by one of two operators and used simple anatomical landmarks. The iliac crest was palpated from anterior to posterior until latissimus dorsi could be identified, a 22-G blunt Plexufix (B Braun) was then passed at right angles to the skin just cephalad to the iliac crest and anterior to latissimus dorsi. First pop indicated passage through external oblique and a second pop passage through internal oblique into the transverses abdominis plane. Following a negative aspiration test the bupivacaine was injected and a dressing applied to the site. Postoperatively the patients were scored for pain, nausea, vomiting and sedation in the postoperative care unit and at 2, 4, 6, and 24 h postoperatively. Results indicated a significantly longer time to first request for morphine (157 min vs 24 min p<0.001) and a reduction in 24-h morphine requirements (22 mg versus 80 mg p <0.01) in the TAP + standard analgesia group compared to standard analgesia alone. Pain scores were significantly reduced in PACU and at 2, 4, and 6 h postoperatively. Sedation scores were significantly reduced at 4 and 6 h and the incidence of postoperative nausea and vomiting was 31% vs 69% in the TAP group compared to standard analgesia-only group (p <0.05).

Citation count

177.

Related references

1 Hebbard P, Fujiwara Y, Shibata Y, *et al.* Ultrasound-guided transversus abdominis plane (TAP) block. *Anaesth Intensive Care* 2007; **35**: 616–18.

2 McDonnell JG Curley G, Carney J, *et al.* The analgesic efficacy of transversus abdominis plane block after cesarean delivery: a randomized controlled trial. *Anesth Analg* 2008; **106**: 186–91.

3 Niraj G, Kelkar A, Fox AJ. Oblique sub-costal transversus abdominis plane (TAP) catheters: an alternative to epidural analgesia after upper abdominal surgery. *Anaesthesia* 2009; **64**: 1137–40.

Key message

The addition of a TAP block significantly reduces postoperative pain scores and opiate requirements in the first 24 h following midline laparotomy compared to a combination of morphine PCAS, paracetamol, and diclofenac used alone.

Strengths

This was a randomized controlled trial using a clinically applicable sample of ASA 1–3 patients. Groups had similar baseline patient characteristics and a power calculation was performed pre trial. The patients, their anaesthetist and the postoperative observer were blinded. TAP block was performed by only one of two operators.

Weaknesses

Only a small sample size and no placebo injection used in the standard analgesia group. This may have made the blinding suboptimal as although both groups had dressings applied over the triangle of Petit, the patients may have known whether they had received bilateral injections. Patient follow-up was limited to 24 h and did not delineate the duration of the TAP block.

Relevance

This is one of the first papers to demonstrate the clinical effectiveness of the TAP block in reducing pain scores and postoperative opiate requirements in patients undergoing abdominal surgery without an epidural. The publication of this small and simple study introduced TAP blocks into everyday clinical use. More recent publications have suggested ultrasound guided blocks may be a more sophisticated technique and that TAP blocks also have a role following lower Caesarean section, upper gastrointestinal surgery and in critical care where epidural analgesia is frequently contraindicated.

Chapter 15

Liver transplantation anaesthesia

RM Planinsic, IA Hilmi, and T Sakai

Introduction

Liver transplantation was first performed and reported by Thomas Starzl in 1963. In the early 1980s, Dr Starzl was recruited to the University of Pittsburgh to develop a liver transplantation programme. This programme quickly grew to become the largest in the world, transplanting more than 500 liver grafts per year into patients at its peak, training most of the surgeons and anaesthetists at that time.

Since that era, numerous advances have been made in caring for patients with end-stage liver disease undergoing liver transplantation. Improved surgical technique, along with advances in anaesthesia care, have allowed this once experimental procedure to become life saving, with 1-year survival of >75% in most patients. There remain, however, several issues in the field of liver transplantation anaesthesia that require a special understanding so as to optimize anaesthetic care of these patients. This section attempts to review a few of the landmark papers in liver transplantation anaesthesia that still have relevance today. Topics of continued interest and debate in the field, and addressed in this chapter, include coagulation issues, post-reperfusion syndrome, hepatopulmonary syndrome, portopulmonary hypertension, fulminant hepatic failure, and renal issues in liver transplantation.

Paper 1: Hemostasis in liver transplantation

Author details

RJ Porte, EAR Knot, FA Bontempo

Reference

Gastroenterology 1989; **97**: 488–501.

Summary

This is a classic paper published in 1989 describing the problems associated with haemostasis in liver transplantation. It describes bleeding complications as the most common cause of death intraoperatively and during the first postoperative week. Patients who received <30 U of red blood cells had a 70% survival rate and those who received >30 U red blood cells had a survival rate of 14%. The haemostasis mechanism is described in general and specifically for liver transplantation. The authors found that the total degree of coagulation disturbances can predict the intraoperative blood usage and survival.

Factors contributing to haemostatic disorders in liver disease are:

- Reduced synthesis of coagulation and fibrinolysis factors and their inhibitors.
- Presence of abnormal molecules (e.g. dysfibrinogenaemia)
- Intravascular coagulation
- Abnormalities in platelet count and function
- Enhanced fibrinolysis
- Loss of haemostasis factors in the enlarged extravascular space
- Portal hypertension with reduced hepatic perfusion, shunt circulation, and sequestration of platelets in the enlarged spleen.

Factors influencing intraoperative blood loss in liver transplantation:

- Primary diagnosis
- Severity of liver disease
- Preoperative haemostatic disorder
- Previous abdominal surgery
- Extent of collateral circulation
- Presence of ascites
- Renal function.

Processes that may affect haemostatic function after graft reperfusion:

- Disseminated intravascular coagulation
- Increased fibrinolytic activity
- Trapping of platelets in the graft
- Release of heparin or heparin-like substances
- Dilutional effect of preservation fluid
- Humoral and metabolic factors
- Graft preservation damage.

Citation count

84.

Related references

1 Warnaar N, Lisman T, Porte RJ. The two tales of coagulation in liver transplantation. *Curr Opin Organ Transpl* 2008; **13**: 298–303.

Key message

The magnitude of bleeding during liver transplantation appears to result from two factors: poor preoperative haemostatic capabilities complicated by specific intraoperative deteriorations, and the technical difficulties of the surgical procedure.

Strengths

This is an excellent overall review of coagulation disorders in liver disease and the haemostatic mechanism.

Weaknesses

The article is a review and surveys the literature available at the time. It is not a report of findings at the then busiest liver transplant centre in the world.

Relevance

This classic paper has been read by most anaesthetists involved with liver transplantation and is still referred to today.

Paper 2: Post-perfusion syndrome: hypotension after reperfusion of the transplanted liver

Author details

S Aggarwal, Y Kang, J Freeman, FL Fortunato, M Pinsky

Reference

Journal of Critical Care 1993; **8**: 154–60.

Abstract

Sixty-nine patients undergoing liver transplantation were evaluated to elucidate the relationship between hypotension and physiological changes seen on reperfusion of the grafted liver. Measured values included hemodynamic profiles, core temperature, serum potassium, ionized calcium levels, arterial blood-gas tensions, and acid-base state. Measurements were taken 60 minutes after skin incision (baseline), 5 minutes before reperfusion, and 30 seconds and 5 minutes after reperfusion. On the basis of changes in mean arterial pressure (MAP) patients were divided in two groups. Group 1 (n = 49) maintained MAP greater than 70% and group 2 (n = 20) had MAP less than 70% of the baseline value for at least 1 minute within 5 minutes after reperfusion. On reperfusion, changes common to both groups were 27% increase in cardiac filling pressures, 23% base deficit, and 30% serum potassium and a decrease of 16% in cardiac output and 9% in temperature. Compared with group 1, group 2 had greater decrease in systemic vascular resistance (SVR) and higher potassium level. Collectively in both groups, there was no correlation between MAP and physiological variables; however, there was a poor correlation with SVR. Reperfusion hypotension seen in group 2 patients correlated only with a decrease in SVR. Acute hyperkalaemia, hypothermia, and acidosis do not appear to be major causes of reperfusion hypotension.

Summary

The authors describe that complex changes occur in the cardiovascular system during liver transplantation, and successful outcome depends on the preservation of cardiovascular homeostasis. Yet despite improvements in the intraoperative anaesthetic and surgical technique, profound hypotension still occurs in some patients immediately after reperfusion of the grafted liver. These haemodynamic changes have collectively been termed the post-reperfusion syndrome (PRS).

The authors discuss two possible causes of PRS:

♦ The acute influx of cold, acidotic, hyperkalaemic blood from the grafted liver into the systemic circulation on reperfusion.

♦ The release of unknown vasoactive substances from the ischaemic graft.

IRB approval was obtained for a prospective study of liver transplant patients. Physiological and haemodynamic parameters were measured at baseline, 60 min after skin incision (I + 60 min), 5 min before reperfusion of the grafted liver during partial bypass (III – 5 min), 30 s after reperfusion (III + 30 seconds), and 5 min after reperfusion (III + 5 min). Results were reported above in the abstract.

Citation count

175.

Related references

1 Hilmi I, Horton CN, Planinsic RM, *et al*. The impact of post-reperfusion syndrome on short-term patient and liver allograft outcome in patients undergoing orthotopic liver transplantation. *Liver Transpl* 2008; **14**: 504–8.

Key message

This classic paper describes and names reperfusion hypotension as the post-reperfusion syndrome (PRS). As defined, PRS occurred in about 29% of patients and was defined as a decrease in MAP of 30%, occurring within 5 min of reperfusion of the grafted liver, and lasting >1 min.

Strengths

This is a systematic prospective evaluation of 69 patients undergoing liver transplantation, describing haemodynamic and physiological changes which occur during reperfusion of the grafted liver.

Weaknesses

This study has a relatively small sample size.

Relevance

This is a classic paper that first described and coined the term PRS for this well-known pheno-menon and explained the changes which occur during this often feared stage of the procedure.

Paper 3: Hepatopulmonary syndrome and portopulmonary hypertension: A report of the multicenter liver transplant database

Author details

MJ Krowka, MS Mandell, MAE Ramsay, SM Kawut, MB Fallon, C Manzarbeitia, M Pardo Jr, P Marotta, S Uemoto, MP Stoffel, JT Benson

Reference

Liver Transplantation 2004; **10**: 174–82.

Summary

In 1996 a cooperative, multicentre effort was initiated to address the issue of orthotopic liver transplantation (OLT) in patients with either hepatopulmonary syndrome (HPS) or portopulmonary hypertension (portoPH). Specifically, by using standardized diagnostic criteria applied to any patient evaluated for OLT. The diagnostic criteria were as follows:
HPS:

- Liver disease that meets minimal listing criteria for liver transplantation; and
- PaO_2 <70 mmHg or alveolar–arterial oxygen gradient >20 mmHg; and
- Pulmonary vascular dilatation documented by either: (a) positive contrast enhanced transthoracic echo or (b) brain uptake >6% following lung perfusion scanning with 99mTc macroaggregated albumin.

PortoPH:

- Liver disease that meets minimal listing criteria for liver transplantation; and
- MPAP 25 mmHg and
- PVR 120 dynes s^{-1} cm^{-5} and
- PCWP 15 mmHg.

During the study period of 1996–2001, there were 106 patients from the 10 liver transplant centres who were deemed to fulfil the diagnostic criteria for either HPS or portoPH. The outcome of these 106 candidates was defined by 1 of 3 mutually exclusive categories: (1) denied OLT, (2) accepted for OLT, underwent OLT and survived transplant hospitalization and (3) accepted for OLT, underwent OLT but died during the transplant hospitalization. The data from this multicentre effort described the relationship among preoperative arterial oxygenation in patients with HPS, preoperative pulmonary haemodynamics in patients with portoPH and liver transplant outcome as categorized by the investigators.

Citation count

176.

Related references

1 Mandell SM, Krowka MJ. National database for hepatopulmonary syndrome and portopulmonary hypertension in liver transplant candidates/recipients. *Anesthesiology* 1997; **87**: 450–1.

Key message

The study reported simple and measurable parameters to assess the impacts of preoperative HPS and portoPH on predefined outcome to address the suitability of patients with HPS or portoPH for liver transplantation.

Strengths

- ◆ Large sample size, multicentre data collection which reflected the differences in practice and the choice of certain selection criteria.
- ◆ Established a link between the outcome of OLT and preoperative haemodynamics in patients with HPS or portoPH.
- ◆ Addressed the need for global practice guidelines to manage patients with liver failure related pulmonary problems.

Weaknesses

The limitations of the study were addressed fully by the authors, as follows:

- ◆ Reporting bias.
- ◆ The selection criteria that were used reflected the study centres experience and preferences, other variables that were not collected may be of equal importance and impact on the outcome.
- ◆ Voluntarily reporting of the adverse events.
- ◆ Lack of addressing the intraoperative adverse events that led to the patient's death.
- ◆ Lack of standardization of the pulmonary vasodilator medication (prostacyclin) dose and regimen and/or its effects on the outcome and patient selection.
- ◆ The study did not document long-term patient and allograft outcome.

Relevance

This study established a relationship between the preoperative variables and postoperative outcome in patients with HPS or PortoPH.

Paper 4: Portopulmonary hypertension: results from a 10-year screening algorithm

Author details

MJ Krowka, KL Swanson, RP Frantz, MD McGoon, RH Wiesner

Reference

Hepatology 2006; **44**: 1502–10.

Abstract

Portopulmonary hypertension (POPH) is the elevation of pulmonary artery pressure due to increased resistance to pulmonary blood flow in the setting of portal hypertension. Increased mortality has occurred with attempted liver transplantation in such patients and thus, screening for POPH is advised. We examined the relationship between screening echocardiography and right heart catheterization determinations of pressure, flow, volume, and resistance. A prospective, echocardiography-catheterization algorithm was followed from 1996 to 2005. Consecutive transplantation candidates underwent Doppler echocardiography to determine right ventricular systolic pressure (RVSP). Of 1,235 patients, 101 with RVSP >50 mmHg underwent catheterization to measure mean pulmonary artery pressure (MPAP), flow via cardiac output (CO), central volume via pulmonary artery occlusion pressure (PAOP), and resistance via calculated pulmonary vascular resistance (PVR). Bland-Altman analysis suggested marked discordance between echocardiography-derived RVSP and catheterization results. All-cause pulmonary hypertension (MPAP >25 mmHg) was documented in 90/101 (90%) patients. Using current pressure and resistance diagnostic guidelines (MPAP >25 mmHg, PVR ≥240 dyne s^{-1} cm^{-5}), POPH was documented in 66/101 (65%) patients. Elevated MPAP was due to increased CO and/or PAOP in 35/101 (35%) patients with normal resistance (PVR <240 dyne s^{-1} cm^{-5}). The transpulmonary gradient (MPAP–PAOP) further characterized POPH in the presence of increased volume. Model for end stage liver disease (MELD) scores correlated poorly with MPAP and PVR. In conclusion, right heart catheterization is necessary to confirm POPH and frequently identifies other reasons for pulmonary hypertension (e.g., high flow and increased central volume) in liver transplantation candidates. Severity of POPH correlates poorly with MELD scores.

Summary

- From July 1996 to December 2005, consecutive patients met minimal listing criteria (Child–Turcotte–Pugh score ≥7) for liver transplantation underwent transthoracic Doppler echocardiography screening and pre-transplantation pulmonary consultation. Transplantation candidates with an increased right ventricular systolic pressure >50 mmHg underwent subsequent right heart catheterization to determine specific pulmonary haemodynamic patterns and document the existence of POPH.

- PortoPH was defined by the European Respiratory Society–European Association for the Study of the Liver Task Force on the Hepatic-Pulmonary Vascular Disorders of portoPH: (1) MPAP ≥25 mmHg; (2) PVR ≥240 dynes s^{-1} cm^{-5}; and (3) PAOP <15 mmHg.
- Transthoracic Doppler echocardiography was performed and the right ventricular systolic pressure was determined by using the modified Bernoulli equation:

$$RVSP \ (mmHg) = 4 \times (TR^2) + \text{right atrial pressure estimate},$$

where TR (m s^{-1}) = tricuspid regurgitant peak velocity. Right atrial pressure estimate was determined via echocardiographic assessment of the inferior vena cava size and degree of collapse with respiration.

- Right heart catheterization was performed in all patients with RVSP >50 mmHg to determine cardiac output, pulmonary artery pressures (systolic, diastolic, and mean), PAOP and PVR.
- The severity of liver disease was determined by MELD score and Child–Turcotte–Pugh score (CTP).
- During the study period there were 1,235 liver transplant candidates had preoperative TEE with 104 patients (10.9%) underwent right heart catheterization that were found to have RVSP >50 mmHg.
- 65% of the patients (66/101, three patients died before transplant) who underwent right-heart catheterization had PVR ≥240 mmHg, while 90/101 (90%) had MPAP ≥25 mmHg and abnormal transpulmonary gradient (TPG) was abnormal in every patient with abnormal PVR.
- There was no significant relationship between the aetiology or the severity of the liver as disease as scored by MELD or CTP and the presence or severity of portoPH.

Related references

1 Krowka MJ, Plevak DJ, Findlay JY, *et al.* Pulmonary hemodynamics and perioperative cardiopulmonary mortality in patients with portopulmonary hypertension undergoing liver transplantation. *Liver Transpl* 2000; **6**: 443–50.

Citation count

87.

Key message

The importance of right heart catheterization in the diagnosis and accurate measurement of portoPH in preoperative evaluation of OLT candidates. No relation between MELD or CTP and the presence or severity of portoPH.

Strengths

- Established a cut off value for portoPH (MPAP ≥50 mmHg) as a contraindication for OLT.
- The importance of right heart catheterization in diagnosis of portoPH. Catheterization allowed calculation of TPG. The importance of the TPG relates to the scenario in which increased

pulmonary venous pressure (measured via PAOP) may exist in addition to and further worsen an increased MPAP.

♦ Documented that the CTP or MELD score had no relation to the existence or severity of portoPH.

Weakness

The weaknesses of the study as documented by the authors are:

♦ No outcome data were included or patients follow-up.

♦ No consideration for any therapeutic intervention or the effects of beta-blocker medication withdrawal on the PVR.

♦ No mention of the aetiology of portoPH.

♦ The choice of RVSP >50 mmHg for screening purposes was based on small series that was studied at the investigator's institution.

Relevance

Screening echocardiography may suggest POPH, but catheterization is vital to accurately diagnose and determine the severity of POPH and to identify other causes for pulmonary hypertension (high flow and/or increased central volume) in the setting of liver disease. MELD scores correlated poorly with all measured parameters of pulmonary haemodynamics in patients with POPH.

Paper 5: Early indicators of prognosis in fulminant hepatic failure

Author details

JG O'Grady, GJ Alexander, KM Hayllar, R Williams.

Reference

Gastroenterology 1989; **97**: 439–45.

Abstract

The successful use of orthotopic liver transplantation in fulminant hepatic failure has created a need for early prognostic indicators to select the patients most likely to benefit at a time when liver transplantation is still feasible. Univariate and multivariate analysis was performed on 588 patients with acute liver failure managed medically during 1973–1985, to identify the factors most likely to indicate a poor prognosis. In acetaminophen-induced fulminant hepatic failure, survival correlated with arterial blood pH, peak prothrombin time, and serum creatinine—a pH less than 7.30, prothrombin time greater than 100 s, and creatinine greater than 300 mmol l^{-1} indicating a poor prognosis. In patients with viral hepatitis and drug reactions three static variables [etiology (non A, non B hepatitis or drug reactions), age less than 11 and greater than 40 yr, duration of jaundice before the onset of encephalopathy greater than 7 days] and two dynamic variables (serum bilirubin greater than 300 mmol l^{-1} and prothrombin time greater than 50 s) indicated a poor prognosis. The value of these indicators in determining outcome was tested retrospectively in a further 175 patients admitted during 1986–1987, leading to the construction of models for the selection of patients for liver transplantation.

Summary

A series of 588 patients with acute liver failure managed medically during 1973–1985 was retrospectively analysed to identify the factors to indicate a poor prognosis.

In paracetamol-induced fulminant hepatic failure, the risk factors were:

◆ Arterial blood pH (pH <7.30).

◆ Peak prothrombin time (>100 s).

◆ Serum creatinine (>300 mmol l^{-1}).

In patients with viral hepatitis and drug reactions, the risk factors were:

◆ Aetiology (non-A, non-B hepatitis or drug reactions).

◆ Age <11 and >40 years.

◆ Duration of jaundice before the onset of encephalopathy >7 days.

◆ Serum bilirubin >300 mmol l^{-1}.

◆ Prothrombin time >50 s.

Citation count

1157.

Related references

1 Farmer DG, Anselmo DM, Ghobrial RM, *et al.* Liver transplantation for fulminant hepatic failure: experience with more than 200 patients over a 17-year period. *Ann Surg* 2003; **237**: 666–75.

Key message

In medical management of acute liver failure, risk factors for poor prognosis should be considered on the two categories of the aetiology: paracetamol-induced fulminant hepatic failure or the others.

Strengths

This is by far one of the largest clinical series of the patients with acute liver failure.

Weaknesses

The retrospective nature of the study is a theoretical weakness; however, the authors provided an additional cohort of 175 patients admitted during 1986–1987, in order to construct models for the selection of patients for liver transplantation.

Relevance

Thanks to this study, the indication for liver transplantation in the patients with fulminant hepatic failure has been established as 'King's College Criteria'. After 20 years of testing of the criteria, the feasibility of the original study has been still demonstrated.

Paper 6: Impact of pre-transplant renal function on survival after liver transplantation

Author details

TA Gonwa, GB Klintmalm, M Levy, LS Jennings, RM Goldstein, BS Husberg

Reference

Transplantation 1995; **59**: 361–5.

Summary

This retrospective study based on 569 consecutive adult patients undergoing liver transplantation concluded as follows:

Pre-transplant renal function other than hepato-renal syndrome has no effect on patient survival after orthotopic liver transplant.

- The recipients with hepato-renal syndrome have a significantly decreased actuarial patient survival after liver transplant at 5 years compared with patients without hepato-renal syndrome (60% vs 68%, P <0.03). Although the renal function recovered after liver transplantation, the patients with hepato-renal syndrome were sicker and required longer stays in the intensive care unit, longer hospitalizations, and more dialysis treatments after transplantation compared with patients who did not have hepato-renal syndrome. The incidence of end-stage renal disease after liver transplantation in patients who had hepato-renal syndrome was 7%, compared with 2% in patients who did not have hepato-renal syndrome.

- Among the non-hepato-renal syndrome patients, the patients with the lowest quartile pre-transplant renal function had the same survival as the patients with the highest quartile pre-transplant renal function. There was no increased incidence of acute or chronic rejection in any of the groups.

Renal function after liver transplant is stable after an initial decline, despite continued administration of CsA.

- The patients with the highest pre-transplant renal function had a 40% decline in renal function in the first year, but maintained stable renal function up to 4 years after transplant.

- The patients with the lower pre-transplant renal function were treated with more azathioprine to maintain renal function and had a negligible decrease in glomerular filtration rate following transplant.

Citation count

275.

Related references

1 Ginès P, Guevar, M, Arroyo V, *et al.* Hepatorenal syndrome. *Lancet* 2003; **362**: 1819–27.
2 Sharma P, Welch K, Eikstadt R, *et al.* Renal outcomes after liver transplantation in the model for end-stage liver disease era. *Liver Transpl* 2009; **15**: 1142–8.

Key message

Preoperative renal assessment should start whether the recipient for liver transplantation has normal renal function or decreased renal function. Then the anaesthetist should determine whether the latter group has hepato-renal syndrome or not. The authors concluded that pre-transplant renal function other than hepato-renal syndrome has no effect on patient survival after orthotopic liver transplant.

Strengths

The large number of cohort was able to provide two different clinical groups of patients with renal dysfunction undergoing liver transplantation. Although the diagnosis of hepato-renal syndrome is based on the exclusion of other causes of renal failure, the study suggests that there is significantly increased mortality and morbidity in this clinical entity.

Weaknesses

There are two weaknesses of the study: retrospective design and a study conducted in 'Pre-MELD (the model for end-stage liver disease) era'. The first point is obvious; however, this study is observational in nature without any intervention. The second point is important. As of 2001, the organ allocation in USA has been conducted based on the MELD score, in which serum creatinine level with or without recent haemodialysis is one of the three major factors (the other two factors are international normalized ratio and total bilirubin). The paper by Sharma et al. (2009) should be read in conjunction with the study.

Relevance

Hepato-renal syndrome is a common complication of end-stage liver disease. It is characterized by renal failure which is caused by intense vasoconstriction of the renal circulation. Not only the renal circulation, most extra-splanchnic vascular beds are vasoconstricted. The prognosis of medical management is very poor, therefore, liver transplantation is the best option in patients without contraindications to the procedure. This study stresses the importance of the diagnosis (hepato-renal syndrome versus non-hepato-renal syndrome) of the renal dysfunction preoperatively.

Paper 7: Orthotopic liver transplantation with preservation of the inferior vena cava

Author details

A Tzakis, S Todo, TE Starzl

Reference

Annals of Surgery 1989; **210**: 649–52.

Summary

'Piggyback' orthotopic liver transplantation was fully described for the first time as the alternative surgical method in implantation of the liver graft. The traditional 'standard' method, which includes resection of the retro-hepatic vena cava, usually necessitates the veno–venous bypass during an-hepatic phase in order to maintain venous return to the heart and decrease venous congestion of the portal and the lower body (including kidneys) systems. The piggyback method is especially beneficial for the paediatric population on whom the veno–venous bypass could be difficult to apply due to the small body size.

Citation count

379.

Related references

1 Shaw BW Jr, Martin DJ, Marquez JM, *et al*. Venous bypass in clinical liver transplantation. *Ann Surg* 1984; **200**: 524–34.

2 Belghiti J, Panis Y, Sauvanet A, *et al*. A new technique of side to side caval anastomosis during orthotopic hepatic transplantation without inferior vena caval occlusion. *Surg Gynecol Obstet* 1992; **175**: 270–2.

3 Sakai T, Matsusaki T, Marsh JW, *et al*. Comparison of surgical methods in liver transplantation: retrohepatic caval resection with veno-venous bypass (VVB) versus piggyback (PB) with VVB versus PB without VVB. *Transpl Int* 2010; **23**: 1247–58.

Key message

The piggyback method can be applied to selected patients undergoing liver transplantation. The new method could decrease blood loss, incidence of vascular and biliary complications, and improve patient outcome.

Strengths

This is the first comprehensive description of the piggyback method in the literature. Based on successive reports with favourable outcomes using this technique over the standard method, the piggyback method has become a new standard for liver transplantation worldwide, not only for the paediatric population but also for the adult population.

Weaknesses

Firstly, in this initial experience, the piggyback operation was only able to be completed in a minority of cases (19%). Over the last 20 years of experience and refinement of the surgical techniques, however, almost all liver transplantations have been performed using the technique. Therefore, the future projection originally made by the authors, who stated that the 19% incidence during the period of the their study was probably a realistic projection, has proved to be an understatement. The contribution they made with the manuscript has turned out to be greater than they predicted. Secondly, the authors used a veno–venous bypass in a majority of the cases with piggyback method. The technique was later perfected by Belghiti *et al.* (1992), who suggested the potential of elimination of veno–venous support.

Relevance

This paper has initiated a change of practice in liver transplantation; the majority of the current liver transplantations are performed with the piggyback method both on paediatric and on adult patients. This method has theoretically and practically eliminated the need for veno–venous bypass during the anhepatic phase. These changes in the surgical technique have had a significant impact on the perioperative anaesthetic management and the outcome (see Sakai *et al.*, 2010). The anaesthetists who are involved in liver transplantation must communicate with the surgical team, and adjust the anaesthetic technique to the surgical option taken.

Paper 8: Cardiovascular depression secondary to citrate intoxication during hepatic transplantation in humans

Author details

J Marquez, D Martin, MA Virji, Y Kang, VS Warty, B Shaw Jr, JJ Sassano, P Waterman, PM Winter, MR Pinsky

Reference

Anesthesiology 1986; **65**: 457–61.

Summary

With the advent of cyclosporine immunosuppression, the number of patients undergoing liver transplantation increased dramatically in the mid 1980s. The procedure was relatively new and blood loss was much more significant than in the current era. This study examined nine patients undergoing liver transplantation. Average blood products transfused were: RBC (39.3 ± 16 units) and FFP (33.4 ± 11 units). Total $CaCl_2$ administered was 4.3 ± 2.2 g. Total $CaCl_2$/total CBP (citrated blood products) transfused (g/unit) was 0.05 ± 0.01. Total $CaCl_2$/kg body weight/CBP transfused (mg/kg-unit) was 0.78 ± 0.15. Although the clinical relationship between ionic hypocalcaemia and cardiovascular function was considered controversial at the time, this study demonstrated that a decrease in Ca^{2+} to 0.56 mmol l^{-1} was associated with depressed cardiovascular function. It was recommended that frequent assessment of haemodynamic function and serum ionized calcium levels was essential in managing the intraoperative care of patients undergoing liver transplantation.

Citation count

69.

Related references

1 Drop L. Ionized calcium, the heart, and hemodynamic function. *Anesth Analg* 1985; **64**: 432–51.

Key message

Measure ionized calcium frequently during liver transplantation. Significant haemodynamic instability may be related to ionized hypocalcaemia. Transfusion of CBP will lead to ionized hypocalcaemia during liver transplantation. Replacement of calcium is essential to avoid this problem.

Strengths

A well-constructed study reporting the results and experiences for the early days of liver transplantation at the University of Pittsburgh.

Weaknesses

The only potential weakness is the small sample size, but the results were quite impressive.

Relevance

Classic landmark article which first described citrate toxicity during liver transplantation and its consequences. A must-read for anaesthetists who provide care for patients undergoing this life-saving procedure.

Paper 9: Ionized hypomagnesaemia in patients undergoing orthotopic liver transplantation: a complication of citrate intoxication

Author details

VL Scott, AM DeWolf, Y Kang, BT Altura, MA Virji, DR Cook, BM Altura

Reference

Liver Transplantation and Surgery 1996; **2**: 343–7.

Summary

This article follows the initial landmark paper (paper 8) describing cardiovascular depression secondary to hypocalcaemia resulting from citrate toxicity published 10 years previously by Marquez *et al*. in *Anesthesiology*. Citrate was also known to chelate magnesium (Mg) ions in a similar fashion, although the presence and magnitude of ionized hypomagnesaemia was not yet known. Scott *et al*. discuss how Mg is an important cofactor for intracellular reactions requiring adenosine triphosphate (ATP) as an energy source, and, as a result, significantly affects maintenance of ion transport, particularly calcium and potassium. In addition, Mg is a smooth muscle relaxant and has anti-arrhythmic as well as positive inotropic effects. During liver transplantation, patients often develop haemodynamic instability and arrhythmias. It is important to delineate whether ionized hypomagnesaemia contributes to these haemodynamic derangements. Finally Scott *et al*. discuss how the prevention of ionized hypomagnesaemia during liver transplantation may attenuate calcium mediated ischemic reperfusion injury of the grafted liver.

Citation count

39.

Related references

1 Altura BM, Altura BT: New prospectives on the role of magnesium in the pathophysiology of the cardiovascular system. I. Clinical Aspects. *Magnesium* 1985; **4**: 226–44.

Key message

Ionized magnesium, similar to ionized calcium, is chelated by citrate. Citrate intoxication resulting from poor or no liver metabolism of citrate present in stored packed red blood cells may also result in ionized hypomagnesaemia. Myocardial depression and irritability during liver transplantation may be in part caused by ionized hypomagnesaemia.

Strengths

Excellent discussion on the importance of magnesium in cardiovascular physiology and its role in maintaining haemodynamic stability during liver transplantation.

Weaknesses

The only potential weakness is the small sample size, but again the results were quite impressive.

Relevance

This is a classic article, still relevant today in liver transplantation and should be read by all who take care of these patients during surgery.

Paper 10: Morbidity and mortality in patients with coronary artery disease undergoing orthotopic liver transplantation

Author details

JS Plotkin, VL Scott, A Pinna, BP Dobsch, AM DeWolf, Y Kang

Reference

Liver Transplantation and Surgery 1996; **2**: 426–30.

Summary

Since advanced age is no longer considered a contraindication to liver transplantation, older patients who are known to have a higher prevalence of coronary artery disease (CAD) are presenting more often for evaluation of candidacy. Although 'significant' CAD may be considered a relative contraindication to liver transplantation, no data existed at the time of this publication documenting the definition of significant CAD or determining the outcome in such patients. This paper attempted to address these issues with results described in the abstract. It was the first study of its kind correlating morbidity and mortality with CAD in liver transplantation patients.

Citation count

95.

Related references

1 Carey WD, Dumont JA, Pimentel RP, *et al*. The prevalence of coronary artery disease in liver transplant candidates over age 50. *Transplantation* 1995; **59**: 859–64.

Key message

Although there is an increased risk of mortality and morbidity of liver transplantation in patients with coexisting coronary artery disease this should not necessarily preclude such patients when for considering liver transplantation.

Strengths

This was a study examining the correlation of CAD with morbidity and mortality in what was at the time of publication, the largest cohort of patients undergoing liver transplantation.

Weaknesses

This was a retrospective study and small sample size.

Relevance

This was a classic paper stressing the importance of appreciating the impact of CAD in liver transplantation recipients.

Chapter 16

Obstetric anaesthesia

G Lyons

Introduction

Much of the literature involving obstetric anaesthesia concerns issues of safety and I make no excuse for the inclusion of such seminal papers. The confidential enquiries into maternal deaths have contributed much to the improved safety in childbirth both in the UK where it originated and indeed the rest of the world. Otherwise my choice of papers to include in this chapter combines some of the best known names in obstetric anaesthesia and illustrates not only their contribution to improvements in obstetric anaesthesia but also the safety of anaesthesia as a whole.

Paper 1: Versuche über cocainisirung des rückenmarkes

Author details

A Bier

Reference

Deustche Zeitschrift für Chirurgie 1899; **51**: 361–8. (Translated by R Fink in Wulf H. The centennial of spinal anesthesia. *Anesthesiology* 1989; **89**: 500–6.)

Summary

Bier is widely credited with performing the world's first spinal anaesthetic, but the New York neurologist Leonard Corning may have got there before. What is not in dispute is that Bier performed the first spinal anaesthetic for a surgical procedure, and was first to describe post dural puncture headache, his own. This translation of his paper gives a fascinating insight into a world where an idea today becomes reality tomorrow, where surgical operations take only a few minutes, where self-experimentation has no rules, and can fill a gap between the day's work and dinner. It also opens an interesting window onto the relationship between Bier and his assistant Hildebrandt.

During his training in Kiel, Bier worked with Esmarch and Quincke. Dr Wulf attributes the development of intravenous regional anaesthesia to an idea that Bier borrowed from Esmarch, and from Quincke he had learnt lumbar puncture. He knew it was desirable to limit loss of cerebrospinal fluid by placing a finger over the needle hub. Cocaine was available then as now, in a white powder. For spinal anaesthesia it was necessary to make a solution to the necessary strength, either by mixing with cerebrospinal fluid, or with water. The source of the water for this was uncertain and neither sterility nor baricity were guaranteed. Bier must have had some idea of the dose required for he was able to achieve mid-thoracic blocks but what is also of interest was that they were not particularly dense. Analgesia with motor-sparing and impaired touch sensation rather than anaesthesia characterized some of his blocks, all of which seemed to have worked at the first attempt.

On 16 August 1898 Bier acting both as anaesthetist and surgeon resected a tuberculous ankle joint. After four more orthopaedic procedures he wrote of 'complications which equalled those that follow general anaesthesia', and 'To reach a well-informed opinion I decided to perform some investigations on my own body'. The inference is that Bier wanted to establish, at least in his own mind, whether the benefit of spinal anaesthesia was worth the risk, by deliberately inflicting post dural puncture symptoms on himself.

On 24 August at around 7pm, Bier persuaded his assistant Hildebrandt to perform the lumbar puncture. Being surgically trained they had not checked their equipment and, awaiting the Luer system, Hildebrandt was unable to fit the syringe onto the hub of the needle. Bier's cerebrospinal fluid must have run freely before Hildebrandt abandoned the experiment. That might have been the end of it. Bier clearly did not feel able to ask Hildebrandt to step in, but instead he volunteered. With Hildebrandt anaesthetized, Bier proceeded to squeeze his testicles, pluck his pubic hair, needle his thighs down to the femur, and hammer his shins. Why Bier wished to do this is unclear. From his surgical experiences with spinal anaesthesia, he already knew what was possible. Perhaps this was his way of exploring differential block.

Because Hildebrandt had no motor block, once Bier was satisfied, the two went out to dine, drink wine, and smoke cigars, 'more than was good for us'. They were both in bed around 11pm, but Hildebrandt developed a headache and vomited in the night. His tibia were bruised and painful where heavy blows had been inflicted. Despite feeling ghastly, he managed to 'perform service duties of operating and changing dressings'. He remained ill for 3–4 days. Bier 'awoke the next morning hale and hearty', and also went to work but during the afternoon he reported that "a 'pressure' developed on my skull and I became rather dizzy". All symptoms disappeared when he lay flat. Presumably he had the luxury of someone else to do his work, possibly Hildebrandt, because he took to his bed and stayed there for 9 days. When he arose, cured, he went on an 8-day hunting trip.

Citation count

223.

Key message

It is probably best not to experiment on oneself.

Strengths

The strength in this manuscript is the quality of description that comes from events in which the author participated and the symptoms which the author experienced. The passage of time has given this the flavour of a period piece, something that can be enjoyed in its own right.

Weaknesses

Bier sought to interpret his experience in the light of the perceived wisdoms of the day, and much of his supposition was wrong. In this he was no different from modern researchers. He had doubts about spinal anaesthesia because those who developed headaches had a more protracted recovery than after chloroform anaesthesia. He reasoned correctly that the post-spinal symptoms were unrelated to cocaine because he had no block. Although he knew that loss of cerebrospinal fluid could cause these symptoms, he suspected a circulatory cause, attributing the postural element to a physiological disturbance rather than the straightforward gravitational behaviour of fluid in a manometer. He saw motor-sparing as a preference of cocaine for blocking pain fibres despite appreciating that larger doses brought on a denser block. The response curve was yet to come.

Relevance

One wonders what Health and Safety would have made of this courageous experiment, and also what became of Hildebrandt, who remains largely overlooked by posterity. In later life Bier wrote disparagingly of 'professional anaesthetists'. He was a surgeon after all.

Paper 2: The aspiration of stomach contents into the lungs during obstetric anaesthesia

Author details

CL Mendelson

Reference

American Journal of Obstetrics and Gynecology 1946; **52**: 191–205. (Read at a meeting of the New York Obstetrical Society, 11 December 1945.)

Summary

Mendelson was a young obstetrician working at the New York Lying-In Hospital when he published the paper that made his name. His case-note review covered the years from 1932–1945. The timing may have some importance since during the First World War chlorine and phosgene gas poisoning introduced hydrochloric acid into the lungs with distressing results (Winternitz *et al.*, 1920), and simultaneously Marie Curie was attempting to make mobile radiography (petites Curies) available to some field hospitals. It is perfectly possible that Mendelson had colleagues who had direct experience of both.

His case-note review found 66 victims of aspiration in association with spontaneously breathing gas, oxygen, and ether anaesthesia. He recognized two broad categories of pathology, the aspiration of solid material and obstructive symptoms, and the aspiration of liquid material that gave rise to an asthma-like syndrome. Of the five women who aspirated solid material, in three the airway was completely blocked, and two of these died immediately from asphyxia. By today's standards these two women were starved; one had eaten her meal 8 h before and the other 6 h before. The third asphyxiated woman coughed and survived. The other two survivors suffered significant unilateral collapse, but physiotherapy alone seems to have led to recovery. Despite the poor reproductive qualities of the images, the unilateral nature of the disorder is clear.

In contrast, those who aspirated liquid had bilateral pulmonary pathology and a different clinical course, with cyanosis, tachycardia, dyspnoea, widespread wheeze, and rales, with progression to cardiac failure and pulmonary oedema. What surprises modern anaesthetists is that none of these women died. Once the acute episode was over, stabilization occurred with resolution of the radiological appearance over 7–10 days. Although he writes of absent laryngeal reflexes in relation to spontaneously breathing ether, it is possible that the profound muscle relaxation of modern anaesthesia offers less protection and gives rise to larger aspirated volumes.

The second half of his paper describes the effects of various installations into the lungs of rabbits. Hydrochloric acid and unneutralized gastric contents both produced a syndrome with bilateral pathology similar to that observed in the women. Accordingly, he identified gastric acid as the cause of the pulmonary syndrome.

Citation count

843.

Related references

1 Winternitz MC. Collected studies on the pathology of war gas poisoning. New Haven, CT: Yale University Press, 1920.

2 Tomkinson J, Turnbull A, Robson G, et al. *Report on confidential enquiries into maternal deaths in England and Wales 1973–1975*. London: Department of Health and Social Security. Her Majesty's Stationery Office, 1979.

3 Marie Curie. Available at: http://en.wikipedia.org/wiki/Marie_Curie (accessed 27 January 2010).

Key message

This is the first paper to describe the effects of aspiration of gastric contents in the labouring woman. Recommendations for safe practice were suggested some of which are still in use today.

Strengths

Mendelson writes simply without embellishment. Half the pages are taken up by images. Time may have passed, but this remains the largest series of aspiration in association with anaesthesia available to us. It is perhaps the only series and it is well worth the read.

Weaknesses

None. This remains a superb observational and investigative study.

Relevance

Mendelson[1] went on to make some recommendations for safe practice. He advised against feeding in labour, and suggested nil-by-mouth for 12 h before elective surgery. As far as solid food is concerned this is largely what happens today. The introduction of nil-by-mouth in UK labour wards was followed by the disappearance of deaths from asphyxia during the course of the 1970s (Tompkinson *et al.*, 1979). Up to that point each triennial enquiry had reported at least one asphyxial maternal death. He commented on the dangers of allowing inexperienced 'interns' to perform emergency obstetric anaesthesia with little or no patient assessment and called for transparent face masks in the hope that detection of aspiration might be improved. It took at least another 40 years before the latter became standard in the UK, but inexperienced anaesthetists still staff labour wards at night.

---

[1] Mendelson may have another lesson for us. At the age of 46 he abandoned his successful New York practice to become the medical officer to Green Turtle Cay, a small Caribbean island. A photograph shows him game fishing. Reports suggest that he thoroughly enjoyed his life there, but at the age of 77 he moved to Florida, where he died in 2002 aged 91.

Paper 3: The confidential enquiries into maternal deaths 1952–2005

Author details

Annonymous

References

Report on Confidential Enquiries into Maternal Deaths in England and Wales 1952–54, 1955–57, 1958–60, 1961–63, 1964–66, 1967–69, 1970–72, 1973–75, 1976–78, 1979–81, 1982–84. London: Her Majesty's Stationery Office, 1957–1989.

Report on Confidential Enquiries into Maternal Deaths in the United Kingdom 1985–87, 1988–90, 1991–93. London: Her Majesty's Stationery Office, 1991–1996.

Why Mothers Die. Report on Confidential Enquiries into Maternal Deaths in the United Kingdom 1994–96. London: The Stationery Office, Royal College of Obstetricians and Gynaecologists, 1997–99.

Why Mothers Die. Report on Confidential Enquiries into Maternal and Child Health 2000–02. London: Royal College of Obstetricians and Gynaecologists, 2004.

Saving Mothers' Lives. Report on Confidential Enquiries into Maternal and Child Health 2003–05. London: Royal College of Obstetricians and Gynaecologists, 2007.

Summary

Billed as the longest running continuous audit, the series of Confidential Enquiries began in the 1920s and stopped during the war years. When it was resumed in 1952, it was in the context of the National Health Service, which must have improved case ascertainment. All aspiring obstetric anaesthetists saw these reports as essential reading, and they were devoured urgently after each publication. The sad and unsettling vignettes with their 'there but for the grace of God . . .' ethos was, and still is, sufficient to keep sleep at bay.

The importance of the Enquiries was in the recommendations they made for practice. Decades of reporting deaths from aspiration and failure of airway management led to the uptake of starvation in labour and antacid therapy across the UK. Warnings of gastric volumes following narcotic administration and the dangers of persisting to intubate without due care for oxygenation, anaesthesia and maternal welfare in general, featured repetitively.

As a trainee, the data was always presented to me to show the steady decline in anaesthetic mortality since 1967–1969. It was not until relatively recently that, in the preparation of a lecture, I undertook to read all the Enquiries since 1952. I then realized that what I had been taught was not the whole truth. According to those despatched to attend labour wards, Mendelson's ether anaesthetic was employed in the UK until the introduction of relaxant anaesthesia with thiopentone, suxamethonium, a tracheal tube, and nitrous oxide, in the early 1960s (Hamer Hodges *et al.*, 1959). What the early Enquiries reveal is that throughout the 1950s maternal anaesthetic mortality declined, but by 1967–1969 not only had the improvement reversed, it had virtually doubled. This presumably was due to the displacement of spontaneously breathing ether by 'gold standard' airway management. There had been a deception. By the time I appreciated this, the trail-blazers of the time were no longer around to explain. Someone did ask my question because a single anecdote gives the explanation by a highly respected luminary of the time. His reply was that, indeed they had been aware of what was happening, but chose to say nothing because for the first time they had the means of preparing a woman for Caesarean section in a matter of moments.

It took another 10 years for maternal anaesthetic mortality to return to the numbers of the 1950s.

Although standards in the administration of general anaesthesia improved, the problems it created on labour wards have never been altogether overcome. Accordingly obstetric anaesthetists progressively abandoned it in favour of regional anaesthesia, and despite lacking incontrovertible scientific proof, it appears that whereas deaths from general anaesthesia are proportional to the numbers given, deaths from regional anaesthesia are not. A possible explanation for this is that the most dangerous part of the general anaesthetic, the administration of muscle relaxant, precedes the most challenging part, the intubation. With epidural and spinal anaesthesia the situation is reversed.

In recent years ownership of the Enquiries has changed, and the drab cover has given way to a larger, glossy publication. Case ascertainment has improved through measures that link the maternal mortality database to the Office for National Statistics, giving access to the second line on the death certificate. This exposed an important number of deaths in the community and identified suicide and post-puerperal depression as a major cause of mortality. Deaths are now placed in a social context, with identification of groups of women who are at increased risk from no specific threat, but who attract morbidity across the board. For today's labour ward anaesthetist there is a need to be aware that the black African has a sixfold increase in mortality risk and that the socially deprived and excluded, the poor, the obese, the victims of domestic violence, drug abusers, and migrants without English skills are also liable to attract problems and experience substandard care. The traditional risk analysis used by anaesthetists must be extended.

Citation count

Not available.

Related references

1 Hamer Hodges RJ, Bennet JR, Tunstall ME, *et al.* General anaesthesia for operative obstetrics. *Br J Anaesth* 1959; **31**: 152–63.

Key message

The rigorous collection of data can result in changes in practice which can have dramatic effects on mortality and morbidity.

Strengths

The overwhelming strength of these reports is in their ability to collect national data. The state's mechanics of data collection now permit detection of virtually all the UK's maternal deaths. The recommendations made over the years are largely common sense, and many of them have been adopted.

Weaknesses

The commentary is necessarily subjective, and some of the comments, and indeed recommendations, reflect purely personal opinions. One example is a preference for central venous monitoring in pre-eclamptic patients, an intervention that has no proven benefit but well-documented risks.

Relevance

The saddest reflection on all of this is that the same mistakes are made over and over again, presumably by anaesthetists who do not read these reports. Mendelson's point regarding 'inexperienced interns' is as apt today as it was then. Obstetric anaesthesia is largely seen as a subspecialty for which practical finesse alone is necessary, and theoretical knowledge is superfluous. Such a philosophy helps feed the vignettes in the Enquiries and maintains several medicolegal practices. Maternal mortality may be small, but it should be an affront to the profession that avoidable deaths occur due to fundamental failures of care.

Paper 4: General anaesthesia for operative obstetrics. With special reference to the use of thiopentone and suxamethonium

Author details

RJ Hamer Hodges, JR Bennet, ME Tunstall, RF Knight

Reference

British Journal of Anaesthesia 1959; **31**: 152–63.

Abstract

It is generally agreed that for obstetric procedures, anaesthesia not only causes particular anxieties for anaesthetist and obstetrician, but embodies inherent dangers for the mother and child. In this unit different methods of general anaesthesia have been studied with these considerations in mind. Following an assessment and comparison of methods in an initial series of 264 patients, a technique based on thiopentone, nitrous oxide, and suxamethonium has now been adopted for all operative obstetric procedures. In this paper the results of these comparisons are presented and discussed. Furthermore, in 600 patients anaesthetized by the adopted technique, the results have been analyzed and are presented and discussed in detail.

Hamer Hodges RJ, Bennet JR, Tunstall ME, Knight RF, 'General anaesthesia for operative obstetrics. With special reference to the use of thiopentone and suxamethonium', *British Journal of Anaesthesia*, 1959, 31, 4, pp. 152–163, by permission of Oxford University Press and British Journal of Anaesthesia.

Summary

This publication is rarely mentioned. Its appearance preceded the change from mask anaesthesia to a relaxant and intubation technique that was accompanied by a marked increase in maternal anaesthetic mortality. My reason for inclusion here is that I suspect it was a catalyst for change and many years passed before its negative influences were overcome.

This was an observational study that involved 704 women over a 3-year period. The analysis began with 264 women on whom four different anaesthetic regimens were used:

1 Thiopentone, suxamethonium, intubation, ventilation with oxygen and nitrous oxide with further relaxation from suxamethonium. No other agent before delivery. Immediately before delivery 100% oxygen was given.

2 As for (1) but with the addition of trilene before delivery.

3 Thiopentone, oxygen, and cyclopropane, with curare and intubation for abdominal surgery.

4 Ether, nitrous oxide, and oxygen, with or without thiopentone for induction.

5 A further analysis was carried out on 600 women who had received anaesthetic number (1).

No particular maternal problems were attributed to anaesthesia. The newborns of mothers receiving anaesthetic number (1) were the most active and were quickest to breathe. Those of mothers receiving the ether sequence were the least active and slowest to breathe. Babies of mothers who were given anaesthetics numbers (2) and (3) occupied intermediate positions.

Anaesthetic mortality associated with vomiting during ether anaesthesia was the reason for changing to a technique with tracheal intubation. Foetal depression from the placental transference of anaesthetic was regarded as a source of morbidity, and a relaxant technique allowed the authors to dispense with a volatile agent before delivery altogether. Delivery within 4 min was recommended. The practice of leaving obstetric anaesthesia to the inexperienced is lamented, and in advocating their relaxant technique, the authors stipulate that experienced anaesthetists are required. They take the view that 'conduction anaesthesia' has little place.

Citation count

33.

Related references

1 Crawford JS. Awareness during operative obstetrics under general anaesthesia. *Br J Anaesth* 1971; **43**: 179–82.

Key message

This was an observational study of four different anaesthetic techniques in the obstetric patient.

Strengths

This was a brave attempt to make a scientific assessment of anaesthetic techniques. By current standards the numbers studied are high. The conviction of the authors and their belief in their message comes over strongly.

Weaknesses

There was a failure to consider maternal welfare adequately. In fairness, at that time, the problems associated with this approach, inability to intubate and maternal awareness, were not apparent. There was recognition that relaxant and intubation required greater skills than spontaneously breathing ether, and in advocating this when obstetric anaesthesia lacked experienced personnel, was, in retrospect, an error of judgement.

Relevance

The impact on maternal mortality has already been considered. The lack of a volatile anaesthetic agent before delivery meant that 26% experienced recall (see Related references).

Paper 5: Inferior vena cava occlusion in late pregnancy and its importance in anaesthesia

Author details

B Scott

Reference

British Journal of Anaesthesia 1968; **40**: 120–8.

Abstract

The effects of posture upon circulatory haemodynamics in late pregnancy and their importance to the anaesthetist are discussed in relation to conscious patients, during general anaesthesia and following epidural or spinal blockade

Scott B, 'Inferior vena cava occlusion in late pregnancy and its importance in anaesthesia', *British Journal of Anaesthesia*, 1968, 40, 2, pp. 120–128, by permission of Oxford University Press and British Journal of Anaesthesia.

Summary

Spinal anaesthesia for Caesarean section had been associated with sporadic unpredictable deaths, and the mechanism was unclear (Macintosh, 1959). During the course of the 1950s, the effects of posture on the circulation in late pregnancy were better understood, and its role in deaths during spinal anaesthesia was under scrutiny (Holmes, 1957). Almost 1 in 2 women in late pregnancy experienced a degree of hypotension in the supine position, and in a few the fall was 30% of baseline and accompanied by unpleasant symptoms. The hypotension and the symptoms disappeared in the lateral position. Measurements of venous pressure in the inferior vena cava (IVC) showed a rise in the supine position that was greatest in the presence of occlusion. Normal values resumed in the lateral position, which restored venous return and cardiac output. With venography, Scott showed that a degree of IVC compression was a normal accompaniment of late pregnancy, and that a collateral circulation involving the internal iliac vein through paravertebral venous plexus to the azygos vein existed in some women. Complete IVC occlusion in a woman who lacked a collateral circulation was likely to be accompanied by a severe, progressive reduction in cardiac output with associated fetal acidosis (Bear and Roberts, 1970).

Scott related this to anaesthesia when sympathetic blockade lowered thresholds for IVC compression. Whilst the beneficial effects of vasopressors were acknowledged, if vasoconstriction persisted beyond delivery of the foetus, when venous return was restored, hypertension and even pulmonary oedema could occur. A safer approach to management was to expedite delivery. A feature of the syndrome of supine hypotension was bradycardia, and the administration of atropine was recommended.

Citation count

36.

Related references

1 Macintosh RR. Spinal anaesthesia and Caesarean section. *Br Med J* 1949; **1**: 409.

2 Holmes F. Spinal analgesia and Caesarean section. *Obstet Gynaec Brit Emp* 1957; **64**: 229.

3 Beard RW, Roberts GM. Supine hypotension syndrome. *Br Med J* 1970; **2**: 297.

4 European Resuscitation Council. Part 8: advanced challenges in resuscitation. Section 3: special challenges in ECC. 3F: cardiac arrest associated with pregnancy. *Resuscitation* 2000; **46**(1–3): 293–5.

Key message

This review brought these issues before anaesthetists for the first time.

Strengths

A picture tells a thousand words. The venograms demonstrated IVC occlusion and the existence of a collateral venous circulation.

Weaknesses

The author's assessment of vasoconstrictors was wrong. Perhaps what was needed was an adjustment of dose. Vasoconstrictors are now regarded as an essential part of spinal anaesthesia for Caesarean section.

Relevance

It took a number of years before left uterine displacement became commonplace. It took longer before guidelines for resuscitation in pregnancy required delivery of the foetus within five minutes of starting cardiopulmonary resuscitation (European Resuscitation Council, 2000). Today resuscitation in pregnancy is not routinely taught to anaesthetists, and the advice that cardiac output can be returned to normal by moving to the lateral position or by expediting delivery is frequently forgotten.

Paper 6: Anaesthesia for Caesarean section: an evaluation of a method using low concentrations of halothane and 50 per cent of oxygen

Author details

DD Moir

Reference

British Journal of Anaesthesia 1970; **42**: 136–42.

Abstract

The addition of 0.5 per cent of halothane vapour to a basic thiopentone, nitrous oxide, muscle relaxant anaesthetic technique does not increase blood loss at Caesarean section, does not affect the incidence of hypotension, and is likely to ensure unconsciousness. By permitting the administration of 50 per cent of oxygen with nitrous oxide, the condition of the newborn infant is likely to be improved. The use of 0.8 per cent of halothane vapour does not increase blood loss but is associated with a high incidence of hypotension and for this reason is not advisable.

Summary

Moir was concerned about maternal anaesthetic mortality, blood loss during Caesarean section, awareness, and the concentration of maternal inspired oxygen before delivery. His study was intended to examine the last three of these.

A total of 245 women were recruited and randomized to receive of four general anaesthetics. These were all based on the thiopentone-suxamethonium-intubation-ventilation sequence, but varying the inspired oxygen concentration between 50–70%. Oxygen was either unsupplemented or 0.5% halothane was added. When 50% oxygen was given, halothane 0.5% or 0.8% was added. A first group of 145 unselected elective and emergency deliveries were used to compare blood loss and blood pressure. Some of these were also included in a second group of 150 Caesarean sections who received either 50% or 70% oxygen in nitrous oxide with 0.5% halothane. Because a comparison of neonatal condition was intended, any women with foetal compromise were excluded. A further 20 women who received epidural anaesthesia, and were not randomized, were also included to permit comparison with regional anaesthesia.

Blood loss was least in the 20 women with epidural anaesthesia; the differences between the general anaesthesia sequences were not statistically different. More women experienced a systolic blood pressure below 90 mmHg in the subgroup who were given 0.8% halothane, to the extent that this group was abandoned after 25 women had been studied. The differences between 0.5% halothane and the unsupplemented group did not reach statistical significance.

Two (4%) women in the unsupplemented group recalled events from anaesthesia and surgery, compared with none in the halothane groups. Apgar scores in the unsupplemented 30% oxygen/nitrous group were impressively lower than when a 50:50 mix was used with 0.5% halothane, but this was not analysed statistically. In his discussion, Moir felt that the 50:50 sequence with 0.5% halothane was the best option for mother and baby, although there was no comparison with 0.5% halothane and a 30:70 sequence.

Citation count

117.

Related references

1 Reynolds F, Seed PT. Anaesthesia for Caesarean section and neonatal acid-base status: a meta analysis. *Anaesthesia* 2005; **60**: 636–53.

2 Paech MJ, Scott KL, Clavisi O, *et al.* The ANZCA Trials Group. A prospective study of awareness and recall associated with general anaesthesia for caesarean section. *Int J Obstet Anesth* 2008; **17**: 298–303.

Key message

This was not the first report to advocate the use of halothane for Caesarean section, but Selwyn Crawford, who was hugely influential, had advised against its use. Moir's paper resolved the debate and laid the foundation for general anaesthesia for Caesarean section as we know it today. It went a long way to reduce the problem of awareness associated with the oxygen and nitrous sequence.

Strengths

With randomization and validated measurement of blood loss and neonatal condition, Moir introduced appropriate scientific method into anaesthesia for Caesarean section.

Weaknesses

There was limited standardization of cases. Statistical analysis was limited to one outcome, and there was no prior calculation of sample size. It seems likely that with a suitable number of cases, blood loss would have been found to be significantly higher in the group without halothane.

Relevance

Moir identified the problems of unsupplemented general anaesthesia before delivery and largely resolved them all, excepting the mortality issue. His recommendations were adopted throughout the UK. Subsequently he found an incidence of recall in the region of 1% with the 50:50 sequence with 0.5% halothane. A more mother-friendly approach still has reduced this to 0.2% (Paech *et al.*, 2008), and a recent meta-analysis of cord blood biochemistry supports his claims of benefit for the neonate (Reynolds *et al.*, 2005).

Paper 7: Anaesthesia for obstetric operations

Author details

ME Tunstall

Reference

Clinics in Obstetrics and Gynaecology 1980; **7**: 665–94.

Summary

To avoid aspiration of gastric contents Tunstall advised the left lateral position with head-down tilt. The aim of this was to position the mouth lower than the larynx so that when gastric contents appeared in the pharynx the natural progression would be towards the floor. He chose the left side because for right-handed individuals using a Mackintosh laryngoscope there would be no need to support the tongue in the flange. His comment was that if aspiration did occur it should only affect the dependent lung. To my knowledge, this has never been tested. He believed in the efficacy of cricoid pressure and advocated this whilst ventilation was performed.

For the next phase a decision was required from the anaesthetist as to whether the woman should be allowed to wake up, and proceed with epidural anaesthesia (spinal anaesthesia was still in the dark ages), or whether an inhalational anaesthetic should be given. Ether and methoxyflurane were preferred for this because of anxieties about halothane and uterine relaxation. So when spontaneous breathing returned, surgical anaesthesia was achieved through spontaneously breathing gas, oxygen, and volatile agent, with the woman still on her side. When the depth of anaesthesia was adequate, an orogastric tube was passed to empty the stomach, and the woman returned to the supine position for surgery with facemask anaesthesia.

Citation count

16.

Related references

1 King TA, Adams AP. Failed tracheal intubation. *Br J Anaesth* 1990; **65**: 400–14.
2 ASA Task Force on Management of the Difficult Airway: Practice guidelines for the management of the difficult airway. *Anesthesiology* 2003; **98**: 1269–77.

Key message

Those who practise regional anaesthesia understand well the need for Plan B. Before Dr Tunstall described his drill for failed intubation, the concept of a Plan B for general anaesthesia did not really exist. He said that the idea for the drill followed his inability to intubate the wife of a colleague for Caesarean section in the early 1970s. The profession in the UK had just completed a decade of the greatest number of maternal airway deaths yet recorded. The maxim for his approach was 'oxygenation without aspiration'. The anecdotal information in the Enquiries identified deaths following failure to oxygenate during persistent attempts to intubate, also associated with deaths from aspiration probably from instrumentation of the pharynx as anaesthesia lightened. He recognized that the key decision was to abandon intubation early, before it became an obsession and before significant hypoxia.

Strengths

The importance of this announcement is conceptual; the details of the drill are less important. Comparisons between anaesthetic and cockpit practice are now commonplace. Dr Tunstall is telling us that certain problems can be anticipated, and by extension, we can train to deal with them. It seems so obvious now, but then it was revolutionary.

Weaknesses

Tunstall asked the photographers of the Aberdeen Hospitals to film the drill. With his customary *sang-froid,* and in what appears to be a clinical setting with a genuine patient, he demonstrates his drill perfectly in what seems to be a single take. Anyone who has attempted to use his drill in earnest will have discovered that it is a clinical *tour de force.* If surgical anaesthesia can be obtained breathing methoxyflurane or ether, the timing of emptying the stomach and progressing to surgical readiness without aspiration or lightening of anaesthesia requires consummate clinical skill. A personal view is that his drill is not for mere mortals, but with adaptation, and without departure from its fundamentals, it is a life-saver.

Relevance

In the years that followed, many others offered their ideas on similar drills, and to these were added the management of difficult laryngoscopy, a failed ventilation drill and the use of airway devices that were unknown at that time, until the modern airway algorithm was built. Earlier in his career Tunstall had persuaded British Oxygen to mix oxygen and nitrous oxide in the same cylinder, to create Entonox, and soon after describing his drill, he was demonstrating his isolated forearm technique to astonished visitors. In retirement he continued research with analgesic concentrations of isoflurane, and windsurfed the North Sea impervious to the climate of North East Scotland.

Paper 8: Cardiac arrest following regional anesthesia with etidocane or bupivacaine

Author details

GA Albright

Reference

Anesthesiology 1979; **51**: 285–7.

Summary

In 1979 from the United States, Albright reported six instances of cardiac collapse following presumed accidental intravenous injection of either etidocaine or bupivacaine. He described rapid onset of ventricular fibrillation, ventricular tachycardia, asystole or complete heart block occurring at the end of injection during a variety of local anaesthetic blocks. Two followed epidural injections in pregnant women and one incident resulted in maternal death. By 1984, Plumer was able to list 35 obstetric cases of accidental intravenous injection of either 0.5% or 0.75% bupivacaine, which included 24 maternal deaths. Of the 11 survivors, three were damaged, and a total of five babies died (Plumer, 1984). From the same period, the North American closed claims study reported 19 instances of convulsions, of which 18 occurred in association with epidural anaesthesia and 17 were attributed to local anaesthetic toxicity. Outcomes were grim, with 83% experiencing neurological injury or death, to the mother, fetus, or both (Chadwick *et al.*, 1991).

The problem identified by Albright was not apparent in obstetric practice in the United Kingdom, but in 1982 Heath reported that a number of deaths had occurred, two in children, during intravenous regional analgesia with bupivacaine. Some of these anaesthetics had been given by surgeons (Heath, 1982).

As a result of the accumulating body count, bupivacaine 0.75% was withdrawn from the market, and a series of research initiatives were taken up. After several years of investigation it was established that pregnant women represented broadly the same risk as non-pregnant, and that bupivacaine toxicity was hard to treat. Pursuit of local anaesthetics with a less toxic profile led to the appearance of the *levo* enatiomers, ropivacaine and levobupivacaine, in clinical practice 25 to 30 years later. A recent development in this field is the concept of lipid rescue (http://lipidrescue.squarespace.com).

Citation count

860.

Related references

1 Thorburn J, Moir D. Epidural analgesia for elective Caesarean section. *Anaesthesia* 1980; **35**: 3–6.

2 Heath ML. Deaths after intravenous regional anaesthesia. *Br Med J* 1982; **285**: 913–4.

3 Plumer M. Appendix B. Obstetric case histories: bupivacaine. *SOAP Newsletter* 1984; **15**(3/4): 8–10.

4 Chadwick HS, Posner K, Caplan RA, Ward RJ, Cheney FW. A comparison of obstetric and nonobstetric anesthesia malpractice claims. *Anesthesiology* 1991; **74**: 242–9.

Key message

The problems associated with general anaesthesia for Caesarean section encouraged greater use of regional, but this was new territory with undeveloped guidelines and recommendations. Albright's editorial alerted the profession to bupivacaine toxicity in conjunction with epidural anaesthesia.

Strengths

Albright had the courage to go to print with just a handful of cases.

Weaknesses

There was no immediate solution on offer. The American experience with epidural anaesthesia for Caesarean section parallels the introduction of relaxant anaesthesia with intubation in the UK.

Relevance

The uptake of epidural anaesthesia in the UK was associated with few adverse events and no deaths. One reason for this was that teaching in the UK advocated incremental doses of local anaesthetic and most of these were given through an epidural catheter (Thorburn and Moir, 1980). Consequently, although the occasional dose was given intravenously, convulsions were the main adverse event; the increments given were too small to be lethal. A modern retrospective notes that these women would have been resuscitated supine, making restoration of venous return unlikely.

Paper 9: Damage to the conus medullaris following spinal anaesthesia

Author details

F Reynolds

Reference

Anaesthesia 2001; **56**: 238–47.

Summary

Imaging shows that termination of the cord is not anatomically constant, terminating at the body of L2 in 11%, and lower than this in 2% (Hogan *et al.*, 1999). The significance of this is that a spinal needle introduced in a cephalad direction at the L2–3 interspace has the potential to enter the conus in a minority of individuals, making L3–4 the most cephalad interspace of choice. Anaesthetists who cannot identify the space accurately are at risk of causing neurological damage, and the evidence suggests that we commonly get this wrong (Broadbent *et al.*, 2000). It was to overcome this problem that Tuffier described his line between the ilia, recognizing that identifying a space in the vertebral column had to involve reference to a fixed anatomical landmark that was independent of the spine (Tuffier, 1901). Classically, Tuffier's line passes through the body of L4, but when imaging is used to identify L4, the line does not have a constant relationship with it, but might lie as high as L3–4 above, and L5–S1 below (Hogan, 1999). Reynolds points out that despite the variability of the termination of the cord, and also of Tuffier's line, there is no overlap between the two in normal individuals (Reynolds, 2000), and this is why it remains useful. If the line passes through a space, then safe practice requires the assumption that the space is L3–4, though L4–5 is more likely. In the other direction is the sacrum, through which spinal anaesthesia cannot be performed. The use of Tuffier's line should ensure that, even given the variability, misidentification should not be more than one space out.

Citation count

163.

Related references

1 Tuffier T. L'analgesie chirurgicale par voie rachidienne. *Oeuvre Médicale et Chirurgicale* 1901; 24.

2 Hogan Q. Anatomy of the epidural space. In: Norris MC (ed) *Obstetric Anesthesia*, 2nd edn., pp. 283–4. Philadelphia, PA: Lippincott Williams & Wilkins, 1999;

3 Broadbent CR, Maxwell WB, Ferrie R, Wilson DJ, Gawne-Cain M, Russell R. Ability of anaesthetists to identify a marked lumbar interspace. *Anaesthesia* 2000; **55**: 1122–6.

4 Reynolds F. Logic in the safe practice of spinal anaesthesia. *Anaesthesia* 2000; **55**: 1045–6.

Key message

Professor Reynolds collected these cases from her medicolegal practice; she had written about safe practice in spinal anaesthesia in an earlier editorial (Reynolds, 2000). Of particular interest was the re-evaluation of Tuffier's line (Tuffier, 1901).

Strengths

Reynolds draws on a handful of old and new publications to support a common sense approach to safer spinal anaesthesia.

Weaknesses

The recommendation that spinal anaesthesia should not be performed above L3–4 loses conviction without an equally strong recommendation for correct identification of the space.

Relevance

This case series is essential reading for all those who practice central neuraxial blocks.

Paper 10: Fetal and maternal effects of phenylephrine and ephedrine during spinal anaesthesia for cesarean delivery

Author details

DW Cooper, M Carpenter, P Mowbray, WR Desira, DM Ryall, MS Kokri

Reference

Anesthesiology 2002; **97**: 1582–90.

Summary

Cooper's idea was to compare the arterio–venous difference between the cord PCO_2 values. The ephedrine group had significantly higher umbilical artery CO_2 tensions than the phenylephrine group, and they correlated with the dose of ephedrine given. There was an inverse relationship between the a–v difference and umbilical artery pH. Up to this moment, the presumption was that the fetal acidosis seen with ephedrine was due to a negative effect on placental flow when compared with phenylephrine. This was despite the fall in cardiac output associated with the lower heart rates seen following phenylephrine. In the Discussion an increase in fetal anaerobic glycolysis and catecholamine production triggered by β-adrenergic effects of ephedrine are given as the source of the acidosis. The same effects have also been shown to reduce the work of breathing and reduce hypoglycaemia in the newborn. Suddenly ephedrine might be moving towards rehabilitation.

Citation count

171.

Key message

There are no clues in the abstract to explain the importance of this paper. Spinal anaesthesia has always been associated with an incidence of fetal acidosis, but as the direct acting α-agonist phenylephrine displaced the indirect acting mixed α and β agonist ephedrine as the vasopressor of choice, fetal biochemistry improved. Many comparisons of these two, in different situations, different doses and different methods of administration had been published, and all tended to confirm that fetal acidosis was greater with ephedrine. Cooper and colleagues repeated this work, but used the data to explore a hypothesis that had been hitherto overlooked. The two vasopressor were the subject of a debate held at the 2004 meeting of the Society for Obstetric Anesthesiologists and Perinatologists, and the speakers took it as given that their audience were familiar with this publication, such was its importance.

Strengths

Cooper saw something that other researchers had missed. His analysis was particularly thorough.

Weaknesses

The clinical importance of Cooper's findings was not clear. It was possible that fetal acidosis of this nature could be beneficial. It was not possible to extrapolate this to situations of fetal compromise.

The animal work still remained in conflict with clinical practice, for reasons that were not altogether understood, and improving fetal biochemistry whilst reducing maternal cardiac output remained unexplained.

Relevance

Cooper conducts clinical research as an interested amateur. He shows us that intellect is more important in ground-breaking clinical research than academic status and well funded departments.

Chapter 17

Airway management

CA Deegan and DJ Buggy

Introduction

Airway management is an essential component of clinical anaesthesia, and involves maintenance of a patent airway to facilitate gas exchange via mask ventilation or airway device. An important aspect of airway management is assessment of the patient's airway to predict the likelihood of ease or difficulty with bag-mask ventilation or with laryngoscopy and intubation. The American Society of Anesthesiology Task Force on the Management of the Difficult Airway has defined a difficult airway as the clinical situation in which a conventionally trained anaesthetist experiences difficulty with face mask ventilation of the upper airway, difficulty with tracheal intubation, or both. Difficulties or failure in airway management are common factors leading to death and brain damage as a direct result of anaesthesia.

Prediction of the difficult airway enables the anaesthetist to prepare for this challenging clinical scenario. However, despite careful airway assessment, direct laryngoscopy sometimes results in unanticipated poor laryngeal views. Difficult laryngoscopy has an incidence of up to 8.5%, and is defined as rigid laryngoscopy resulting in a grade III view (just the epiglottis is seen) or a grade IV view (just part of the soft palate is seen). Glottic visualization can generally be improved with application of additional force, external laryngeal manipulation, the use of airway adjuncts such as articulated laryngoscopes and bougies, or alternative techniques such as an intubating laryngeal mask airway. The American Society of Anesthesiologists difficult airway algorithm provides guidelines on the management of difficult laryngoscopy and difficult intubation but does not provide management guidelines on the more immediately life-threatening clinical situation of difficult mask ventilation. Despite the large amount of research into the prediction of difficult laryngoscopy and difficult intubation, data on difficult or impossible mask ventilation are limited.

Difficult mask ventilation may be predicted in the presence of a beard, a history of snoring, obesity, advanced age, and absence of teeth. Difficult laryngoscopy may be predicted by careful clinical examination, using the Mallampati classification, thyromental distance, and several other anatomical measurements. Managing a difficult airway is a clinical decision based on the patient's clinical status and the anaesthetist's experience. Supraglottic devices, such as the laryngeal mask airway, have emerged as important rescue ventilation devices. Intubation techniques include blind nasal intubation, the intubating laryngeal mask airway, use of a gum-elastic bougie, flexible fibreoptic intubation and a variety of rigid fibreoptic techniques. Rigid fibreoptic laryngoscopes offer the advantages of ease of use and high success rates, while providing direct visualization of the airway and advancement of the endotracheal tube.

Papers 1–4 concentrate on the preoperative assessment of the patient's airway in order to identify clinical signs which would assist the anaesthetist in predicting difficulty with mask ventilation, laryngoscopy, or both. One of these studies describes the best way to elucidate these clinical findings to increase sensitivity and specificity of these tests. Paper 5 highlights the importance of simulation and training in potentially reducing perioperative morbidity and mortality, with the author simulating the difficult laryngoscopy scenario with obstetric anaesthesia trainees. Paper 6 was the first description of the use of cricoid pressure to control regurgitation of gastric contents in patients at high risk of aspirating during general anaesthesia. The final four papers describe the use of different airway devices, including the laryngeal mask airway, the intubating laryngeal mask airway, the laryngeal mask airway CTrach, the Glidescope videolaryngoscope, and the Airwayscope which may be used routinely or in the management of the difficult airway.

Paper 1: Prediction of difficult mask ventilation

Author details

O Langeron, E Masso, C Huraux, M Guggiari, A Bianchi, P Coriat, B Riou

Reference

Anesthesiology 2000; **92**: 1229–36.

Summary

Difficult mask ventilation is an important cause of perioperative morbidity and mortality. Difficult airway management algorithm highlight the importance of preoperative airway assessment, with particular focus on predicting difficult intubation. However, difficulty with mask ventilation has far more serious consequences. This prospective non-randomized study identified predictive factors associated with difficult mask ventilation, including body mass index >26 kg m^{-2}, age >55 years, macroglossia, beard, lack of teeth, history of snoring, increased Mallampati grade, and lower thyromental distance. Presence of two criteria was the most accurate predictor of difficult mask ventilation. The incidence of difficult mask ventilation was 5%. Difficult mask ventilation was associated with a four-fold increased risk of difficult intubation and a 12-fold increased risk of impossible intubation. Difficult mask ventilation was only predicted preoperatively in 17% of patients who proved difficult to ventilate by mask.

Citation count

369.

Related references

1 Kheterpal S, Han R, Tremper KK, *et al.* Incidence and predictors of difficult and impossible mask ventilation. *Anesthesiology* 2006; **105**: 885–91.

2 Kheterpal S, Martin L, Shanks AM, *et al.* Prediction and outcomes of impossible mask ventilation. A review of 50,000 anesthetics. *Anesthesiology* 2009; **110**: 891–7.

Key message

Potential risk factors for DMV in the general adult population include body mass index >26 kg m^{-2}, age >55 years, macroglossia, beard, lack of teeth, history of snoring, increased Mallampati grade, and lower thyromental distance.

Strengths

This was a large well-designed prospective study (n=1502). All patients were managed by experienced consultant anaesthetists.

Weaknesses

This was a non-randomized study. The investigators used a subjective definition of DMV, including signs of inadequate ventilation and requirement for alternative methods to assist mask ventilation. The investigators excluded emergency surgical patients, ear/nose/throat patients, and paediatric patients, so the results can not be extrapolated to include this patient population.

Relevance

Difficulties or failure in management of the difficult airway is a major cause of morbidity and mortality resulting from hypoxia or anoxia during anaesthesia. Recognition of the difficult airway is one of the key components in difficult airway management, in particular difficulty with mask ventilation, which may ultimately decrease morbidity and mortality associated with failed ventilation. This paper identified several factors associated with DMV, and also reported that anaesthetists in this study only predicted DMV in 17% of cases highlighting the need to identify predicting factors for DMV.

Paper 2: A clinical sign to predict difficult intubation: a prospective study

Author details

SR Mallampati, SP Gatt, LD Gugino, SP Desai, B Waraksa, D Freiberger

Reference

Canadian Anaesthesia Society Journal 1985; **32**: 429–34.

Abstract

It has been suggested that the size of the base of the tongue is an important factor determining the degree of difficulty of direct laryngoscopy. A relatively simple grading system which involves preoperative ability to visualize the faucial pillars, soft palate and base of uvula was designed as a means of predicting the degree of difficulty in laryngeal exposure. The system was evaluated in 210 patients. The degree of difficulty in visualizing these three structures was an accurate predictor of difficulty with direct laryngoscopy (p <0.001).

Summary

This prospective study was carried out to determine if the visibility of the faucial pillars and uvula in a seated patient with mouth fully open and tongue protruded is a predictor of difficult laryngoscopy. The authors hypothesized that concealment of the faucial pillars and uvula was related to a disproportionately large tongue, which may cause difficult laryngoscopy due to overshadowing of the larynx. The authors found that when faucial pillars, soft palate and uvula were visible (Class I), there were no difficult laryngoscopies (all Grade I or II). In patients whose uvula was masked (Class II), laryngoscopy was difficult in 35% (Grade III or IV). Laryngoscopy was difficult in over 93% of patients in whom only part of the soft palate was visible (Class III).

Citation count

1276.

Related references

1 Samsoon GL, Young JR. Difficult tracheal intubation: a retrospective study. *Anaesthesia* 1987; **42**: 487–90.

2 Butler PJ, Dhara SS. Prediction of difficult laryngoscopy: an assessment of the thyromental distance and Mallampati predictive tests. *Anaesth Intensive Care* 1992; **20**: 139–42.

3 L'Hermite J, Nouvellon E, Cuvillon P, *et al*. The Simplified Predictive Intubation Difficulty Score: a new weighted score for difficult airway assessment. *Eur J Anaesthesiol* 2009; **26**: 1003–9.

Key message

When faucial pillars, soft palate and uvula are visible with patient's mouth open widely and tongue protruding (Class I) difficult laryngoscopy is unlikely. If soft palate and uvula are obscured in this view due to a disproportionately large tongue (Class III), difficult laryngoscopy should be anticipated.

Strengths

This was a prospective study of 210 consecutive patients, enabling statistical significance to be calculated. The methodology for determining the Mallampati class was well described.

Weaknesses

The grading system used by the authors differs from the commonly used Cormack and Lehane system for laryngoscopy views. Mallampati's Grade 3 view, regarded as difficult laryngoscopy, correlates with a Cormack and Lehane Grade 2b, which is considered an easy laryngoscopic view. This may account for the high positive predictive value of an oropharyngeal Class 2 and 3 view, which has not been validated in any subsequent study. The same investigators who graded the oropharyngeal class also graded the laryngoscopy view, and this may be a source of bias.

Relevance

This study was the first to describe three classes of oropharyngeal view which assist in predicting difficulty with laryngoscopy preoperatively. The Mallampati classification was subsequently modified by Samsoon and Young, by adding a fourth class. This classification is used routinely as part of the preoperative assessment to predict a difficult airway. The original Mallampati classification predicted difficult laryngoscopy with a high degree of specificity. However, this high positive predictive value has not been validated in subsequent larger studies, which demonstrated only modest degrees of accuracy using the original classification. The Mallampati test is insufficient to use alone to predict a difficult airway, and it is recommended by the American Society of Anesthesiologists Task Force on the management of difficult airways as one part of the airway assessment.

Paper 3: Preoperative airway assessment: predictive value of a multivariate risk index

Author details

AR El-Ganzouri, RJ McCarthy, KJ Tuman, EN Tanck, AD Ivankovich

Reference

Anesthesia and Analgesia 1996; **82**: 1197–204.

Summary

The investigators developed a multivariate model for risk stratification of difficult laryngoscopy using objective airway risk criteria. Data were collected prospectively on 10,507 consecutive patients receiving general anaesthesia and endotracheal intubation. Objective data recorded from preoperative airway assessment included body weight, history of difficult intubation, mouth opening, Mallampati classification, head/neck movement, ability to prognath, and thyromental distance. Each airway assessment variable was stratified into 'risk categories'. Ease of mask ventilation following induction of anaesthesia was documented, as was the laryngeal view using the Cormack and Lehane grading system. Grade IV laryngoscopy was present in 1% of patients, and difficult mask ventilation in 0.07%. All seven criteria were identified as independent predictors of difficulty with laryngoscopic visualization. The investigators showed that using this preoperative scoring system resulted in a higher positive predictive value for laryngoscopy Grade IV at scores with similar sensitivity to Mallampati Class III, as well as higher sensitivity at scores with similar positive predictive value. The higher positive predictive value results in fewer unanticipated episodes of difficult laryngoscopy, while the lower false positive rate results in less unnecessary airway manoeuvres.

Citation count

267.

Related references

1 Arné J, Descoins P, Fusciardi J, *et al*. Preoperative assessment for difficult intubation in general and ENT surgery: predictive value of a clinical multivariate risk index. *Br J Anaesth* 1998; **80**: 140–6.

2 Karkouti K, Rose DK, Wigglesworth D, *et al*. Predicting difficult intubation: a multivariable analysis. *Can J Anaesth* 2000; **47**: 730–9.

3 Cattano D, Panicucci E, Paolicchi A, *et al*. Risk factors assessment of the difficult airway: an Italian survey of 1956 patients. *Anesth Analg* 2004; **99**: 1774–9.

4 Shiga T, Wajima Z, Inoue T, *et al*. Predicting difficult intubation in apparently normal patients. A meta-analysis of bedside screening test performance. *Anesthesiology* 2005; **103**: 429–37.

Key message

Use of a simple scoring system preoperatively results in reliable risk stratification of patients for difficult laryngoscopy/intubation.

Strengths

The population size studied (n=10,507) was sufficiently large to enable multivariate modelling for derivation of a predictive index for difficult intubation, which occurs in approximately 1% of patients.

Weaknesses

Patients with known airway malformations scheduled for awake intubation were excluded from the study, so one cannot extrapolate the results to include this patient population. In addition, the study was underpowered to detect multivariate predictors of difficult mask ventilation, requiring over 100,000 patients.

Relevance

Difficult endotracheal intubation may increase morbidity and mortality related to anaesthesia. Preoperative airway assessment is essential to recognize a potentially difficult airway. Several studies have identified various individual clinical signs which are associated with difficult laryngoscopy and/or intubation, but the sensitivity and positive predictive value of these are low. This study demonstrates that improved risk stratification for difficult laryngoscopy can be obtained by using a simplified preoperative multivariate airway risk index, with better accuracy compared to oropharyngeal (Mallampati) classification at both low- and high-risk levels. This may lead to less unanticipated difficult airways and less unnecessary airway manoeuvres.

Paper 4: What is the best way to determine oropharyngeal classification and mandibular space length to predict difficult laryngoscopy?

Author details

M Lewis, S Keramati, JL Benumof, CC Berry

Reference

Anesthesiology 1994; **81**: 69–75.

Summary

This study investigates the optimum way to determine oropharyngeal class and mandibular space length to assist in predicting difficult laryngoscopy. They assessed 48 different combinations of head and body position, tongue position, specific part of mentum to measure, measurement of thyroid versus hyoid, and phonation to determine oropharyngeal class and mandibular space length. The authors found that using oropharyngeal class and mandibular space length together can accurately predict difficult laryngoscopy. However, the false positive rate is up to 50%. For determination of oropharyngeal class, the optimum position is sitting with full head extension, tongue out with phonation. For mandibular space length, the patient should be sitting with sniff position and full head extension. The inner mentum should be used as a proximal landmark.

Citation count

103.

Related references

1 Tse JC, Rimm EB, Hussain A. Predicting difficult endotracheal intubation in surgical patients scheduled for general anesthesia: a prospective blind study. *Anesth Analg* 1995; **81**: 254–8.

2 Khan ZH, Mohammadi M, Rasouli MR, *et al.* The diagnostic value of the upper lip bite test combined with sternomental distance, thyromental distance, and interincisor distance for prediction of easy laryngoscopy and intubation: a prospective study. *Anesth Analg* 2009; **109**: 822–4.

Key message

Use of mandibular space length and oropharyngeal class together can predict difficult laryngoscopy with reasonable degree of accuracy, although false positive rates are high (up to 50%). Ideal positioning for oropharyngeal class is sitting with full head extension, tongue out and phonation. For mandibular space length, the patient should be sitting with head in sniff position and full extension and inner mentum used as anatomical landmark.

Strengths

The study was a well-designed prospective controlled trial. The study (n=213) was sufficiently powered to enable statistical significance to be determined.

Weaknesses

There were a few sources of potential bias, including use of several different intubators who were assessing laryngoscopy difficulty, and use of two different observers to record oropharyngeal class and mandibular space length under the 48 different conditions tested.

Relevance

Oropharyngeal class and mandibular space length were used in countless studies on prediction and management of difficult airways. However, no one study determined the best way for assessing these anatomical characteristics. The authors sought to describe the best way to determine these measurements to better predict difficult laryngoscopy clinically. This would also assist in improving uniformity and objectivity in these measurements in subsequent clinical trials.

Paper 5: Difficult tracheal intubation in obstetrics

Author details
RS Cormack, J Lehane

Reference
Anaesthesia 1984; **39**: 1105–11.

Summary
The confidential enquiry into maternal deaths demonstrated that the most common cause of perioperative death was related to difficult or failed intubation. As grade 3 or 4 laryngoscopy views are uncommonly encountered in normal clinical practice, anaesthetic trainees may be inexperienced in the management of this potentially life-threatening clinical scenario. Simulation of a grade 3 or 4 laryngoscopy view may be achieved by performing laryngoscopy as usual, but then lowering the blade so that the epiglottis descends and thus obscures the vocal cords. Following practicing this drill, the authors report that their trainees had little difficulty in managing a real difficult intubation.

Citation count
1294.

Related references
1 Samsoon GLT, Young JRB. Difficult tracheal intubation: a retrospective study. *Anaesthesia* 1987; **42**: 487–90.

2 Rocke DA, Murray WB, Rout CC, *et al.* Relative risk analysis of factors associated with difficult intubation in obstetric anesthesia. *Anesthesiology* 1992; **77**: 67–73.

3 Rahman K, Jenkins JG. Failed tracheal intubation in obstetrics: no more frequent but still managed badly. *Anaesthesia* 2005; **60**: 168–71.

4 Djabatey EA, Barclay PM. Difficult and failed intubation in 3430 obstetric general anaesthetics. *Anaesthesia* 2009; **64**: 1168–71.

Key message
Simulation of the difficult airway may assist anaesthetic trainees in becoming proficient in managing this uncommon, but potentially life-threatening, clinical situation.

Strengths
This was a novel idea to simulate a difficult clinical scenario that is uncommonly encountered in order to improve the clinical skills of trainees.

Weaknesses
There are no data presented regarding the number of trainees included, or their level of seniority, or the number of simulated difficult airways they practised on. As a result, there is no statistical analysis performed to demonstrate any significant improvement in practice, other than to report that management of the difficult airway in clinical practice improved.

Relevance

Difficulty with management of the difficult airway in obstetrics is a known cause of maternal morbidity and mortality. Quite often, in obstetrical anaesthesia practice, junior anaesthetic trainees are managing difficult airways alone while on-call. To confound this problem, difficult airways are infrequently encountered in normal clinical practice, so that trainees may be inexperienced in the management of this serious condition, with potentially disastrous consequences. The authors describe a technique of simulating a difficult airway in patients with normal airway anatomy, to improve trainee's clinical skills. The mannequin-based fully interactive patient simulator was first developed over 20 years after this paper was published, and the benefits of simulation-based training in anaesthesia are now well recognized.

Paper 6: Cricoid pressure to control regurgitation of stomach contents during induction of anaesthesia

Author details

BA Sellick

Reference

Lancet 1961; **2**: 404–6.

Abstract

Backward pressure of the cricoid cartilage against the cervical vertebrae can be used to occlude the oesophagus (a) to control regurgitation of stomach or oesophageal contents during induction of anaesthesia, or (b) to prevent gastric distension from positive-pressure ventilation applied by facepiece or mouth-to-mouth respiration. It is contraindicated during active vomiting.

Summary

This study is the first to describe the use of cricoid pressure in high-risk patients for the prevention of aspiration of gastric contents during induction of anaesthesia. Sellick suggested that following emptying of the stomach with a nasogastic tube, and subsequent removal of this tube, the patient should be positioned with the cervical spine extended, to stretch the oesophagus and prevent its lateral displacement when cricoid pressure is applied. Following preoxygenation and intravenous rapid sequence induction in 26 high-risk cases, cricoid pressure was applied by an assistant. Light cricoid pressure was applied as anaesthesia began, by exerting pressure with the thumb and index finger. As soon as consciousness was lost, firm pressure was applied without obstructing the patient's airway. Pressure was maintained until intubation and inflation of the cuff of the endotracheal tube was completed. In 23 of the 26 cases, no regurgitation or vomiting occurred before, during, or after cricoid pressure. In three cases, reflux of gastric contents occurred following release of cricoid pressure after intubation, suggesting that it had been effective.

Citation count

605.

Related references

1 Brimacombe JR, Berry AM. Cricoid pressure. *Can J Anaesth* 1997; **44**: 414–25.

2 Hartsilver EL, Vanner RG. Airway obstruction with cricoid pressure. *Anaesthesia* 2000; **55**: 208–11.

Key message

Cricoid pressure is effective in reducing reflux of gastric or oesophageal contents during induction of anaesthesia in high-risk cases. During cricoid pressure the lungs may be ventilated by intermittent positive-pressure without risking gastric distension. Cricoid pressure cannot be used to control active vomiting as there is a risk of oesophageal rupture.

Strengths

Sellick described a simple and seemingly effective manoeuvre to reduce regurgitation and aspiration during induction of anaesthesia in high-risk patients.

Weaknesses

Sellick recommended application of cricoid pressure in the presence of neck extension, however, this usually distorts the glottic view during laryngoscopy. All patients were anaesthetized in a head-down position with the head slightly turned. The supine position with the neck in the 'sniffing position' has subsequently been recommended as the standard during cricoid pressure. The force to be applied to the cricoid cartilage was not alluded to.

Relevance

Aspiration of stomach contents can have disastrous consequences, thus its prevention could significantly reduce anaesthetic morbidity and mortality. Risk of aspiration is especially high during obstetrics and emergency general surgery. The 'gold standard' for prevention of aspiration during anaesthesia is endotracheal intubation, although micro-aspirations may still occur. Protective airway reflexes are lost during induction of anaesthesia, and this is a period where patients are at risk for aspiration. This study was the first to demonstrate that cricoid pressure is effective in reducing the risk of pulmonary aspiration of gastric contents during emergency surgery. This report revolutionized the practice of anaesthesia and application of cricoid pressure during a rapid sequence induction in a patient at high risk of aspirating is now a standard of care. However, there is ongoing debate in the literature as to the effectiveness of cricoid pressure, and there is evidence that it may increase the risk of regurgitation and difficult intubation. A randomized control trial to investigate the appropriateness and effectiveness of cricoid pressure would be unethical.

Paper 7: The laryngeal mask—a new concept in airway management

Author details

AIJ Brain

Reference

British Journal of Anaesthesia 1983; **55**: 801–5.

Abstract

A new type of airway is described, which may be used as an alternative to either the endotracheal tube or the face-mask with either spontaneous or positive pressure ventilation. The results of a pilot study involving 23 patients are presented and the possible merits and disadvantages of the device are discussed, bearing in mind that the study is of a preliminary nature.

Summary

This paper is the first paper describing the clinical use of the laryngeal mask airway (LMA) devised by the British anaesthetist Archie Brain. A prototype LMA was inserted blindly into the hypopharynx of 23 patients undergoing elective surgery, with six of these patients breathing spontaneously and the remainder receiving positive pressure ventilation. In all patients, ventilation was adequate, leaks were easily abolished, and insertion and pharyngeal suction was easy. There were no documented respiratory complications, and less than 20% of patients complained of mild sore throat.

Citation count

654.

Related references

1 Brain AI. Three cases of difficult intubation overcome by the laryngeal mask airway. *Anaesthesia* 1985; **40**: 353–5.

2 Brain AIJ, McGhee TD, McAteer EJ, *et al*. The laryngeal mask airway. Development and preliminary trials of a new type of airway. *Anaesthesia* 1985; **40**: 356–61.

3 Pennant JH, White PF. The laryngeal mask airway. Its uses in anesthesiology. *Anesthesiology* 1993; **79**: 144–63.

Key message

The LMA is a new supraglottic airway device which is easy to use and has minimal side effects. It possesses some of the advantages of endotracheal intubation while avoiding the need for neuromuscular blockade and visualization of the vocal cords.

Strengths

The prototype LMA was well designed, easy to insert, and enabled successful ventilation in all study patients with minimal side effects.

Weaknesses

It is not possible to draw definitive conclusions from this study as the study size is too small (n=23).

Relevance

This paper is the first of many papers describing the use of the LMA which has revolutionized the delivery of anaesthesia. The LMA has been proven in numerous trials to be a safe and effective airway device for patients who are not at risk for aspiration of gastric contents. It is introduced blindly into the hypopharynx thus forming a seal around the larynx, permitting spontaneous or positive pressure ventilation. It is also a valuable airway device in cases of difficult intubation and thereby may add to the safety of general anaesthesia. Side effects from the use of the device are minimal.

Paper 8: Use of the intubating LMA-Fastrach™ in 254 patients with difficult-to-manage airways

Author details

DZ Ferson, WH Rosenblatt, MJ Johansen, I Osborn, A Ovassapian

Reference

Anesthesiology 2001; **95**: 1175–81.

Summary

The authors conducted a retrospective review of patient charts with known difficult airways that were managed electively or emergently with the LMA- Fastrach™ over a 3-year period in four different institutions.

Citation count

203.

Related references

1 Combes X, Sauvat S, Leroux B, *et al.* Intubating laryngeal mask airway in morbidly obese and lean patients: a comparative study. *Anesthesiology* 2005; **102**: 1106–19.

2 Caponas G. Intubating laryngeal mask airway. *Anaesth Intensive Care* 2002; **30**: 551–69.

3 Baskett PJ, Parr MJ, Nolan JP. The intubating laryngeal mask. Results of a multicentre trial with experience of 500 cases. *Anaesthesia* 1998; **53**: 1174–9.

4 Brain AI, Verghese C, Addy EV, *et al.* The intubating laryngeal mask. II: A preliminary clinical report of a new means of intubating the trachea. *Br J Anaesth* 1997; **79**: 704–9.

Key message

The LMA- Fastrach™ is a useful airway device in the elective management of difficult airways and in patients with immobilized cervical spines. It is also useful in the emergency management of failed intubation with a rigid laryngoscope.

Strengths

The investigators included a large patient cohort (n=254) in their analysis. All investigators were highly trained in the use of the LMA- Fastrach™.

Weaknesses

One limitation of the study is the study design. It is a retrospective chart review, which leads to difficulties in controlling study bias and confounders. A second potential weakness is that the investigators cut out the chin portion of the rigid cervical collar to aid insertion of the LMA-Fastrach™, but this may have reduced the efficacy of the collar.

Relevance

This paper was one of the first reports of the use of the intubating LMA in a large patient cohort with difficult airways. The devastating consequences of difficulty in managing a patient's airway are well known, and the intubating LMA or LMA- Fastrach™ was devised to incorporate the ventilatory advantages of the classic LMA with an improved method of tracheal intubation. The investigators reported a high (92%) success rate for blind intubation in patients in whom intubation failed with rigid laryngoscopy, and an overall success rate for blind intubation of 96% in all cases. There was no evidence of consequent airway or oesophageal trauma. Therefore, the results suggest that the LMA- Fastrach™ has much to offer in the management of patients with difficult airways.

Paper 9: The GlideScope® Video Laryngoscope: randomized clinical trial in 200 patients

Author details

DA Sun, CB Warriner, DG Parsons, R Klein, HS Umedaly, M Moult

Reference

British Journal of Anaesthesia 2005; **94**: 381–4.

Abstract

Background: The GlideScope® Video Laryngoscope is a new intubating device. It was designed to provide a view of the glottis without alignment of the oral, pharyngeal and tracheal axes. The aim of the study was to describe the use of the GlideScope® in comparison with direct laryngoscopy for elective surgical patients requiring tracheal intubation.

Methods: Two hundred patients were randomly assigned to intubation by direct laryngoscopy using a Macintosh size 3 blade (DL, n=100) or intubation using the GlideScope® (GS, n=100). Prior to intubation all patients were given a Cormack and Lehane (C&L) grade by a separate anaesthetist using a Macintosh size 3 blade. The patient was then intubated, using direct laryngoscopy or the GlideScope®, by a different anaesthetist during which the larynx was inspected and given a laryngoscopy score. Time to intubate was measured.

Results: In the GS group, laryngoscopy grade was improved in the majority (28/41) of patients with C&L grade >1 and in all but one of patients who were grade 3 laryngoscopy (P<0.001). The overall mean time to intubate was 30 (95% CI 28–33) s in the DL group and 46 (95% CI 43–49) s in the GS group. The time to intubate for C&L grade 3 was similar in both groups, being 47 s for the DL group and 50 s for the GS group respectively.

Conclusion: In most patients, the GlideScope® provided a laryngoscopic view equal to or better than that of direct laryngoscopy, but it took an additional 16 s (average) for tracheal intubation. It has potential advantages over standard direct laryngoscopy for difficult intubations.

Summary

The GlideScope® video laryngoscope is designed to allow a view of the glottis with a camera without aligning oral, pharyngeal, and tracheal axes. In this study, 200 elective surgical patients requiring endotracheal intubation were randomly assigned to intubation using the GlideScope® or to intubation using the Macintosh laryngoscope. This study demonstrated an improvement in C&L grade with the GlideScope® in comparison to the Macintosh laryngoscope in 68% of patients with C&L grade >1. The investigators demonstrated that the laryngoscopic view was improved with the GlideScope®, but the time taken to intubate was longer and more attempts were required.

Citation count

194.

Related references

1 Cooper RM, Pacey JA, Bishop MJ, *et al.* Early clinical experience with a new videolaryngoscope (GlideScope®) in 728 patients. *Can J Anaesth* 2005; **52**: 191–8.

2 Rai MR, Dering A, Verghese C. The Glidescope system: a clinical assessment of performance. *Anaesthesia* 2005; **60**: 60–4.

3 Kim JT, Na HS, Bae JY, *et al.* GlideScope video laryngoscope: a randomized clinical trial in 203 paediatric patients. *Br J Anaesth* 2008; **101**: 531–4.

4 Serocki G, Bein B, Scholz J, *et al.* Management of the predicted difficult airway: a comparison of conventional blade laryngoscopy with video-assisted blade laryngoscopy and the GlideScope. *Eur J Anaesthesiol* 2010; **27**: 24–30.

Key message

The GlideScope® can provide a laryngoscopic view equal to or better than that of direct laryngoscopy in adults. The time to intubation is longer as is the number of attempts required using the GlideScope®.

Strengths

The study was adequately powered to detect a statistically significant difference in laryngoscopic view obtained with the GlideScope® compared to direct laryngoscopy with a Macintosh laryngoscope.

Weaknesses

Emergency surgical cases and patients with known airway pathology or cervical spine injury were excluded from the study. Therefore the results cannot be extrapolated to this patient population. The study was not adequately powered to demonstrate statistical equivalence using time to intubate as an outcome measure between intubation using direct laryngoscopy and the GlideScope®.

Relevance

This is the first randomized controlled trial investigating the use of the GlideScope® in comparison to the Macintosh laryngoscope in an adult surgical population. A major advantage of the GlideScope® is that it allows a view of the larynx without having to align oral, pharyngeal or laryngeal axes. It is designed in such a way as to be able 'to look around the corner'. The GlideScope® has subsequently been shown in other studies to have a role in the management of the difficult airway.

Paper 10: Tracheal intubation in patients with cervical spine immobilization: a comparison of the Airwayscope®, LMA CTrach®, and the Macintosh laryngoscopes

Author details

MA Malik, R Subramaniam, S Churasia, CH Maharaj, BH Harte, JG Laffey

Reference

British Journal of Anaesthesia 2009; **102**: 654–61.

Abstract

Background: The purpose of this study was to evaluate the effectiveness of the Pentax AWS®, and the LMA CTrach®, in comparison with the Macintosh laryngoscope, when performing tracheal intubation in patients with neck immobilization using manual in-line axial cervical spine stabilization.

Methods: Ninety patients undergoing anaesthesia who required tracheal intubation were randomly assigned to undergo intubation using a Macintosh (n=30), LMA CTrach® (n=30), or AWS® (n=30) laryngoscope. All patients were intubated by one of the three anaesthetists familiar with the use of each laryngoscope.

Results: The intubation difficulty scores were significantly higher with the Macintosh laryngoscope and were significantly lower with the AWS® compared with the LMA CTrach®. All 30 patients were successfully intubated with the Macintosh and the AWS® device, compared with 27 patients with the LMA CTrach®. The duration of both the first and the successful tracheal intubation attempts was significantly longer with the LMA CTrach® compared with the AWS® and Macintosh laryngoscopes. A greater number of optimization manoeuvres were required to facilitate tracheal intubation with the LMA CTrach® compared with the AWS® laryngoscope. The AWS® group had a significantly better Cormack and Lehane glottic view obtained at laryngoscopy compared with both other devices.

Conclusions: The AWS® laryngoscope has several advantages over the Macintosh laryngoscope, or LMA CTrach®, in patients undergoing cervical spine immobilization.

Summary

This study compares the effectiveness of two airway devices—the Pentax AWS® and the LMA CTrach®, and the Macintosh laryngoscope. The Pentax AWS® and the LMA CTrach® are indirect laryngoscopes that do not require alignment of the oral-pharyngeal-tracheal axes. They were developed in an attempt to reduce the difficulty of endotracheal intubation potentially encountered by conventional laryngoscopy during cervical spine immobilization. Cervical spine immobilization, necessary in cases of suspected cervical spinal cord injury, creates difficulty with glottic visualization during laryngoscopy thereby making intubation more difficult. This can increase perioperative morbidity and mortality. Thirty patients were randomized to undergo intubation with each of the three airway devices. This study demonstrated that the Pentax AWS® laryngoscope performed better than both the LMA CTrach® and the Macintosh laryngoscope in patients undergoing cervical immobilization, but the LMA CTrach® offered no advantage.

Citation count

18.

Related references

1 Timmermann A, Russo S, Graf BM. Evaluation of the CTrach—an intubating LMA with integrated fibreoptic system. *Br J Anaesth* 2006; **96**: 516–21.

2 Enomoto Y, Asai T, Arai T, *et al*. Pentax-AWS, a new videolaryngoscope, is more effective than the Macintosh laryngoscope for tracheal intubation in patients with restricted neck movements: a randomized comparative study. *Br J Anaesth* 2008; **100**: 544–8.

3 Malik MA, Maharaj CH, Harte BH, *et al*. Comparison of Macintosh, Truview EVO2®, Glidescope®, and Airwayscope® laryngoscope use in patients with cervical spine immobilization. *Br J Anaesth* 2008; **101**: 723–30.

Key message

The Pentax AWS® improved endotracheal intubation conditions compared to the LMA CTrach® and conventional laryngoscopy with a Macintosh laryngoscope in patients with cervical spine immobilization.

Strengths

The study, a prospective randomized controlled trial, has a strong design.

Weaknesses

The study design is such that the investigators were unblinded to the airway device used, thereby potentially introducing bias. In addition, as the investigators mention, certain measurements used in the study are subjective rather than objective.

Relevance

Endotracheal intubation with conventional laryngoscopy in patients with spinal cord immobilization poses a significant challenge to even experienced anaesthetists. Several airway devices have been devised in an attempt to reduce this difficulty and this study evaluated the effectiveness of two novel devices—the Pentax AWS® and the LMA CTrach®. Improving intubating conditions in this patient population by the use of new and effective airway devices could improve perioperative morbidity or mortality in patients with suspected spinal cord injury.

Chapter 18

Paediatric anaesthesia

P-A Lönnqvist

Introduction

To appropriately care for our smallest patients is one of the most demanding tasks bestowed upon anaesthetists. Fortunately the body of scientific evidence and data regarding the safest and best care in paediatric anaesthesia has increased immensely during the last couple of decades and the foundation on which to base our practice is now on much more solid ground. The current text has targeted ten key publications that the author feels has had, or will have, considerable impact on how paediatric anaesthesia is best practised, both by the occasional and the more seasoned paediatric anaesthetist.

Paper 1: Early exposure to common anesthetic agents causes widespread neurodegeneration in the developing rat brain and persistent learning deficits

Author details

V Jevtovic-Todorovic, RE Hartman, Y Izumi, ND Benshoff, K Dikranian, CF Zorumski, JW Olney, DF Wozniak

Reference

Journal of Neuroscience 2003; **23**: 876–82.

Summary

This ground-breaking publication set off an avalanche of further research within this field. This study in neonatal rats clearly shows that common anaesthetic agents do not only cause increased apoptotic neurodegeneration but also that the enhanced apoptosis results in later cognitive impairment. This and later studies have sparked a large interest and have resulted in several reviews and editorials. Maybe the most interesting commentary on this new field are some recent editorials in *Anesthesiology*. In these editorials different aspects of this complex problem are discussed by researchers who by various approaches try to investigate the clinical relevance of the apoptotic changes seen in animal studies. Perhaps the most interesting data that has already been partially verbally communicated at scientific meetings are large-scale epidemiological national registry data from Denmark. These preliminary data from Hansen *et al.* did not show any convincing evidence that exposure to anaesthesia in early life is in fact associated with any more substantial, negative, long-term cognitive effects. Anand also has published interesting reading regarding potential flaws in various animal studies and also pointed to the negative effects of insufficient anaesthesia and analgesia in neonates that can result from not providing adequate anaesthesia to children in early life. Preliminary data show that newer anaesthetic alternatives, e.g. xenon and alpha-2 adrenoceptor agonists, may provide a better and safer alternative since these agents do not seem to be associated with the same degree of apoptotic cell death in neonatal animals as other commonly used anaesthetics are.

Citation count

559.

Related references

1 Anand KJ, Soriano SG. Anesthetic agents and the immature brain: are these toxic or therapeutic? *Anesthesiology* 2004; **101**: 527–30.

2 Ma D, Williamson P, Januszewski A, *et al.* Xenon mitigates isoflurane-induced neuronal apoptosis in the developing rodent brain. *Anesthesiology* 2007; **106**: 746–53.

3 Davidson AJ, McCann ME, Morton NS, *et al.* Anesthesia and outcome after neonatal surgery: the role for randomized trials. *Anesthesiology* 2008; **109**: 941–4.

4 Hansen TG; Danish Registry Study Group, Flick R; Mayo Clinic Pediatric Anesthesia and Learning Disabilities Study Group. Anesthetic effects on the developing brain: insights from epidemiology. *Anesthesiology* 2009; **110**: 1–3.

5 McCann ME, Bellinger DC, Davidson AJ, *et al.* Clinical research approaches to studying pediatric anesthetic neurotoxicity. *Neurotoxicology* 2009; **30**: 766–71.

6 Patel P, Sun L. Update on neonatal anesthetic neurotoxicity: insight into molecular mechanisms and relevance to humans. *Anesthesiology* 2009; **110**: 703–8.

Key message

Anaesthetic exposure in young animals has detrimental effects in the brain.

Strengths

The fact that more than one common anaesthetic drug that is frequently used in neonatal anaesthesia was investigated is clearly an advantage. However, the most important feature of the study is that that it also have investigated the potential cognitive long-term effects of the apoptotic changes cause by the anaesthetic agents.

Weaknesses

A number of later editorials and reviews on this topic have criticized the dosages of the investigated drugs and the lack of proper monitoring during the anaesthetic. Furthermore the 6-h exposure of the neonatal rats to the anaesthetic agents may also be inappropriate due to the fact that such an exposure may represent many days of anaesthesia if translated to the human context.

Relevance

This pioneering study has focused relevant interest on the possible negative effects of exposure to anaesthetic agents to young individuals. Currently there are insufficient data to support general guidelines but, if possible, elective or semi-elective surgical procedures that require general anaesthesia should be postponed until after 6 months of age. Future clinical data will most likely result in alternative ways of providing anaesthesia to this vulnerable age group.

Paper 2: The minimum effective dose of lignocaine to prevent injection pain due to propofol in children

Author details
E Cameron, G Johnston, S Crofts, NS Morton

Reference
Anaesthesia 1992; **47**: 604–6.

Summary
The commercial availability of dermal anaesthetic creams and patches (e.g. EMLA and Ametop) has made intravenous induction of anaesthesia a common alternative in paediatric practice. However, it is very illogical to do everything possible to avoid pain and discomfort when establishing intravenous access and then subsequently inject a drug (propofol) that is associated with a very high incidence of injection pain (40–80%). Based on the positive effects of mixing the propofol solution with lidocaine in adults this study does, in a very nice way, define the role of this practice in children. The results nicely show that the addition of lidocaine is very effective in reducing the incidence of propofol injection pain in children but that a substantially larger dose of lidocaine is needed in order to get the positive effect seen in adults.

A new and effective way of reducing the incidence of propofol injection pain in children is to use a more dilute preparation of propofol. In a prospective, randomized, double-blind study Soltész *et al.* (2007) has shown that the use of a 0.5% propofol solution is associated with a significantly reduced incidence of injection pain as compared to the use of the standard 1% solution (23% vs 70%, respectively). Based on the results of this study the 0.5% propofol solution is now marketed as a commercially available product. An alternative strategy in order to almost completely avoid the occurrence of injection pain in association with intravenous induction of anaesthesia in children is to use a new commercially available lipid-based preparation of etomidate (Etomidate-Lipuro R). If using this alternative the incidence is of injection pain is only 5% as compared to 37.5% if using 1% propofol with added lidocaine, as has been reported by Nyman *et al.* (2006).

Citation count
71.

Related references
1 Nyman Y, Von Hofsten K, Palm C, *et al.* Etomidate-Lipuro is associated with considerably less injection pain in children compared with propofol with added lidocaine. *Br J Anaesth* 2006; **97**: 536–9.

2 Soltész S, Silomon M, Gräf G, *et al.* Effect of a 0.5% dilution of propofol on pain on injection during induction of anesthesia in children. *Anesthesiology* 2007; **106**: 80–4.

Key message
Higher concentrations of lignocaine need to be used to minimize the pain of propofol administration in children than in adults.

Strengths

The study design, the number of patients included, as well as the quite large number of patients studied indicate that the results of the study are valid and generally applicable.

Weaknesses

The study does not answer the question on how best the mixing should be performed or if some ways of lidocaine addition, e.g. premixing prior to induction, will affect the efficacy of this practice. Such considerations are clinically valid since later studies using the recommended amount of lidocaine have not been able to reproduce the good efficacy reported in this study.

Relevance

The results of the study show that the serious problem of propofol injection pain in children can be handled in such a way that this otherwise excellent anaesthetic alternative can be used in paediatric practice. This has also made it possible for children of all ages to benefit from the advantages associated with intravenous induction of anaesthesia.

Paper 3: The effect of intranasal administration of remifentanil on intubating conditions and airway response after sevoflurane induction of anesthesia in children

Author details

ST Verghese, RS Hannallah, M Brennan, JL Yarvitz, KA Hummer, KM Patel, J He, R McCarter

Reference

Anesthesia and Analgesia 2008; **107**: 1176–81.

Summary

The paediatric anaesthetist is regularly involved in situations where either intravenous access is difficult or the duration of the surgical procedure is too short to mandate the insertion of an intravenous catheter. An effective analgesic alternative of short duration that does not require intravenous administration would, thus, be of great benefit in this setting. The present study nicely show that the nasal administration of remifentanil $4 \, \mu g \, kg^{-1}$ within 3 min provides good quality analgesia that facilitates endotracheal intubation after sevoflurane induction of anaesthesia.

Citation count

9.

Related references

1 Karl HW, Keifer AT, Rosenberger JL, *et al*. Comparison of the safety and efficacy of intranasal midazolam or sufentanil for preinduction of anesthesia in pediatric patients. *Anesthesiology* 1992; **76**: 209–15.

2 Galinkin JL, Fazi LM, Cuy RM, *et al*. Use of intranasal fentanyl in children undergoing myringotomy and tube placement during halothane and sevoflurane anesthesia. *Anesthesiology* 2000; **93**: 1378–83.

3 Borland M, Jacobs I, King B, *et al*. A randomized controlled trial comparing intranasal fentanyl to intravenous morphine for managing acute pain in children in the emergency department. *Ann Emerg Med* 2007; **49**: 335–40.

Key message

Nasal administration of synthetic opioids to children is effective for short duration anaesthesia.

Strengths

The large number of patients studied, taken together with adequate determinations of plasma levels make the data highly reliable.

Weaknesses

The lack of data regarding neonates and infants may be seen as limiting but hopefully the authors may be be undertaking a study to present such complementary information.

Relevance

The option to provide fast and high-quality analgesia of short duration in situations where intravenous access is not present is of great benefit for the paediatric anaesthetist. The short and predicable action of remifentanil must be seen as a significant advantage when compared to the use of other synthetic opioids, e.g. fentanyl or sufentanil. Nasal administration of remifentanil will not only be useful in the context of paediatric endotracheal intubation but can most likely be successfully used in a wide variety of situations associated with intraoperative nociceptive stimulation and could potentially also be useful in the context of procedural pain in children.

Paper 4: Prospective randomized controlled multi-centre trial of cuffed or uncuffed endotracheal tubes in small children

Author details

M Weiss, A Dullenkopf, JE Fischer, C Keller, AC Gerber; European Paediatric Endotracheal Intubation Study Group.

Reference

British Journal of Anaesthesia 2009; **103**: 867–73.

Abstract

Background: The use of cuffed tracheal tubes (TTs) in small children is still controversial. The aim of this study was to compare post-extubation morbidity and TT exchange rates when using cuffed vs uncuffed tubes in small children.

Methods: Patients aged from birth to 5 yr requiring general anaesthesia with TT intubation were included in 24 European paediatric anaesthesia centres. Patients were prospectively randomized into a cuffed TT group (Microcuff PET) and an uncuffed TT group (Mallinckrodt, Portex, Rüsch, Sheridan). Endpoints were incidence of post-extubation stridor and the number of TT exchanges to find an appropriate-sized tube. For cuffed TTs, minimal cuff pressure required to seal the airway was noted; maximal cuff pressure was limited at 20 cm H_2O with a pressure release valve. Data are mean (SD).

Results: A total of 2246 children were studied (1119/1127 cuffed/uncuffed). The age was 1.93 (1.48) yr in the cuffed and 1.87 (1.45) yr in the uncuffed groups. Post-extubation stridor was noted in 4.4% of patients with cuffed and in 4.7% with uncuffed TTs (P=0.543). TT exchange rate was 2.1% in the cuffed and 30.8% in the uncuffed groups (P<0.0001). Minimal cuff pressure required to seal the trachea was 10.6 (4.3) cm H_2O.

Conclusions: The use of cuffed TTs in small children provides a reliably sealed airway at cuff pressures of <or=20 cm H_2O, reduces the need for TT exchanges, and does not increase the risk for post-extubation stridor compared with uncuffed TTs.

Summary

Ever since routine endotracheal (ET) intubation was introduced in paediatric anaesthesia there has been an ongoing debate regarding the use of cuffed or uncuffed ET tubes in small children. This debate has almost exclusively been based on personal or institutional opinion and the lack of appropriate scientific data to base a more evidence-based consensus has been apparent. Following the development of a new and more appropriately designed paediatric cuffed ET tube, the Zürich paediatric anaesthetists group has managed to perform this large-scale, prospective, randomized, multicentre study. The primary aim was to compare the incidence of post-extubation stridor between their new cuffed ET tube and conventional uncuffed alternatives. The results of the study clearly show that there is no difference in post-extubation stridor whether cuffed or the uncuffed alternatives were used. As may have been expected, the need for ET tube exchanges were significantly lower if a cuffed tube was used and the quality of the end-tidal carbon dioxide reading was also enhanced.

Citation count

43.

Related references

1 Lönnqvist PA. Cuffed or uncuffed tracheal tubes during anaesthesia in infants and small children: time to put the eternal discussion to rest? *Br J Anaesth* 2009; **103**: 783–5.

Key message

Cuffed ET tubes can be safely used in small children.

Strengths

The very meticulous study protocol is impressive as is the very substantial number of patients that were included in the study (>2200). The multicentre nature of the study also makes it very reasonable to expect that the results can be extrapolated to be true also in every day clinical practice regardless of the hospital environment (i.e. equally true both in the district general hospital as in the university setting).

Weaknesses

The fact that the study was stopped before reaching the initially projected number of included patients is, from a purely scientific point of view, a slight concern but the study still managed to recruit a very respectable number of patients and the conclusions of the study must still be regarded as highly valid. It can obviously be argued that this study does not address the incidence of more rare but very troublesome long-term sequelae of ET intubations, e.g. laryngeal damage or tracheal stenosis. However, to design adequately sized prospective studies that address these issues will be very difficult, not to say almost impossible. It is also important to remember that the conclusions of the study is only valid if the Microcuff PET tube is used and the cuff-pressure is continuously monitored and the pressure kept at <20 cmH$_2$O.

Relevance

The results of this study have provided solid data to show that a cuffed ET tube can not only can be safely used in small paediatric patients but that it also does provide some advantages over the conventional use of uncuffed alternatives. It is likely that data generated from this study will change common practice to more routine use of the Microcuff PET tube when ET intubation in needed in babies, infants, and toddlers.

Paper 5: Lactated Ringer with 1% dextrose: an appropriate solution for peri-operative fluid therapy in children

Author details

MC Dubois, L Gouyet, I Murat, C Saint-Maurice

Reference

Paediatric Anaesthesia 1992; **2**: 99–104.

Summary

Prior to this publication it had been shown that even babies and infants could be treated with balanced electrolyte solutions without added glucose in the majority of cases. However, a certain risk for devastating intraoperative hypoglycaemia exists in at-risk babies if this regimen is used. At the same time the very common practice of effectively administering hypotonic intravenous solution may be associated with serious and even potentially life-threatening postoperative hyponatraemia.

Citation count

22.

Related references

1 Söderlind M, Salvignol G, Izard P, *et al.* Use of albumin, blood transfusion and intraoperative glucose by APA and ADARPEF members: a postal survey. *Paediatr Anaesth* 2001; **11**: 685–9.

2 Cunliffe M, Potter F. Four and a fifth and all that. *Br J Anaesth* 2006; **97**: 274–7.

3 Lönnqvist PA. Inappropriate perioperative fluid management in children: time for a solution?! *Paediatr Anaesth* 2007; **17**: 203–5.

4 Murat I, Dubois MC. Perioperative fluid therapy in pediatrics. *Paediatr Anaesth* 2008; **18**: 363–70.

Key message

The use of a 'golden compromise' that contains 1% glucose in a balanced electrolyte solution appears to result in both protection against hypoglycaemia and at the same time preserves safe and normal plasma levels of sodium in children.

Strengths

The three-group design, where the new 'golden compromise' solution is compared to the two most commonly used alternatives, provides a clinically very relevant scenario.

Weaknesses

The relatively limited number of patients included in the study is slightly concerning, especially with regards to the results concerning glucose homeostasis. Plasma determinations of antidiuretic hormone (ADH) would have been helpful but is unfortunately lacking.

Relevance

This study represents the foundation for the development of more appropriate fluids for use in the perioperative period in children. A new solution containing 1% glucose and 140 mmol l^{-1} of sodium has recently been made commercially available in Germany and may soon be accessible within the whole of the European Union. As a result of the discussions sparked by this study new national UK guidelines regarding the appropriate choice of intravenous solutions in the paediatric perioperative have also been issued. If the inappropriate use of suboptimal high-glucose low-sodium solutions can be generally replaced by the new, more appropriate alternatives then paediatric lives will be saved since the risk of serious postoperative hyponatraemia will, for practical reasons, be abolished.

Paper 6: Emergence agitation in paediatric patients after sevoflurane anaesthesia and no surgery: a comparison with halothane

Author details

J Cravero, S Surgenor, K Whalen

Reference

Paediatric Anaesthesia 2000; **10**: 419–24.

Summary

The introduction of sevoflurane has been one of the most important developments ever in paediatric anaesthesia. This non-pungent agent allows fast and smooth induction of anaesthesia combined with stable haemodynamics and a rapid and predictable emergence from anaesthesia. However, a crucial discussion point has been if this agent is associated with an increased incidence of emergence agitation. Despite the publication of numerous randomized studies this issue remain unanswered since these studies have not adequately been controlled for the inevitable postoperative pain that is associated with even minor surgical procedures. This study unequivocally shows that sevoflurane in a situation where no pain component is present, in fact is associated with both a statistical and clinically relevant increase in emergence agitation as compared to halothane.

Citation count

152.

Related references

1 Bergendahl HT, Lönnqvist PA, Eksborg S, *et al.* Clonidine vs. midazolam as premedication in children undergoing adeno-tonsillectomy: a prospective, randomized, controlled clinical trial. *Acta Anaesthesiol Scand* 2004; **48**: 1292–300.

2 Sikich N, Lerman J. Development and psychometric evaluation of the pediatric anesthesia emergence delirium scale. *Anesthesiology* 2004; **100**: 1138–45.

3 Shibata S, Shigeomi S, Sato W, *et al.* Nitrous oxide administration during washout of sevoflurane improves postanesthetic agitation in children. *J Anesth* 2005; **19**: 160–3.

4 Aouad MT, Yazbeck-Karam VG, Nasr VG, *et al.* A single dose of propofol at the end of surgery for the prevention of emergence agitation in children undergoing strabismus surgery during sevoflurane anesthesia. *Anesthesiology* 2007; **107**: 733–8.

5 Dahmani S, Stany I, Brasher C, *et al.* Pharmacological prevention of sevoflurane- and desflurane-related emergence agitation in children: a meta-analysis of published studies. *Br J Anaesth* 2010: **104**: 216–23.

Key message

Sevoflurane causes more emergence agitation than halothane.

Strengths

Using a study design that excludes any confounding pain component is ingenious.

Weaknesses

The optimal tool to assess emergence reactions in children has been debated and the varied results from different studies may, to a large part, be explained by the use of different assessment scales. Sikich and Lerman (2004) published a validated tool, the Pediatric Anesthesia Emergence Delirium (PAED) scale, which is specifically designed for use in this context (A). The fact that this scale was not used in this study is a minor concern but since the study was performed before the PAED scale was published this must be seen as only a minor concern.

Relevance

The clear insight that sevoflurane is in fact associated with an increased risk of emergence agitation has made it possible to provide effective strategies on how to minimize the only clinically relevant side effect of sevoflurane in paediatric practice. Following the publication of the unequivocal results of this study it has been possible to adequately address the issue of post-sevoflurane agitation in children in a way that has resulted in several options on how to minimize this clinical problem. Effective ways to reduce the incidence of emergence agitation are premedication with clonidine, replacement of sevoflurane by nitrous oxide during the final stage of surgery, or the administration of a small dose of intravenous propofol in association with the transfer of the child from the operating room to the post-anaesthesia care unit.

Paper 7: I.V. acetaminophen pharmacokinetics in neonates after multiple doses

Author details

GM Palmer, M Atkins, BJ Anderson, KR Smith, TJ Culnane, CM McNally, EJ Perkins, GA Chalkiadis, RW Hunt

Reference

British Journal of Anaesthesia 2008; **101**: 523–30.

Abstract

Background: Pharmacokinetics of an i.v. prodrug of acetaminophen (propacetamol) in neonates after repeat dosing are reported, with scant data for i.v. acetaminophen formulation.

Methods: Neonates from an intensive care unit received 6-hourly prn i.v. acetaminophen dosed according to postmenstrual age (PMA): 28–32 weeks, 10 mg kg^{-1}; 32–36 weeks, 12.5 mg kg^{-1}; and ≥36 weeks, 15 mg kg^{-1}. A maximum of five blood samples for assay and liver function tests (LFTs) were collected. A one-compartment linear disposition model (zero-order input; first-order elimination) was used to describe time-concentration profiles using population modelling (NONMEM).

Results: Fifty neonates, median (range) PMA 38.6 (32–45) weeks, mean (SD) weight 2.9 (0.7) kg, received a mean of 15 doses over a median 4 days with 189 serum acetaminophen and 231 LFT measurements. Standardized population parameter estimates for a term neonate were clearance (CL) 5.24 (CV 30.5%) litre h^{-1} 70 kg^{-1} and volume of distribution (V) 76 (29.6%) litre 70 kg^{-1}. CL increased with PMA from 4.4 litre h^{-1} 70 kg^{-1} at 34 weeks to 6.3 litre h^{-1} 70 kg^{-1} at 46 weeks. The presence of unconjugated hyperbilirubinaemia was associated with reduced CL: 150 µmol litre^{-1} associated with 40% CL reduction. Acetaminophen concentrations between 10 and 23 mg litre^{-1} at steady state are predicted after 15 mg kg^{-1} 6-hourly for a neonate of PMA 40 weeks. Hepatic enzyme analysis of daily samples changed significantly for one patient whose alanine aminotransferase concentration tripled.

Conclusions: The parameter estimates are similar to those described for propacetamol. There was no evidence of hepatotoxicity. Unconjugated hyperbilirubinaemia impacts upon CL, dictating dose reduction.

Summary

This study represents the latest addition to a long list of publications from Anderson and co-workers that delineate the pharmacology of paracetamol in children. After previous population pharmacokinetic studies of regular paracetamol preparations as well as the pro-drug pro-paracetamol this study nicely demonstrates that the recent intravenous paracetamol preparation can be safely used in even neonatal patients. If 15 mg kg^{-1} is administered 6-hourly to the newborn, safe and clinically effective plasma concentrations will be achieved. The study also shows that the presence of hyperbilirubinaemia necessitates a dose reduction in this patient category.

Citation count

25.

Related references

1 Anderson BJ, Woolard GA, Holford NH. Pharmacokinetics of rectal paracetamol after major surgery in children. *Paediatr Anaesth* 1995; **5**: 237–42.

2 Anderson BJ, Holford NH. Rectal acetaminophen pharmacokinetics. *Anesthesiology* 1998; **88**: 1131–3.

3 Anderson BJ, Holford NH, Woollard GA, *et al.* Perioperative pharmacodynamics of acetaminophen analgesia in children. *Anesthesiology* 1999; **90**: 411–21.

4 Anderson BJ, van Lingen RA, Hansen TG, *et al.* Acetaminophen developmental pharmacokinetics in premature neonates and infants: a pooled population analysis. *Anesthesiology* 2002; **96**: 1336–45.

5 Allegaert K, Anderson BJ, Naulaers G, *et al.* Intravenous paracetamol (propacetamol) pharmacokinetics in term and preterm neonates. *Eur J Clin Pharmacol* 2004; **60**: 191–7.

6 Anderson BJ, Pons G, Autret-Leca E, *et al.* Pediatric intravenous paracetamol (propacetamol) pharmacokinetics: a population analysis. *Paediatr Anaesth* 2005; **15**: 282–92.

7 Prins SA, Van Dijk M, Van Leeuwen P, *et al.* Pharmacokinetics and analgesic effects of intravenous propacetamol vs rectal paracetamol in children after major craniofacial surgery. *Paediatr Anaesth* 2008; **18**: 582–92.

Key message

The adequate and safe dosage of this paracetamol preparation in neonates is described.

Strengths

The number of patients included in the study (n = 50) must be seen as clearly adequate and the stratification according to degree of prematurity is a nice feature. The use of population pharmacokinetics must also be perceived as a considerable strength.

Weaknesses

A comparison with some other form of paracetamol preparation would have further enhanced the informative value of the study.

Relevance

This chosen study, taken together with the multitude of previous paracetamol studies by Anderson *et al.* have made it possible to use paracetamol in children of all age groups. Paracetamol represents an effective basic analgesic therapy with few significant side effects and the definition of pharmacokinetic and pharmacodynamic data has made it possible to issue safe and effective dosage regimens even for premature babies. These accumulated data have had a major impact on the care of neonatal children.

Paper 8: Ultrasound guidance for infraclavicular brachial plexus anaesthesia in children

Author details

P Marhofer, C Sitzwohl, M Greher, S Kapral

Reference

Anaesthesia 2004; **59**: 642–6.

Summary

This study represents the first randomized study in children where the novel technique of real-time ultrasound-guided regional anaesthesia was compared to the traditional use of nerve stimulation for infraclavicular brachial plexus blocks. This study was able to verify many of the advantages of this new technique, e.g. higher degree of patient comfort during the block procedure, a more rapid onset, a longer duration, and better sensory and motor block scores.

Citation count

197.

Related references

1 Marhofer P, Frickey N. Ultrasonographic guidance in pediatric regional anesthesia Part 1: Theoretical background. *Paediatr Anaesth* 2006; **16**: 1008–18.

2 Roberts S. Ultrasonographic guidance in pediatric regional anesthesia. Part 2: techniques. *Paediatr Anaesth* 2006; **16**: 1112–24.

Key message

Real-time ultrasound guidance can be used successfully in children.

Strengths

The study design is solid and the new technique of ultrasound guidance is adequately compared to the previous gold standard.

Weaknesses

The data concerning better sensory and motor block scores should be viewed with a certain degree of caution since it is difficult to properly examine such parameters in children.

Relevance

The introduction of ultrasound-guidance into paediatric regional anaesthesia represents maybe the biggest single break-through in recent years within the subspecialty of paediatric anaesthesia in general. At present ultrasound-guided techniques have been described for almost all types of peripheral nerve blocks both in adults and children and will soon represent standard of care in the more effluent part of the world. However, the usefulness of this new technique with regards to central nerve blocks is less clear and further studies are needed to prove its utility in this setting.

Paper 9: The national pediatric epidural audit

Author details

N Llewellyn, A Moriarty

Reference

Paediatric Anaesthesia 2007; **17**: 520–33.

Abstract

Background: This paper describes a prospective audit of children receiving epidural infusion analgesia (EIA) in Great Britain and Ireland. The aim was to quantify the risks associated with this technique.

Methods: In order to obtain sufficient data on the number of pediatric epidurals performed and the incidence of unwanted events, a decision was taken, at an Annual Meeting of Great Britain and Ireland Paediatric Pain Services, to establish a national audit of EIA practice in these centers. Each site sent a monthly return of the numbers of EIA performed to the coordinating center. If an incident occurred then the referring site completed a more detailed form and the child was followed up for 1 year if possible. Incidents were graded by severity 13, serious to minor. These data were collected over the 5-year period (2001–2005).

Results: (i) Ninety six incidents were reported in 10 633 epidurals performed. (ii) Fifty six were associated with the insertion or maintenance of EIA; most were of low severity (1:189). (iii) Five incidents were graded as 1 (serious) (approximately 1:2000). (iv) Nine incidents were graded as 2 (approximately 1:1100). (v) Only one child has residual effects from a grade 1 incident 12 months after surgery (approximately 1:10 000). (vi) Forty incidents were also reported that were felt to be associated with the use of EIA; 33 of these incidents were the development of pressures sores. Four incidents of compartment syndrome were reported, in each of these cases the presence of EIA did not mask the condition.

Conclusions: Epidural infusion analgesia in children does have risks associated with the technique. The occurrence of compartment syndrome does not appear to be masked by the presence of working EIA. As a result of this audit we can now provide parents with better information, thereby improving the process of informed consent.

Summary

This prospective, multicentre, large-scale audit delineates the complications associated with the use of epidural blockade in children. The most relevant findings were that neonates, centres performing <100 epidurals per year and the caudal approach to the epidural space were all associated with a slight increased incidence of complications. The most frequently encountered complications that could be related to the epidural block were localized cutaneous infection and drug errors. However, the overall incidence of serious incidents was reassuringly low at 1 in 2000 and the incidence of persistent problems at 12 months as low as 1 in 10,000.

Citation count

58.

Related references

1 Marhofer P, Sitzwohl C, Greher M, *et al.* Ultrasound guidance for infraclavicular brachial plexus anaesthesia in children. *Anaesthesia* 2004; **59**: 642–6.

2 Morton NS, Errera A. APA national audit of pediatric opioid infusions. *Paediatr Anaesth* 2010; **20**: 119–25.

Key message

The risks associated with epidurals in children are presented.

Strengths

The prospective data collection and the large number of cases included in the audit is to be applauded and provides excellent data for bench marking as well as for preoperative information to children and their parents.

Weaknesses

The major weakness of the study is that it does not deal with the analgesic efficacy of the epidural blocks. This makes it difficult to perform a clinically valid risk:benefit assessment regarding the use of paediatric epidural blocks.

Relevance

This study provides very important and useful information regarding the incidence of complications associated with paediatric epidural blockade. Thus, there is no relevant argument for withholding this excellent method of postoperative pain relief in children and parents can now be presented with an adequate and reassuring risk assessment regarding this analgesic method.

Paper 10: APA national audit of pediatric opioid infusions

Author details

NS Morton, A Errera

Reference

Paediatric Anaesthesia 2010; **20**: 119–25.

Abstract

Introduction: A prospective audit of neonates, infants, and children receiving opioid infusion techniques managed by pediatric acute pain teams from across the United Kingdom and Eire was undertaken over a period of 17 months. The aim was to determine the incidence, nature, and severity of serious clinical incidents (SCIs) associated with the techniques of continuous opioid infusion, patient-controlled analgesia, and nurse-controlled analgesia (NCA) in patients aged 0–18.

Methods: The audit was funded by the Association of Paediatric Anaesthetists (APA) and performed by the acute pain services of 18 centers throughout the United Kingdom. Data were submitted weekly via a web-based return form designed by the Document Capture Company that documented data on all patients receiving opioid infusions and any SCIs. Eight categories of SCI were identified in advance, and the reported SCIs were graded in terms of severity (Grade 1 (death/permanent harm); Grade 2 (harm but full recovery and resulting in termination of the technique or needing significant intervention); Grade 3 (potential but no actual harm). Data were collected over a period of 17 months (25/06/07-25/11/08) and stored on a secure server for analysis.

Results: Forty-six SCIs were reported in 10 726 opioid infusion techniques. One Grade 1 incident (1: 10 726) of cardiac arrest occurred and was associated with aspiration pneumonitis and the underlying neurological condition, neurocutaneous melanosis. Twenty-eight Grade 2 incidents (1: 383) were reported of which half were respiratory depression. The seventeen Grade 3 incidents (1: 631) were all drug errors because of programming or prescribing errors and were all reported by one center.

Conclusions: The overall incidence of 1: 10 000 of serious harm with opioid infusion techniques in children is comparable to the risks with pediatric epidural infusions and central blocks identified by two recent UK national audits. Avoidable factors were identified including prescription and pump programming errors, use of concurrent sedatives or opioids by different routes and overgenerous dosing in infants. Early respiratory depression in patients with specific risk factors, such as young age, neurodevelopmental, respiratory, or cardiac comorbidities, who are receiving nurse-controlled analgesia or continuous opioid infusion suggests that closer monitoring for at least 2 h is needed for these cases. As a result of this audit, we can provide parents with better information on relative risks to help the process of informed consent.

Summary

This represents the second and most recent large-scale, multicentre audit by the Association of Paediatric Anaesthetists of Great Britain and Ireland. Using a similar design as for paediatric epidurals (see Paper 9) this audit prospectively registered the problems and complications associated with the use of various postoperative modalities of morphine administration (e.g. continuous intravenous infusion, PCA, and NCA) in more than 10,000 children of different ages. An overall risk of serious complication was found to be 1 in 10,000, an incidence which is identical to the risk for a serious incident following the use of epidural anaesthesia in children.

Citation count

17.

Related references

1 Llewellyn N, Moriarty A. The national pediatric epidural audit. *Paediatr Anaesth* 2007; **17**: 520–33.

2 Howard RF. Audits of postoperative analgesia: what have we learned and what should we do now? *Paediatr Anaesth* 2010; **20**: 119–25.

Key message

The risk of serious complication associated with morphine in children is the same as the risk after epidurals, 1 in 10,000.

Strengths

The prospective data collection and the large number of cases included in the audit is definitely a major merit of the study.

Weaknesses

As with the epidural audit the study does not evaluate the analgesic efficacy of the opioid infusion strategies, something that make a clinically valid risk benefit assessment difficult.

Relevance

This study provides very important and useful information regarding the incidence of complications associated with paediatric postoperative morphine infusion regimens. As for epidural blockade there is no relevant argument for withholding this excellent method of postoperative pain relief in children if adequate prescribed and monitored. The generated data will provide substantial help when informing parents about the relative risks of postoperative morphine infusions in children.

Chapter 19

Malignant hyperthermia

PM Hopkins and A Urwyler

Introduction

To select just ten papers from 50 years of literature, in which more than 10,000 papers have been published on the subject of malignant hyperthermia, is indeed a challenge. There are, therefore, many worthy contributions that we have not been able to include and to the authors of these papers we apologize. In tackling this challenge it soon became apparent to us that we had to focus our choices. This means that although much has been learnt about the human condition from work on animals, especially the porcine model of malignant hyperthermia, we decided to restrict ourselves to human studies where possible. The one notable exception to this was the paper by Harrison and colleagues that led to the demonstration of the efficacy of dantrolene in treating malignant hyperthermia. We have chosen also to exclude the vast literature that has examined the relationship between malignant hyperthermia and other disorders. These relationships now range from the well established, such as with central core disease, to the extremely tenuous such as with sudden infant death syndrome. For many other conditions, such as exertional heat stroke, the debate remains more balanced and it would be difficult to do justice to these debates without diluting the impact of research that is focused purely on malignant hyperthermia and hence our decision not to include such work.

Paper 1: Anaesthetic deaths in a family

Author details

MA Denborough, RRH Lovell

Reference

Lancet 1960; **II**: 45.

Summary

This paper is the first description of what became known subsequently as malignant hyperthermia or malignant hyperpyrexia, the condition was not known to exist before 1960. This letter to *The Lancet* was essentially a request to the journal's readers for any knowledge of cases similar to the one reported in the letter. At that time, death during or immediately after anaesthesia was not uncommon but it would have been remarkable bad luck for the family of the patient described in this report for ten of its members to succumb to anaesthesia by chance. The family affected were aware in fact that they were unusual and sought to avoid general anaesthesia if at all possible. By the time of this case in April 1960, however, they had come to the view that the problem was caused by ether. When the patient was therefore admitted with compound fractures of the tibia and fibula he agreed to a general anaesthetic as long as ether was avoided.

In just five paragraphs Denborough and Lovell set out a series of observations that illustrate many of the key features of malignant hyperthermia. The patient, who received premedication with pethidine and atropine, was given thiopentone for induction of anaesthesia followed by maintenance with halothane in nitrous oxide and oxygen. Within 10 min the patient's blood pressure started to fall and despite reduction of the inspired concentration of halothane, the blood pressure fell further and was accompanied by a tachycardia and cyanosis. At this stage the halothane was discontinued and the surgery concluded within 10 min but the patient remained unconscious and was now hot and sweaty to the touch. He was given a blood transfusion and packed in ice and after half an hour the patient opened his eyes but he could not move. Fortunately he recovered completely over the next 90 min and there were no sequelae.

Subsequent investigation of the family tree suggested a dominantly inherited genetic disorder. Where information was available on the ten relatives who had died, the course of the reaction seemed to follow the same pattern as the patient described by Denborough and Lovell, with sudden high temperature occurring during or soon after the operation followed by convulsions and death. As postmortem examination had not revealed any consistent abnormality the cause remained a mystery. There had been several reports of convulsions following ether anaesthesia in the literature and fever was noted in some of these but, as Denborough and Lovell state, ether could not be implicated in this case.

Citation count

Not available.

Related references

1 Denborough MA, Forster JF, Lovell RR, *et al.* Anaesthetic deaths in a family. *Br J Anaesth* 1962; **34**: 395–6.

2 Ball C. Unravelling the mystery of malignant hyperthermia. *Anaesth Intensive Care* 2007; **35**(Supp 1): 26–31.

Key message

This is the first case report of malignant hyperthermia.

Strengths

The importance of this publication was that the clarity of the description of events led to further cases of a similar nature to be reported. What was not apparent in this brief report was the role played by the anaesthetist, J. Villiers, in averting the patient's death and recording the details of the reaction. This was revealed partly in the full description of the case and the family history published in the *British Journal of Anaesthesia* (Denborough et al., 1962) but was further revealed in an article by Ball in 2007.

Weaknesses

The role of the anaesthetist in preventing the death of the patient was not detailed.

Relevance

The collection of cases and families stimulated by Denborough and Lovell's letter thus began the systematic study of malignant hyperthermia and probably also had an immediate impact in saving lives from a condition that prior to this date probably was universally lethal.

Paper 2: Metabolic error of muscle metabolism after recovery from malignant hyperthermia

Author details

W Kalow, BA Britt, ME Terreau, C Haist

Reference

Lancet 1970; **2**: 895–8.

Summary

Prior to this publication malignant hyperthermia (MH) was well known as a genetic predisposition to a life-threatening reaction triggered by volatile anaesthetics and succinylcholine. The incidence of MH was estimated to be about 1:15,000 general anaesthetics with an extremely high mortality of about two-thirds of the affected patients. There was no presymptomatic test to identify patients at risk. Only within a few families with a history of MH episodes could individuals be labelled as potentially at risk for MH. Although the aetiology was not known and opinion-leaders were almost always against a single entity theory of MH, several findings were in favour of skeletal muscle playing a central role in this uncommon disease:

◆ Myopathies and elevated levels of creatine kinase (CK) had been observed in some affected families.

◆ Muscle rigidity and muscle breakdown with elevated CK levels, hyperkalaemia, and 'cola' coloured urine caused by myoglobinuria were found during or after an MH crisis.

◆ A similar or identical syndrome was known in MH-susceptible (MHS) pigs, in which halothane caused an MH reaction with rapid loss of adenosine triphosphate (ATP) in excised skeletal muscle.

The major advance imparted by this paper was the finding that freshly biopsied muscle strips from two patients having survived MH with muscle rigidity were more sensitive to caffeine and halothane *in vitro* compared to muscle strips from patients with no history of MH. Freshly isolated muscle strips about 2 cm long and 3 mm thick were mounted for measurements of isometric contractions in a tissue bath with an isotonic solution bubbled with oxygen containing 5% carbon dioxide (CO_2). Dose–response curves were obtained using caffeine alone and in the presence of 1% halothane in the gas phase during the whole experiment. Caffeine was increased stepwise from 0.1 up to 32 mM. The increase in caffeine sensitivity of muscle strips from potentially MHS subjects compared to normal controls was documented with a shift of a dose–response curve to the left. Halothane was shown to have modulating properties on this phenomenon by increasing the sensitivity to caffeine (see Fig. 19.1).

Citation count

273.

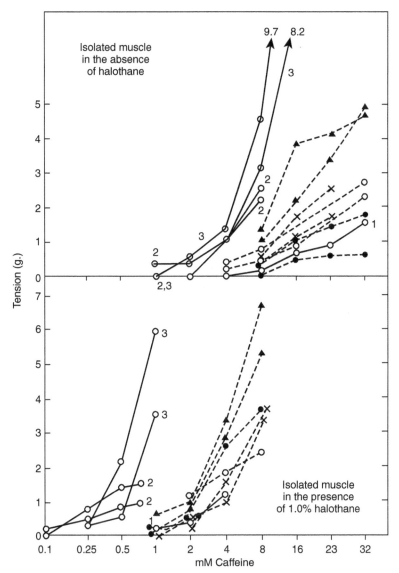

Fig. 19.1 Caffeine contracture of isolated muscle from volunteers disposed to malignnant hyperthermia and from controls. Reprinted from *The Lancet*, **296**, 7679, W. Kalow, B.A. Britt, M.E. Terreau, C. Haise, Metabolic error of muscle metabolism after recovery from malignant hyperthermia, pp. 895–898, 1970, with permission from Elsevier.

Key message

The first report of potential *in vitro* testing to allow detection of MH susceptibility.

Strengths

The scientific strength of this paper is its simplicity and robust technical approach. The idea of using biopsied muscle strips to perform diagnostic *in vitro* challenges and to demonstrate an altered calcium control in skeletal muscle was relatively simple, straightforward, and safe for patients at risk for MH.

Weaknesses

The scientific weakness of the paper is the small number of investigated individuals with an MH history. From the three potentially MHS individuals only two had abnormal *in vitro* muscle contractures. With current knowledge and experience it is easy to conclude that 'Volunteer A', who had normal *in vitro* test results, had a clinical event that is not consistent with MH. Unfortunately, the authors did not question or discussed the clinical MH diagnosis of 'Volunteer A' after having obtained the test results. Their conclusion that there are two different forms of MH, one with and another without muscle rigidity which requires different treatment, was of course a possible explanation for the findings, but obviously not the right one.

Relevance

This publication presented for the first time the potential use of freshly excised skeletal muscle, a process now referred to as *in vitro* muscle contracture testing, in the diagnosis of MH susceptibility. In addition, in the knowledge that caffeine induces muscle contracture by stimulating the release of calcium, it could be deduced that at least some MHS individuals had an underlying altered calcium control mechanism in skeletal muscle.

The impact of this publication is that it led to the development of a variety of protocols for the use of *in vitro* muscle contracture testing for the laboratory diagnosis of MH susceptibility. The simultaneous use of halothane and caffeine to challenge a muscle strip in this work and the subsequent experience with this approach in the MH research unit in Toronto played a major part in distinguishing the MH test protocol in North America from that subsequently developed in Europe.

Paper 3: A protocol for the investigation of malignant hyperpyrexia susceptibility

Author details

European Malignant Hyperpyrexia Group.

Reference

British Journal of Anaesthesia 1984; **56**: 1267–9.

Abstract

A European Malignant Hyperpyrexia Group has been formed to facilitate exchange of information between centres performing in vitro muscle testing for malignant hyperpyrexia susceptibility. Data have been collected according to a protocol agreed by the Group. Based on these results, test criteria have been established to allow the following diagnoses to be made: MH susceptible (MHS), MH normal (MHN) or MH equivocal (MHE). It is accepted that MHE classified patients will be under permanent review, pending the collection of further data.

European Malignant Hyperpyrexia Group, 'A protocol for the investigation of malignant hyperpyrexia suscepti-bility', *British Journal of Anaesthesia*, 1984, 56, 11, pp. 1267–1269, by permission of Oxford University Press and British Journal of Anaesthesia.

Summary

The state of knowledge concerning the investigation of MH susceptibility prior to this publication was based on the observation by several researchers in various countries, particularly in Europe and North America, that muscle strips form MHS individuals had increased sensitivity to *in vitro* halothane and caffeine challenge. Furthermore, similar results had been reported using a variety of other drugs or combinations of substances. However, the different findings and parallel research in several MH investigation units worldwide led to the development of different test protocols and did not allow comparison of diagnostic results between different MH investigation units.

The major advances imparted by this paper are the formation of the European Malignant Hyperthermia Group and the standardization of *in vitro* muscle contracture testing (IVCT) in Europe. In 1983, physicians from eight European countries (UK, Denmark, Sweden, Ireland, Germany, Austria, France, Netherlands) met in Lund and in Leeds to establish the European MH Group with the following aims:

♦ To provide a forum for discussion between the various European centres.

♦ To standardize the investigation of MH subjects to allow comparisons between centres.

♦ To establish a common data bank.

♦ To allow for combined research facilities.

The Group agreed upon a specific, standardized protocol for *in vitro* screening of MH susceptibility using separate applications of caffeine and halothane as the test drugs.

Citation count

Not available.

Key message

The paper suggested a standardization for the investigation of MH subjects.

Strengths

The scientific strength of this paper is the robustness of the diagnostic approach using two test drugs and using a classification system with three diagnostic groups:

- MH susceptible (MHS) group: abnormal muscle contractures to both halothane and caffeine.
- MH normal (MHN) group: no abnormal muscle contractures.
- MH equivocal (MHE) group: abnormal muscle contractures to only one of the applied test drugs (either halothane or caffeine).

The introduction of the MHE group was a wise solution to increase the specificity of the protocol. Because the MHE group was regarded clinically as MHS and to be under permanent review, the European MH Group found a solution to incorporate the fact that almost all biological tests have some overlap between the affected and the non-affected groups in their responses.

Weaknesses

The scientific weakness of the paper is that it did not recommend complete standardization of the procedures used. Financial considerations dictated that the test equipment was not standardized. Other variances, such as in handling of the muscle biopsies, perhaps were not apparent at that stage. However, the future and successful genetic findings that crucially depended on the IVCT test results, particularly in the European countries, demonstrate that the protocol of the European MH Group has been a cornerstone for the scientific and clinical advances in MH.

Relevance

The impact of this manuscript may be addressed as the breakthrough of establishing MH screening using a standardized approach in Europe. The introduction of the European protocol led over the coming years to comparable laboratory data of hundreds of MH family pedigrees in 20 European countries, Australia, and New Zealand. These laboratory data subsequently proved crucial for the successful detection of genetic loci causing MH susceptibility.

Paper 4: Control of the malignant hyperpyrexic syndrome in MHS swine by dantrolene sodium

Author details

GG Harrison

Reference

British Journal of Anaesthesia 1975; **47**: 62–5.

Abstract

Experiments are described which demonstrate that dantrolene sodium effectively terminates the syndrome of malignant hyperpyrexia induced in susceptible swine by exposure to halothane. Dantrolene is also shown to block initiation of the syndrome of malignant hyperpyrexia by halothane in MHS swine. Therapeutic use of this drug in patients with anaesthetic-induced malignant hyperpyrexia appears to be indicated.

Harrison GG, 'Control of the malignant hyperpyrexic syndrome in MHS swine by dantrolene sodium', *British Journal of Anaesthesia*, 1975, 47, 1, pp. 62–65, by permission of Oxford University Press and British Journal of Anaesthesia.

Summary

The state of knowledge prior to this publication was that malignant hyperthermia (MH) was an uncommon, almost always fatal syndrome, which results from a hereditary underlying defect of calcium regulation in skeletal muscle. The syndrome could be triggered with volatile anaesthetics and succinylcholine in MH-susceptible (MHS) humans and pigs. Whilst the basic pathophysiology of MH was quite well understood, successful treatment was limited due to the lack of a specific antidote. The major components of MH treatment at that time were:

◆ Early diagnosis.

◆ Rapid elimination of volatile anaesthetics using hyperventilation with 100% oxygen (O_2).

◆ Cooling with surface ice and ice water application to the stomach and the bladder.

◆ Suggestions that dexamethasone and procainamide might have some value.

The major advance imparted by this paper is the finding that dantrolene sodium is an effective antidote for MH treatment. Dantrolene sodium was synthesized together with a series of hydanto-ins by Norwich Pharmacal Company Laboratories, New York, and in 1967, Snyder and colleagues (Snyder *et al.*, 1967) reported the muscle relaxant properties of this drug. Harrison developed an experimental protocol to test the effects of dantrolene sodium in MH pigs, which developed MH following anaesthesia with halothane, and as a preventive drug before the application of halothane in MH pigs. He performed eight experiments in five pigs. In one pig three experiments, in a second pig two, and once each in the remaining three pigs. Pigs were monitored with:

◆ Electrocardiogram (ECG).

◆ Clinical observation of rigor.

◆ Temperature measurement in skeletal muscle.

◆ Repeated sampling of mixed venous blood from a right atrial cannula.

Anaesthesia was induced using ketamine or ketamine/thiopentone and MH was initiated by the administration of 2.5% halothane. Figure 2 in the publication (see Fig. 19.2) gives detailed information about the performed animal experiments. One out of five pigs died during the experiment. Interestingly, this animal was treated with 1 mg kg^{-1} dantrolene sodium only. A second animal treated with 1 mg kg^{-1} survived, but all other experiments with surviving animals were performed with higher doses (2.5, 6, 7 or 10 mg kg^{-1}). Harrison describes the effect of dantrolene with the following three statements:

◆ Rapid loss of muscle rigor commencing within 5 min and usually complete within 20 min.

◆ Immediate cessation of the increase in deep muscle temperature followed by a rapid decrease.

◆ Termination of the progressive, inexorable acidosis characteristic of the syndrome rendering easy the buffering of acidosis developed until the dantrolene administration.

Dantrolene pretreatment of one MHS pig blocked initiation of MH by halothane (described time of halothane application is 90 min).

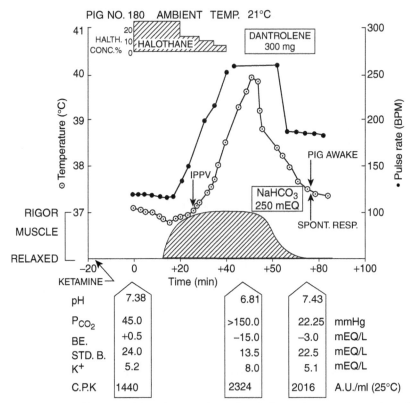

Fig. 19.2 Temperature (deep muscle) and events chart of typical experiment on MHS pig weighing 45 kg. Dantrolene administered as i.v. drip infusion for duration of square so marked. Biochemical values from mixed venous blood. Reproduced from G.G. Harrison, Control of the malignant hyperpyrexic syndrome in MHS swine by dantrolene sodium, *British Journal of Anaesthesia*, 1975, **47**, pp. 62–65, Oxford University Press, by permission of British Journal of Anaesthesia.

Citation count

164.

Related references

1 Snyder HR, Davis CS, Bickerton RK, *et al.* 1 (5-Arylfurfurylidene) amino hydantoins: a new class of muscle relaxants. *J Med Chem* 1967; **10**: 807–10.

Key message

The first description of an effective treatment for MH.

Strengths

The scientific strength of this paper is the finding that dantrolene sodium is indeed an effective drug for successful treatment of MH. Due to the high mortality of the syndrome in pigs (nearly 100%) and the convincing effects of dantrolene sodium in this study, the therapeutic use of this drug was proposed for patients with anaesthetic-induced MH.

Weaknesses

The scientific weakness of the paper is an extensive variability of the protocol for the experiments. The publication is much more a case series of different but similar experiments in MH pigs. However, the combination of the well-known high mortality of the syndrome and the convincing effect of dantrolene sodium in the presented experiments underline the importance of this publication.

Relevance

The impact that the paper has had is the demonstration that dantrolene sodium effectively terminates the MH syndrome in MH pigs triggered by halothane and that this drug is also able to block the initiation of MH by halothane in pigs.

Paper 5: Ryanodine receptor gene is a candidate for predisposition to malignant hyperthermia

Author details

DH MacLennan, C Duff, F Zorzato, J Fujii, M Phillips, RG Korneluk, W Frodis, BA Britt, RG Worton

Reference

Nature 1990; **343**: 559–61.

Abstract

Malignant hyperthermia (MH) is a potentially lethal condition in which sustained muscle contracture, with attendant hypercatabolic reactions and elevation in body temperature, are triggered by commonly used inhalational anaesthetics and skeletal muscle relaxants. In humans, the trait is usually inherited in an autosomal dominant fashion, but in halothane-sensitive pigs with a similar phenotype, inheritance of the disease is autosomal recessive or co-dominant. A simple and accurate non-invasive test for the gene is not available and predisposition to the disease is currently determined through a halothane- and/or caffeine-induced contracture test on a skeletal muscle biopsy. Because Ca^{2+} is the chief regulator of muscle contraction and metabolism, the primary defect in MH is believed to lie in Ca^{2+} regulation. Indeed, several studies indicate a defect in the Ca^{2+} release channel of the sarcoplasmic reticulum, making it a prime candidate for the altered gene product in predisposed individuals. We have recently cloned complementary DNA and genomic DNA encoding the human ryanodine receptor (the Ca^{2+} -release channel of the sarcoplasmic reticulum) and mapped the ryanodine receptor gene (*RYR*) to region q13.1 of human chromosome 19, in close proximity to genetic markers that have been shown to map near the MH susceptibility locus in humans and the halothane-sensitive gene in pigs. As a more definitive test of whether the *RYR* gene is a candidate gene for the human MH phenotype, we have carried out a linkage study with MH families to determine whether the MH phenotype segregates with chromosome 19q markers, including markers in the *RYR* gene. Co-segregation of MH with *RYR* markers, resulting in a lod score of 4.20 at a linkage distance of zero centimorgans, indicates that MH is likely to be caused by mutations in the *RYR* gene.

Summary

In the late 1980s, several pieces of information came together to implicate the sarcoplasmic reticulum calcium release channel of skeletal muscle as the site of the defect in porcine MH. The sarcoplasmic reticulum calcium release channel was alternatively known as the ryanodine receptor because the plant alkaloid ryanodine had been used to isolate and characterize the channel in the 'heavy' fraction of the sarcoplasmic reticulum. Mickelson and colleagues (Mickelson *et al.*, 1988) subsequently demonstrated that the heavy sarcoplasmic reticulum fraction from MH susceptible pigs had an increased affinity for ryanodine compared with the same fraction from normal pigs.

Also by that time the genetic locus implicated in the porcine condition, the *HAL* (for halothane) locus, had been genetically linked to the glucose phosphate isomerase, alpha-1 B-glycoprotein and H-blood group antigen loci on porcine chromosome 6. This linkage group is highly conserved through mammalian evolution and maps to the long arm of chromosome 19 (chromosome

19q12–13.2) in humans. MacLennan's group then cloned complementary and genomic DNA of the ryanodine receptor and mapped this to human chromosome 19q13.1 (Zorzato *et al.*, 1990). All they needed to do now was demonstrate linkage between genetic markers in this region and the MH trait to confirm the likely role of the ryanodine receptor in the aetiology of MH.

Citation count

391.

Related references

1 Mickelson JR, Gallant EM, Litterer LA, *et al.* Abnormal sarcoplasmic reticulum ryanodine receptor in malignant hyperthermia. *J Biol Chem* 1988; **263**: 9310–15.

2 McCarthy TV, Healy JM, Heffron JJ, *et al.* Localization of the malignant hyperthermia susceptibility locus to human chromosome 19q12-13.2. *Nature* 1990; **342**: 562–4.

3 Zorzato F, Fujii J, Otsu K, *et al.* Molecular cloning of cDNA encoding human and rabbit forms of the Ca^{2+} release channel (ryanodine receptor) of skeletal muscle sarcoplasmic reticulum. *J Biol Chem* 1990; **265**: 2244–56.

4 Gillard EF, Otsu H, Fujii J, Khanna VK, *et al.* A substitution of cysteine for argentine 614 in the ryanodine receptor is potentially causative of human malignant hyperthermia. *Genomics* 1991; **11**: 751–5.

Key message

The ryanodine receptor and its mutations are important in determining susceptibility to MH.

Strengths

The strength of this paper is the state of the art (for the time) molecular genetics used to identify polymorphic markers within the ryanodine receptor gene and to characterize these markers in Canadian malignant hyperthermia families.

Weaknesses

The weakness of the paper emanates from the clinical material MacLennan's group had to work with. Firstly, segregation data in the paper are presented on ten small pedigrees. Furthermore, for several of these pedigrees it is not possible to make any comment about the likely pattern of inheritance within the family and yet the paper states 'families who did not fit the standard criteria for autosomal dominant inheritance were not used for the linkage study'. This clearly raises the suspicion of selection bias which is important as the results depend on the combination of results from all the pedigrees. The problem with using combined data from small pedigrees is that it assumes that there is no locus heterogeneity for the condition, which we now know does exist.

The problem of these small pedigrees was compounded by the methods used for phenotyping the MH trait. Unlike the standardized contracture test protocol used by the European MH Group, at that time no such standardization process had taken place in North America. Indeed, it would appear that there was even a lack of standardization within the Toronto MH Diagnostic Centre. In several cases the diagnosis of MH is dependent on a combined halothane and caffeine test which has subsequently been shown to have an unacceptably high false positive rate leading to its abandonment. Without the rigour of phenotyping data the reliability of genetic linkage studies is dubious.

In conclusion, therefore, one does get the feeling that despite its profile, this paper actually added very little evidence to support the theory. This is not to belittle the contribution made by MacLennan's group firstly in cloning and localizing the human *RYR1* gene and subsequently demonstrating mutations in this gene associated with malignant hyperthermia.

Relevance

Although this paper claims to demonstrate such linkage, the methodological approach is somewhat contentious. Indeed, if it were not for the simultaneous publication of a more rigorous linkage study carried out on large Irish pedigrees by McCarthy *et al.* (1990), it is doubtful whether MacLennan's paper would have achieved such a high profile.

The combined impact of the two papers, however, at the time led many to conclude that the problem of MH was solved and that a genetic screening test for the condition could be rapidly developed and applied. Although this proved not to be the case, even after MacLennan's group identified the first of many mutations in the *RYR1* gene, McCarthy *et al.*'s 1990 *Nature* paper is now widely regarded as confirmation of *RYR1* as the major genetic influence in human MH.

Paper 6: Evidence for genetic heterogeneity of malignant hyperthermia susceptibility

Author details

T Deufel, A Golla, D Iles, A Meindl, T Meitinger, D Schindelhauer, A De Vries, D Pongretz, DH MacLennan, KJ Johnson, F Lehmann-Horn

Reference

American Journal of Human Genetics 1992; **50**: 1151–61.

Abstract

A locus for malignant hyperthermia susceptibility (MHS) has been localized on chromosome 19q12–13.2, while at the same time the gene encoding the skeletal muscle ryanodine receptor (RYR1) also has been mapped to this region and has been found to be tightly linked to MHS. RYR1 was consequently postulated as the candidate for the molecular defect causing MHS, and a point mutation in the gene has now been identified and is thought to be the cause of MH in at least some MHS patients. Here we report the results of a linkage study done with 19q12-13.2 markers, including the RYR1 cDNA, in two Bavarian families with MHS. In one of the families, three unambiguous recombination events between MHS and the RYR1 locus were found. In the second family only one informative meiosis was seen with RYR1. However, segregation analysis with markers for D19S75, D19S28, D19S47, CYP2A, BCL3, and APOC2 shows that the crossovers in the first family involve the entire haplotype defined by these markers flanking RYR1 and, furthermore, reveals multiple crossovers between these haplotypes and MHS in the second family. In these families, pairwise and multipoint lod scores below −2 exclude MHS from an interval spanning more than 26 cM and comprising the RYR1 and the previously described MHS locus. Our findings thus strongly suggest genetic heterogeneity of the MHS trait and prompt the search for another MHS locus.

Summary

Prior to publication of this paper many workers assumed that malignant hyperthermia (MH) was a monogenic disorder caused by mutations in the ryanodine receptor gene, *RYR1*, although it should be noted that Gillard *et al.* (1991) had demonstrated allelic heterogeneity in that they identified an *RYR1* mutation in one Canadian family but not in a further 34 families. This paper was paradigm-shifting as it added a new dimension to MH genetic research, that is the search for new candidate genes in addition for further mutations in the *RYR1* gene. In fact Deufel and colleagues were not the first to publish a paper along these lines. Levitt *et al.* (1991) working in the USA published a report with a similar message detailing genetic studies in three American families which showed a lack of segregation between chromosome 19q markers and MH susceptibility. However Levitt's paper did not convince the heterogeneity sceptics as no details of the phenotyping (clinical reaction of the index cases and *in vitro* muscle contracture data) were published.

Citation count

67.

Related references

1 Gillard EF, Otsu H, FujiiJ, Khanna VK, *et al.* A substitution of cysteine for argentine 614 in the ryanodine receptor is potentially causative of human malignant hyperthermia. *Genomics* 1991; **11**: 751–5.

2 Levitt RC, Nourl N, Jedlicka AE, *et al.* Evidence for genetic heterogeneity in malignant hyperthermia susceptibility. *Genomics* 1991; **11**: 543–7.

3 MacKenzie AE, Allen G, Lahey D, *et al.* A comparison of the caffeine halothane muscle contracture test with the molecular genetic diagnosis of malignant hyperthermia. *Anesthesiology* 1991; **75**: 4–8.

Key message

There is more than one gene involved in MH.

Strengths

The weight of the evidence for heterogeneity in Deufel's paper resisted all attempts to challenge its integrity. Indeed, the number of recombination events was such that no attempt at manipulating the data could change the interpretation. This paper therefore represents a real triumph for the scientific virtue of allowing new data to challenge preconceptions rather than only accepting data that are compatible with those preconceptions.

Weaknesses

None.

Relevance

The discussion section of Deufel's paper indeed strongly suggests that the journal reviewers were reluctant to accept the robust contracture test data presented for the two Bavarian families. This is quite remarkable when one considers the lack of scrutiny that was given to the phenotyping data used to demonstrate linkage to the ryanodine receptor locus in the first place. Indeed, the previous year MacKenzie and colleagues (MacKenzie *et al.*, 1991), in attempting to demonstrate the use of chromosome 19 linkage for molecular genetic diagnosis of MH, resorted to post hoc manipulation of the North American caffeine–halothane contracture test results in order to achieve segregation between genotype and phenotype.

Paper 7: Malignant hyperthermia susceptibility is associated with a mutation of the alpha 1-subunit of the human dihydropyridine-sensitive L-type voltage-dependent calcium-channel receptor in skeletal muscle

Author details

N Monnier, V Procaccio, P Stieglitz, J Lunardi

Reference

American Journal of Human Genetics 1997; **60**: 1316–25.

Abstract

Malignant hyperthermia susceptibility (MHS) is characterized by genetic heterogeneity. However, except for the MHS1 locus, which corresponds to the skeletal muscle ryanodine receptor (RYR1) and for which several mutations have been described, no direct molecular evidence for a mutation in another gene has been reported so far. In this study we show that the CACNL1A3 gene encoding the alpha 1-subunit of the human skeletal muscle dihydropyridine-sensitive L-type voltage-dependent calcium channel (VDCC) represents a new MHS locus and is responsible for the disease in a large French family. Linkage analysis performed with an intragenic polymorphic microsatellite marker of the CACLN1A3 gene generated a two-point LOD score of 4.38 at a recombinant fraction of 0. Sequence analysis of the coding region of the CACLN1A3 gene showed the presence of an Arg-His substitution at residue 1086, resulting from the transition of A for G3333, which segregates perfectly with the MHS phenotype in the family. The mutation is localized in a very different part of the alpha 1-subunit of the human skeletal muscle VDCC, compared with previously reported mutations found in patients with hypokalemic periodic paralysis, and these two diseases might be discussed in terms of allelic diseases. This report is the first direct evidence that the skeletal muscle VDCC is involved in MHS, and it suggests a direct interaction between the skeletal muscle VDCC and the ryanodine receptor in the skeletal muscle sarcoplasmic reticulum.

Malignant hyperthermia susceptibility is associated with a mutation of the alpha 1-subunit of the human dihydropyridine-sensitive L-type voltage-dependent calcium-channel receptor in skeletal muscle, Monnier N, Procaccio V, Stieglitz P, Lunardi J, American Journal of Human Genetics 1997; 60: 1316-25.

Summary

With the publication by Deufel and colleagues (see paper 6) of clear evidence for genetic hetero-geneity the search for new candidate genes began in earnest. Two main approaches to this challenge were taken. The first of these is termed the candidate gene approach. Here, physiologically plausible candidate genes were selected whose genetic locus is known. Polymorphic markers in the vicinity of the locus were selected and typed in malignant hyperthermia (MH) pedigrees. At the time this paper was published the voltage sensor of the skeletal muscle T-tubular system, which was presumed to interact with the ryanodine receptor in excitation-contraction coupling, had been identified as structurally similar to the dihydropyridine-sensitive calcium channels of the heart and endovas-cular smooth muscle. This skeletal muscle DHPR was found to comprise of products of four genes, an alpha-1 subunit on chromosome 1q, a beta subunit on chromosome 17q, an alpha-2/delta subunit on chromosome 7q, and a gamma subunit also localized on chromosome 17q. Levitt and colleagues (Levitt *et al.*, 1992) were the first to publish a candidate gene linkage study. They had selected the chromosome 17q region containing the beta and gamma subunit genes and reported linkage with the MH trait. Their paper was however subsequently criticized because of the lack of phenotype data and also because their linkage was derived from combined data from several small American and South African pedigrees. As mentioned before, this approach is inappropriate for a condition displaying locus heterogeneity. It is interesting to note that no mutations in either the gamma or beta subunits have been reported in the pedigrees included in this study and neither have any other workers confirmed linkage to this region.

Iles and colleagues (Iles *et al.*, 1994) subsequently reported linkage in a single German family to the chromosome 7q21–22 region which incorporates the alpha-2/delta subunit gene. Surprisingly, no mutations in this gene were found in this family.

The second approach available at that time was to do a genome-wide linkage study. Here, one or more large pedigrees are genotyped for markers across the entire genome spaced approximately every 300 kilobases. The power of this approach depends on the size and structure of the pedigree. In the current era of genome-wide sequencing it is worth emphasizing the time and resources required to carry out a genome-wide linkage study. Nevertheless, two such studies were tackled by the European Malignant Hyperthermia Group. The first of these found suggestive linkage to a region of chromosome 3q (Sudbrak *et al.*, 1995) but follow-up fine mapping of the region failed to identify a likely candidate gene. The second European genome-wide linkage study did however bear fruit in that one of two loci identified in separate families not only demonstrated good linkage but was also in the chromosome 1q region known to be the locus of the alpha-1 subunit of the skeletal muscle DHPR (Robinson *et al.*, 1997). In the knowledge of these preliminary results Monnier and colleagues, who had provided the French family linked to chromosome 1q progressed rapidly to undertake fine mapping of the chromosome 1q region and subsequently generated cDNA which was used for direct sequencing of the alpha-1 subunit gene. It is these results that Monnier and colleagues report in the *American Journal of Human Genetics* in 1997.

Citation count

250.

Related references

1 Levitt RC, Olckers A, Meyers S, *et al* Evidence for the localization of a malignant hyperthermia susceptibility locus (MHS2) to human chromosome 17q. *Genomics* 1992; **14**: 562–6.

2 Iles DE, Lehmann-Horn F, Scherer SW, *et al.* Localization of the gene encoding the alpha 2/delta-subunits of the L-type voltage-dependent calcium channel to chromosome 7q and analysis of the segregation of flanking markers in malignant hyperthermia susceptible families. *Hum Mol Genet* 1994; **3**: 969–75.

3 Sudbrak R, Procaccio V, Klausnitzer M, *et al.* Mapping of a further malignant hyperthermia susceptibility locus to chromosome 3q13.1. *Am J Hum Genet* 1995; **3**: 684–91.

4 Robinson R, Monnier N, Wolz W, *et al.* A genome-wide search for susceptibility loci in two European malignant hyperthermia pedigrees. *Hum Mol Genet* 1997; **6**: 953–61.

Key message

The first and only paper to show a gene mutation which can cause MH susceptibility.

Strengths

The demonstration of this mutation (p.R1086H) finally removed any possible objection to the classification of MH as a disorder with locus heterogeneity. It is interesting, however, that subsequently very few families with MH have been found to contain a mutation in the alpha-1 subunit of DHPR. Furthermore, no mutations in other genes have been reported since Monnier's paper.

Weaknesses

None.

Relevance

It was a testament to their speed and skill that Monnier and colleagues actually found a mutation in the alpha-1 DHPR subunit gene and demonstrated its segregation in their family before the European Group subsequently published the genome-wide linkage study on which Monnier's work depended.

Paper 8: Discordance in a malignant hyperthermia pedigree, between in vitro contracture-test phenotypes and haplotypes for the MHS1 region on chromosome 19q12–13.2, comprising the C1840T transition in the RYR1 gene

Author details

T Deufel, R Sudbrak, Y Feist, B Rübsam, I Du Chesne, K-L Schäfer, N Roewer, T Grimm, F Lehmann-Horn, EJ Hartung, CR Müller

Reference

American Journal of Human Genetics 1995; **56**: 1334–42.

Abstract

A point mutation in the gene encoding the skeletal muscle calcium release channel (RYR1) has been proposed as the probable cause of malignant hyperthermia (MH) in swine, where it segregates with the disease in all MH-prone strains investigated. The same C-to-T exchange in nucleotide position 1840 of the human RYR1 cDNA sequence was found in a few human MH pedigrees. We report a German MH pedigree where in vitro contracture test (IVCT) results and haplotypes of markers for the MHS1/RYR1 region including this base transition have yielded several discrepancies. The MH-susceptible phenotype was defined by IVCT performed according to the European standard protocol. Haplotypes were constructed for markers for the MHS1/RYR1 region on chromosome 19 and include the C1840T base exchange. Discussing the probabilities for a number of hypotheses to explain these data, we suggest that our results may challenge the causative role of this mutation— and possibly the role of the RYR1 gene itself—in human MH susceptibility, at least in some cases.

Summary

The state of knowledge prior to this publication was evidence that a point mutation in the gene encoding the skeletal muscle calcium release channel of the sarcoplasmic reticulum (ryanodine receptor; *RYR1*) had been proposed as the cause of MH in pigs, because it segregates with the disease in all MH-prone strains investigated. The analogous exchange (c.C1840T) of the human *RYR1* cDNA sequence was also found in 5–10% of human MH pedigrees previously investigated using IVCT. At this time no individual presenting an MHN phenotype with IVCT in an MH pedigree had been described as carrying this mutation. It was of greatest interest therefore to compare MH diagnosis obtained by IVCT with genetic findings in pedigrees with the c.C1840T mutation in the *RYR1* gene.

The major advance imparted by this paper is the finding that IVCT results and genetic analyses may produce discordant results. The authors investigated a large MH pedigree with a fatal MH index case (patient 401 in the pedigree on Fig. 19.3) previously investigated by IVCT for the c.C1840T using *Rsa*I digestion of an amplified genomic DNA fragment. In addition alleles of the genetic region were characterized with microsatellite markers for the loci D19S75, D19S191, RYR1, D19S190, and D19S47. This pedigree (see Fig. 19.3) is of particular interest for three specific reasons:

- One individual of the left branch of the pedigree, tested MHS using IVCT (408), is homozygous for the c.C1840T mutation.

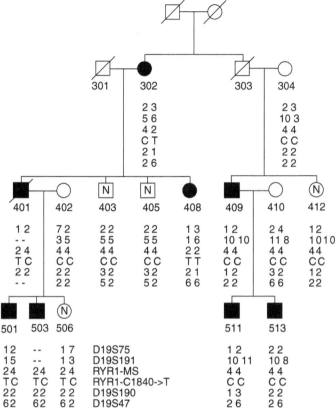

Fig. 19.3 Pedigree MH011 with MHS. The results of the IVCT are indicated by blackened symbols (designating MHS) and by symbols with "N" (designating MHN); blank symbols denote untested individuals. The index case 401 died as a consequence of a fulminant MH crisis. Also given are the alleles found with microsatellite markers for the loci D19S75, D19S191, RYR1, D19S190, and D19S47, as well as the results of analysis for the C1840T base transition in the RYR1gene. In the latter, "C" denotes the wild-type sequence, and "T" denotes the mutated base. This article was published in *American Journal of Human Genetics*, **56**, 6, T. Deufel, R. Sudbrak, Y. Feist, B. Rübsam, I. Du Chesne, K-L. Schäfer, N. Roewer, T. Grimm, F. Lehmann-Horn, E.J. Hartung, C.R. Müller, Discordance, in a Malignant Hyperthermia Pedigree, between in Vitro Contracture-Test Phenotypes and Haplotypes for the MHS1 Region on Chromosome 19q12–13.2, Comprising the C1840T Transition in the RYR1 Gene. pp. 1334–1342, Copyright Elsevier, 1995.

♦ One individual of the left branch of the pedigree, tested MHN using IVCT (506), is a carrier of the c.C1840T mutation (discordant finding).

♦ Three individuals of the right branch of the pedigree, tested MHS using IVCT (409, 511, and 513), do not carry the c.C1840T mutation.

The authors give three potential hypotheses that might explain these findings:

♦ MH susceptibility is caused by two independent *RYR1*-c.C1840T mutations in one branch of the family and by a third mutation that is unrelated to *RYR1* in the other branch; in addition, one false-negative IVCT must have occurred in individual 506.

- *RYR1*-c.C1840T mutations are the cause of MH susceptibility in the entire pedigree. Individual 506 would still have to be a false-negative IVCT result, whilst individuals 409, 511, and 513 must be false positive IVCT results.
- A single dominant mutation accounts for all observed MHS phenotypes in the family; this mutation then would most likely be unlinked to the *RYR1* locus.

Citation count

62.

Key message

Genetic testing and *in vitro* contracture testing may provide differing results in determining MH susceptibility.

Strengths

The reliability of IVCT was questioned at these times from an increasing number of experts. However, the scientific strength of this paper lies within the careful presentation of the data and a wise interpretation of the findings. The presented hypotheses and the potential significance of the c.C1840T mutation for MH diagnosis were an important scientific contribution supporting further MH research.

Weaknesses

None.

Relevance

The impact that this paper has had was scientific evidence that the inheritance of MH susceptibility must be much more complex than previously suspected by the majority of geneticists.

Paper 9: Guidelines for molecular genetic detection of susceptibility to malignant hyperthermia

Author details

A Urwyler, T Deufel, T McCarthy, S West; European Malignant Hyperthermia Group

Reference

British Journal of Anaesthesia 2001; **86**: 283–7.

Abstract

Malignant hyperthermia (MH) is a potentially fatal pharmacogenetic disease triggered by several anaesthetic agents. The *in vitro* muscle contracture test (IVCT) is the standard test to establish an individual's risk of susceptibility to MH. Clinical practitioners and geneticists of the European MH Group have agreed on the present guidelines for the detection of MH susceptibility using molecular genetic techniques and/or IVCT to predict the risk of MH.

Summary

Prior to the publication of this paper there was no consensus on the role for DNA analysis in MH diagnostics. At this time 15 mutations in the *RYR1* gene had been studied in heterologous expression systems and been found to impart an increased sensitivity of intracellular calcium release on exposure of the cells to caffeine and/or halothane. These data confirmed the functional significance of these particular *RYR1* mutations. The problem was, however, the accumulating number of cases of discordance between *RYR1* mutation genotype and IVCT phenotype in families where these mutations had been found.

Citation count

177.

Key message

Demonstration of absence of a familial *RYR1* mutation requires an *in vitro* test to exclude the possibility of other unidentified mutations—phenotyping is more sensitive than genotyping.

Strengths

The scientific advance offered by these guidelines was the application of scientific data in a pragmatic way such that the use of the invasive muscle biopsy required for IVCT could be reduced without comprising patient safety. This was achieved by recognizing that the real value of any laboratory diagnosis of MH is related to its ability to demonstrate that an individual with increased risk of susceptibility was in fact not at risk. The main take home message of the guidelines therefore is that a demonstration of absence of a familial *RYR1* mutation should be followed-up by an IVCT to exclude the possibility of the presence of another, unidentified mutation being present (Fig. 19.4); this was the presumed mechanism for the 5% incidence of discordance between *RYR1* genotype and IVCT phenotype.

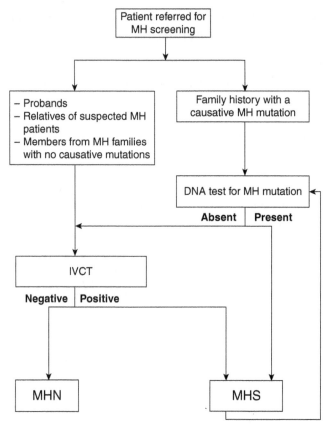

Fig. 19.4 Suggested route for MH susceptibility testing. IVCT, *in vitro* muscle contracture test; MHN, malignant hyperthermia negative; MHS, malignant hyperthermia susceptible. Reproduced from A. Urwyler, T. Deufel, T. McCarthy, S. West, Guidelines for molecular genetic detection of susceptibility to malignant hyperthermia, *British Journal of Anaesthesia*, 2001, **86**, pp. 283–287, Oxford University Press, by permission of British Journal of Anaesthesia.

Weaknesses

The weakness of the paper is that it is inevitably based on the consensus views of experts because of a lack of evidence for a complete understanding of the genetics of malignant hyperthermia in all cases. However, the impact of the publication of these guidelines was immediate with adoption of the guidelines into clinical services across Europe enabling confirmation of MH susceptible status by DNA analysis. Initially the restriction of the use of DNA testing within the guidelines to *RYR1* mutations that had been demonstrated to be functionally important meant that only about 20% of MH families benefited. However, with subsequent efforts to screen further families for the known *RYR1* mutations and demonstration of the functional importance of further *RYR1* mutations, almost 50% of MH families in some countries are now suitable for testing according to these guidelines.

Relevance

The significance of discordant results at this time was disputed. One view was that the genetic data must be correct and that discordance must therefore be attributed to errors in the IVCT phenotyping. Fortunately, a more informed view was offered by the geneticists who had been collaborating as part of the European Malignant Hyperthermia Group since 1990. By 2001 they were at least doubtful that the discordance could be explained by phenotyping or even genotyping errors. While some in the European MH Group considered the best course to be to confine DNA analysis to research, there was a growing concern that this latter approach might lead to *RYR1* mutation screening being offered by DNA diagnostic facilities that could not provide the expertise in MH genetics required to safely interpret the data.

Paper 10: Genetic variation in *RYR1* and malignant hyperthermia phenotypes

Author details

D Carpenter, RL Robinson, RJ Quinnell, C Ringrose, M Hogg, F Casson, P Booms, DE Iles, PJ Halsall, DS Steele, MA Shaw, PM Hopkins

Reference

British Journal of Anaesthesia 2009; **103**: 538–48.

Abstract

Background: Malignant hyperthermia (MH) is associated, in the majority of cases, with mutations in *RYR1*, the gene encoding the skeletal muscle ryanodine receptor. Our primary aim was to assess whether different *RYR1* variants are associated with quantitative differences in MH phenotype.

Methods: The degree of *in vitro* pharmacological muscle contracture response and the baseline serum creatine kinase (CK) concentration were used to generate a series of quantitative phenotypes for MH. We then undertook the most extensive *RYR1* genotype–phenotype correlation in MH to date using 504 individuals from 204 MH families and 23 *RYR1* variants. We also determined the association between a clinical phenotype and both the laboratory phenotype and *RYR1* genotype.

Results: We report a novel correlation between the degree of *in vitro* pharmacological muscle contracture responses and the onset time of the clinical MH response in index cases (P<0.05). There was also a significant correlation between baseline CK concentration and clinical onset time (P=0.039). The specific *RYR1* variant was a significant determinant of the severity of each laboratory phenotype (P<0.0001).

Conclusions: The MH phenotype differs significantly with different *RYR1* variants. Variants leading to more severe MH phenotype are distributed throughout the gene and tend to lie at relatively conserved sites in the protein. Differences in phenotype severity between *RYR1* variants may explain the variability in clinical penetrance of MH during anaesthesia and why some variants have been associated with exercise-induced rhabdomyolysis and heat stroke. They may also inform a mutation screening strategy in cases of idiopathic hyperCKaemia.

Summary

Prior to this publication genetic mutations affecting the RyR1 protein that forms the calcium release channel of the sarcoplasmic reticulum of skeletal muscle were estimated to be present in at least 50% of MH susceptible individuals. A total of 178 non-synonymous changes with potentially functional significance were described across the whole *RYR1* gene, 72 of these with documented recurrence, and 29 showing functional abnormality using *in vitro* calcium experiments at the cellular level with either transfected cells or immortalized B-lymphocytes, which express the RyR1 protein. Based on preliminary assessment, the authors hypothesized that different *RYR1* variants confer differential sensitivity to the triggering agents and thereby may contribute to the known variability in clinical presentation of MH during anaesthesia. Alternatively, this variability was also

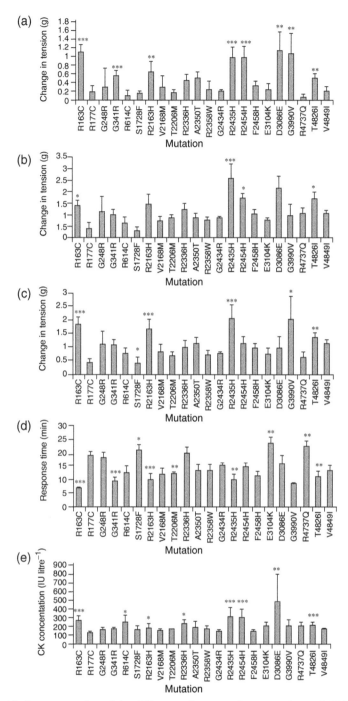

Fig. 19.5 Graphical representation of the differences between the means for each *RYR1* variant type for every MH IVCT phenotype. (a) Static caffeine (*n*=502), (b) static halothane (*n*=502), (c) dynamic halothane (*n*=502), (d) static ryanodine response time (*n*=446), and (e) CK levels (*n*=463). Values shown are the mean and SD of back transformed date for each variant. Asterisks represent significant defferences from G2434R; *P<0.05, **P<0.01, and ***P<0.001. Reproduced from D. Carpenter, R.L. Robinson, R.J. Quinnell, C. Ringrose, M. Hogg, F. Casson, P. Booms, D.E. Iles, P.J. Halsall, D.S. Steele, M.A. Shaw, P.M. Hopkins, Genetic variation in RYR1 and malignant hyperthermia phenotypes, *British Journal of Anaesthesia*, 2009, **103**, pp. 538–548, Oxford University Press, by permission of British Journal of Anaesthesia.

attributed to various other genetic and environmental factors, particularly genetic background and delayed diagnosis, resulting in severe morbidity and mortality.

The major advance imparted by this paper is a careful analysis of data from the largest resource worldwide of phenotypically (clinical presentation of MH, CK concentration, IVCT results) and genotypically characterized MH patients to present the most extensive *RYR1* genotype–IVCT phenotype correlation in MH using 504 individuals from 204 MH families and 23 *RYR1* variants. The most prevalent variant in the UK, p.G2434R was used for comparisons with 22 other variants for *RYR1* genotype–IVCT phenotype correlation.

The following results of importance were obtained:

◆ Analysis of IVCT and clinical onset: there was no significant relationship between variants and time to clinical onset of MH.

◆ *RYR1* genotype–IVCT phenotype correlation: comparison between p.G2434R showed that the variants p.R163C, p.R2163H, p.R2435H, and p.T4826I were associated with more severe reactions (stronger contractures, shorter response times) and higher CK concentrations than p.G.2434R (see Fig. 19.5), whilst p.S1728F was significantly associated with weaker IVCT phenotypes.

Citation count

13.

Key message

RYR1 variants affect the severity of MH.

Strengths

The scientific strength of this paper is the large number of MH families investigated in the same MH investigation unit.

Weaknesses

The scientific weakness is that the important factors in the individual genetic background that may impact on the MH phenotype remain unknown.

Relevance

The impact of this paper is that it provided evidence that different *RYR1* variants vary in the severity of MH phenotype (IVCT response and CK concentration) that they are associated with. Because these phenotypes are associated with the speed of onset of clinical MH episodes, the data is in line with a 'threshold' model of MH susceptibility in which the inheritance of certain *RYR1* variants with weaker effects on calcium dysregulation under anaesthesia may be insufficient to cause clinical MH risk without coinheritance of other genetic factors.

Appendix

Table A.1 The 25 most highly cited papers published in *Anaesthesia*

Rank	Author(s)	Article title	Year	Reference	Times cited
1	Cormack RS, Lehane J	Difficult tracheal intubation in obstetrics.	1984	**39**: 1105–11.	889
2	Revill SI, Robinson JO, Rosen M, Hogg MIJ	Reliability of a linear analog for evaluating pain.	1976	**31**: 1191–8.	746
3	Samsoon GLT, Young JRB	Difficult tracheal intubation – a retrospective study.	1987	**42**: 487–90.	480
4	Bromage PR, Robson JG	Concentrations of lignocaine in blood after intravenous, intramuscular, epidural and endotracheal administration.	1961	**16**: 461–78.	259
5	Henderson JJ, Popat MT, Latto IP, Pearce AC	Difficult Airway Society guidelines for management of the unanticipated difficult intubation.	2004	**59**: 675–94.	257
6	Dawkins CJM	An analysis of complications of extradural and caudal block.	1969	**24**: 554–63.	233
7	Koivuranta M, Laara E, Snare L, Alahuhta S	A survey of postoperative nausea and vomiting.	1997	**52**: 443–9.	207
8	Vickers MD, O'Flaherty D, Szekely SM, Read M, Yoshizumi J	Tramadol – pain relief by an opioid without depression of respiration	1992	**47**: 291–6.	200
9	Whittaker M	Plasma cholinesterase variants and the anaesthetist	1980	**35**: 174–97.	192
10	Cummings GC, Dixon J, Kay NH, Windsor JPW, Major E, Morgan M, Sear JW, Spence AA, Stephenson DK	Dose requirements of ICI 35,868 (propofol, Diprivan) in a new formulation for induction of anaesthesia.	1984	**39**: 1168–71.	169
11	Gillies GWA, Kenny GNC, Bullingham RES, McArdle CS	The morphine sparing effect of ketorolac tromethamine: a study of a new, parenteral nonsteroidal anti-inflammatory agent after abdominal surgery.	1987	**42**: 727–31.	161
12	Grounds RM, Twigley AJ, Carli F, Whitwam JG, Morgan M	The haemodynamic effects of intravenous induction – comparison of the effects of thiopentone and propofol.	1985	**40**: 735–40.	160
13	English ICW, Frew RM, Pigott JF, Zaki M	Percutaneous catheterisation of internal jugular vein.	1969	**24**: 521–31.	158
14	Scott RPF, Saunders DA, Norman J	Propofol: clinical strategies for preventing the pain of injection.	1988	**43**: 492–4.	155
15	Morgan M	Amniotic fluid embolism.	1979	**34**: 20–32.	152

	Authors	Title	Year	Volume: Pages	Citations
16	Hall GM, Young C, Holdcroft A, Alaghbandzadeh J	Substrate mobilization during surgery: comparison between halothane and fentanyl anaesthesia.	1978	**33**: 924–30.	146
17=	Brain AIJ, McGhee TD, McAteer EJ, Thomas A, Abu-Saad MA, Bushman JA	The laryngeal mask airway: development and preliminary trials of a new type of airway.	1985	**40**: 356–61.	142
17=	Khan ZP, Ferguson CN, Jones RM	Alpha-2 and imidazoline receptor agonists: their pharmacology and therapeutic role.	1999	**54**: 146–65.	142
19	Brodrick PM, Webster NR, Nunn JF	The laryngeal mask airway: a study of 100 patients during spontaneous breathing.	1989	**44**: 238–41.	140
20	McKeating K, Bali IM, Dundee JW	The effects of thiopentone and propofol on upper airway integrity.	1988	**43**: 638–40.	137
21	Mason DG, Bingham RM	The laryngeal mask airway in children.	1990	**45**: 760–3.	136
22	Eason MJ, Wyatt R	Paravertebral thoracic block: reappraisal.	1979	**34**: 638–42.	133
23	Odoom JA, Sih IL	Epidural analgesia and anticoagulant therapy: experience with 1000 cases of continuous epidurals.	1983	**38**: 254–9.	132
24=	Liu WHD, Thorp TAS, Graham SG, Aitkenhead AR	Incidence of awareness with recall during general anaesthesia.	1991	**46**: 435–7.	131
24=	Venn RM, Bradshaw CJ, Spencer R, Brealey D, Caudwell E, Naughton C, Vedio A, Singer M, Feneck R, Treacher D, Willatts SM, Grounds RM	Preliminary UK experience of dexmedetomidine, a novel agent for postoperative sedation in the intensive care unit.	1999	**54**: 1136–42.	131

The citation scores are all-time and were accessed via Web of Science on 16 September, 2011.

Table A.2 The 25 most highly cited papers published in *Anesthesia and Analgesia*

Rank	Author(s)	Article title	Year	Reference	Times cited
1	Woolf CJ, Chong MS	Preemptive analgesia treating postoperative pain by preventing the establishment of central sensitization.	1993	**77**: 362–79.	704
2	Scott DB, Lee A, Fagan D, Bowler GMR, Bloomfield P, Lundh R	Acute toxicity of ropivacaine compared with that of bupivacaine.	1989	**69**: 563–9.	403
3	Kehlet H, Dahl JB	The value of multimodal or balanced analgesia in postoperative pain treatment.	1993	**77**: 1048–56.	400
4	Vandermeulen EP, Van Aken H, Vermylen J	Anticoagulants and spinal epidural anesthesia.	1994	**79**: 1165–77.	391
5	Bromage PR, Camporesi E, Chestnut D	Epidural narcotics for postoperative analgesia.	1980	**59**: 473–80.	378
6	Ballantyne JC, Carr DB, deFerranti S, Suarez T, Lau J, Chalmers TC, Angelillo IF, Mosteller F	The comparative effects of postoperative analgesic therapies on pulmonary outcome: Cumulative meta analyses of randomized, controlled trials.	1998	**86**: 598–612.	371
7	Roberts RB, Shirley MA	Reducing risk of acid aspiration during Cesarean section.	1974	**53**: 859–68.	353
8	Craig DB	Postoperative recovery of pulmonary function.	1981	**60**: 46–52.	348
9	Rigler ML, Drasner K, Krejcie TC, Yelich SJ, Scholnick FT, DeFontes J, Bohner D	Cauda equina syndrome after continuous spinal anesthesia.	1991	**72**: 275–81.	347
10	Tuman KJ, McCarthy RJ, March RJ, Delaria GA, Patel RV, Ivankovich AD	Effects of epidural anesthesia and analgesia on coagulation and outcome after major vascular surgery.	1991	**73**: 696–704.	335
11	Kang YG, Martin DJ, Marquez J, Lewis JH, Bontempo FA, Shaw BW, Starzl TE, Winter PM	Intraoperative changes in blood coagulation and thrombelastographic monitoring in liver transplantation.	1985	**64**: 888–96.	333
12	Tverskoy M, Cozacov C, Ayache M, Bradley EL, Kissin I	Postoperative pain after inguinal herniorrhaphy with different types of anesthesia.	1990	**70**: 29–35.	322
13	Stein C	Peripheral mechanisms of opioid analgesia.	1993	**76**: 182–91.	317
14	Gepts E, Camu F, Cockshott ID, Douglas EJ	Disposition of propofol administered as constant rate intravenous infusions in humans.	1987	**66**: 1256–63.	290

			Year	Vol: Pages	Citations
15	Glass PSA, Hardman D, Kamiyama Y, Quill TJ, Marton G, Donn KH, Grosse CM, Hermann D	Preliminary pharmacokinetics and pharmacodynamics of an ultra-short-acting opioid, remifentanil (GI87084B).	1993	**77**: 1031–40.	282
16	Stanley TH, Webster LR	Anesthetic requirements and cardiovascular effects of fentanyl-oxygen and fentanyl-diazepam-oxygen anesthesia in man.	1978	**57**: 411–16.	281
17	Bowman WC	Prejunctional and postjunctional cholinoceptors at the neuromuscular junction.	1980	**59**: 935–43.	271
18	Gan TJ, Meyer T, Apfel CC, Chung F, Davis PJ, Eubanks S, Kovac A, Philip BK, Sessler DI, Temo J, Tramer MR, Watcha M	Consensus guidelines for managing post-operative nausea and vomiting.	2003	**97**: 62–71.	264
19	Shore-Lesserson L, Manspeizer HE, DePerio M, Francis S, Vela-Cantos F, Ergin MA	Thromboelastography-guided transfusion algorithm reduces transfusions in complex cardiac surgery.	1999	**88**: 312–19.	259
20	Winnie AP, Ramamurt S, Durrani Z	Inguinal paravascular technique of lumbar plexus anesthesia: 3 in 1 block.	1973	**52**: 989–96.	249
21	DeLoach LJ, Higgins MS, Caplan AB, Stiff JL	The visual analog scale in the immediate postoperative period: Intrasubject variability and correlation with a numeric scale.	1998	**86**: 102–6.	247
22	Wallin RF, Regan BM, Napoli MD, Stern IJ	Sevoflurane – new inhalational anesthetic agent.	1975	**54**: 758–66.	244
23	Murkin JM, Farrar JK, Tweed WA, McKenzie FN, Guiraudon G	Cerebral autoregulation and flow metabolism coupling during cardiopulmonary bypass – the influence of PaCO2.	1987	**66**: 825–32.	242
24	Johnston RR, Eger EI, Wilson C	Comparative interaction of epinephrine with enflurane, isoflurane, and halothane in man.	1976	**55**: 709–12.	239
25	Apfelbaum JL, Chen C, Mehta SS, Gan TJ	Postoperative pain experience: Results from a national survey suggest postoperative pain continues to be undermanaged.	2003	**97**: 534–40.	237

The citation scores are all-time and were accessed via Web of Science on 16 September, 2011.

Table A.3 The 25 most highly cited papers published in *Anesthesiology*

Rank	Author(s)	Article title	Year	Reference	Times cited
1	White PF, Way WI, Trevor, AL	Ketamine: its pharmacology and therapeutic uses.	1982	**56**: 119–36.	829
2	Cousins MJ, Mather LE	Intrathecal and epidural administration of opioids.	1984	**61**: 276–310.	806
3	Watcha MF, White PF	Postoperative nausea and vomiting – its etiology, treatment, and prevention.	1992	**77**: 162–84.	750
4	Eger EI, Saidman LJ,Brandstater B	Minimum alveolar anesthetic concentration – a standard of anesthetic potency.	1965	**26**: 756–63.	688
5	Mangano DT	Perioperative cardiac morbidity.	1990	**72**: 153–84.	685
6	Owens WD, Felts A, Spitznagel EI	ASA physical status classifications: a study of consistency of ratings.	1978	**49**: 239–43.	644
7	Glass PS, Bloom M, Kearse L, Rosow C, Sebel P, Manberg P	Bispectral analysis measures sedation and memory effects of propofol, midazolam, isoflurane, and alfentanil in healthy volunteers.	1997	**86**: 836–47.	614
8	Albright GA	Cardiac arrest following regional anesthesia with etidocaine or bupivacaine.	1979	**51**: 285–7.	592
9	Wang JK, Nauss LA,Thomas JE	Pain relief by intrathecally applied morphine in man.	1979	**50**: 149–51.	560
10	Yeager MP, Glass DD, Neff RK, Brinck-Johnsen T	Epidural anesthesia and analgesia in high-risk surgical patients.	1987	**66**: 729–36.	547
11	Gronert GA	Malignant hyperthermia.	1980	**53**: 395–423.	539
12	Rampil IJ	A primer for EEG signal processing in anesthesia.	1998	**89**: 980–1002.	495
13	Yaksh TI, Reddy SVR	Studies in the primate on the analgesic effects associated with intrathecal actions of opiates, alpha-adrenergic agonists and baclofen.	1981	**54**: 451–67.	490
14	Butterworth JF, Strichartz GR	Molecular mechanisms of local anesthesia: a review.	1990	**72**: 711–34.	478
15	Reves JG, Fragen RJ, Vinik HR, Greenblatt DJ	Midazolam: pharmacology and uses.	1985	**62**: 310–24.	468
16=	Melzack R, Torgerson WS	On the language of pain.	1971	**34**: 50–9	465

16=	Quasha AI, Eger EI, Tinker JH	Determination and applications of MAC.	1980 **53**: 315–34	465
18	Maze M, Tranquilli W	Alpha-2 adrenoceptor agonists – defining the role in clinical anesthesia.	1991 **74**: 581–605	451
19	Froese AB, Bryan AC	Effects of anesthesia and paralysis on diaphragmatic mechanics in man.	1974 **41**: 242–55	448
20	Benumof JL	Management of the difficult adult airway – with special emphasis on awake tracheal intubation.	1991 **75**: 1087–110	443
21	Stehling LC, Doherty DC, Faust RJ, Greenburg AG, Harrison CR, Landers DF, Laros RK, Pierce EC, Prust RS, Rosenberg AD, Weiskopf RB, Woolf SH, Zeiger JF	Practice guidelines for blood component therapy – A report by the American Society of Anesthesiologists Task Force on blood component therapy.	1996 **84**: 732–47	435
22	Caplan RA, Benumof JI, Berry FA, Blitt CD, Bode RH, Connis RT, Guidry OF, Nickinovich DG, Ovassapian A, Arens JF	Practice guidelines for management of the difficult airway – an updated report by the american society of anesthesiologists task force on management of the difficult airway.	2003 **98**: 1269–77	431
23	Liu S, Carpenter RL, Neal JM	Epidural anesthesia and analgesia: their role in postoperative outcome.	1995 **82**: 1474–506	429
24	Slogoff S, Keats AS	Does perioperative myocardial ischemia lead to postoperative myocardial-infarction?	1985 **62**: 107–14	428
25	Auroy Y, Narchi P, Messiah A, Litt L, Rouvier B, Samii K	Serious complications related to regional anesthesia: Results of a prospective survey in France.	1997 **87**: 479–86	407

The citation scores are all-time and were accessed via Web of Science on 16 September, 2011.

Table A.4 The 25 most highly cited papers published in *British Journal of Anaesthesia*

Rank	Author(s)	Article title	Year	Reference	Times cited
1	Brain AIJ	The laryngeal mask: a new concept in airway management.	1983	**55**: 801–5.	397
2	Marsh B, White M, Morton N, Kenny GNC	Pharmacokinetic model driven infusion of propofol in children.	1991	**67**: 41–8.	396
3	Knudsen K, Suurkula MB, Blomberg S, Sjovall J, Edvardsson N	Central nervous and cardiovascular effects of i.v. infusions of ropivacaine, bupivacaine and placebo in volunteers.	1997	**78**: 507–14	361
4=	Gustafsson LL, Schildt B, Jacobsen K	Adverse effects of extradural and intrathecal opiates: report of a nationwide survey in Sweden.	1982	**54**: 479–86.	307
4=	Kehlet H	Multimodal approach to control postoperative pathophysiology and rehabilitation.	1997	**78**: 606–17.	307
6	Mallett SV, Cox DJA	Thrombelastography.	1992	**69**: 307–13.	304
7	Prys-Roberts C, Greene LT, Meloche R, Foex P	Studies of anaesthesia in relation to hypertension. 2. Haemodynamic consequences of induction and endotracheal intubation.	1971	**43**: 531–47.	290
8	Dahl JB, Kehlet H	Nonsteroidal antiinflammatory drugs: rationale for use in severe postoperative pain.	1991	**66**: 703–12.	266
9	Wilson ME, Spiegelhalter D, Robertson JA, Lesser P	Predicting difficult intubation.	1988	**61**: 211–16.	264
10	Woolf CJ	Recent advances in the patho-physiology of acute pain.	1989	**63**: 139–46.	258
11	Steward A, Allott PR, Cowles AL, Mapleson WW	Solubility coefficients for inhaled anaesthetics for water, oil and biological media.	1973	**45**: 282–93.	255
11	Denborough MA, Lovell RRH, Forster JFA, Villiers JD, Maplestone PA	Anaesthetic deaths in a family.	1962	**34**: 395–6.	250
12	Dray A	Inflammatory mediators of pain.	1995	**75**: 125–31.	226
13	Claeys MA, Gepts E, Camu F	Haemodynamic changes during anaesthesia induced and maintained with propofol.	1988	**60**: 3–9.	223

Rank	Authors	Title	Year	Volume: Pages	Citations
14	Tucker GT, Mather LE	Pharmacology of local anaesthetic agents: pharmacokinetics of local anaesthetic agents.	1975	**47**: 213–4.	217
15	Kehlet H	Surgical stress: the role of pain and analgesia.	1989	**63**: 189–95.	216
16	Idvall J, Ahlgren I, Aronsen KF, Stenberg P	Ketamine infusions: pharmacokinetics and clinical effects.	1979	**51**: 1167–73.	213
17=	Johnstone M	The human cardiovascular response to fluothane anaesthesia.	1956	**28**: 392–410.	209
17=	Prys-Roberts C, Meloche R, Foex P	Studies of anaesthesia in relation to hypertension. 1. Cardiovascular responses of treated and untreated patients.	1971	**43**: 122–37.	209
17=	Payne, JP; Hughes, R	Evaluation of atracurium in anesthetized man.	1981	**53**: 45–54.	209
17=	Desborough, JP	The stress response to trauma and surgery.	2000	**85**: 109–17.	209
21=	Child KJ, Currie JP, Davis B, Dodds MG, Pearce DR, Twissell DJ	Pharmacological properties in animals of CT1341 – new steroid anaesthetic agent.	1971	**43**: 2–13.	208
21=	Joris J, Cigarini I, Legrand M, Jacquet N, De Groote D, Franchimont P, Lamy M	Metabolic and respiratory changes after cholecystectomy performed via laparotomy or laparoscopy.	1992	**69**: 341–5.	208
21=	McClure JH	Ropivacaine.	1996	**76**: 300–7.	208
24=	Kelman GR, Swapp GH, Smith I, Benzie RJ, Gordon NLM	Cardiac output and arterial blood gas tension during laparoscopy.	1972	**44**: 1155–62.	205
24=	Dahl JB, Kehlet H	The value of pre-emptive analgesia in the treatment of postoperative pain	1993	**70**: 434–9.	205

The citation scores are all-time and were accessed via Web of Science on 16 September, 2011.

Author Index

A

Adami, J. 170
Adams, H.P. 268–9
Adams, J. 160
Aggarwal, S. 358
Ahn, H.J. 292
Albret, R. 162–3
Albright, G.A. 393
Alexander, G.J. 365
Ali, H.H. 11–12, 109–10
Altura, B.M. 372
Altura, B.T. 372
Anderson, B.J. 438
Anderson, J. 347
Andresen, C. 96
Antkowiak, B. 190–1
Anton, J. 240–1
Appel, P.L. 131–2
Arango, B. 270–1
Arlt, M. 299
Arras, M. 190–1
Aaslid, R. 99
Asgeirsson, B. 265–7
Atkins, M. 438
Avezum, A. 242–4

B

Baird, W.L.M. 8–9
Baldwin, N. 261
Banning, A.P. 258
Barclay, G.R. 147–8, 344–6
Barthel, H. 226
Basse, L. 342
Bauer, M. 232–3
Beck, D.W. 268–9
Beecher, H.K. 78
Beier-Holgersen, R. 166
Bein, B. 232–3
Bendtsen, A. 164–5
Benefiel, D.J. 122
Bennet, J.R. 385–6
Bennett, E.D. 133–4, 149, 334–5
Benshoff, N.D. 426
Benson, J.T. 360–1
Benumof, J.L. 281–2, 408–9
Berg, H. 25–7
Berry, C.C. 408–9
Bestle, M. 162–3
Bestmann, L. 230–1
Bianchi, A. 402
Bie, P. 347–9
Bier, A. 378–9
Bigelow, H.J. 60–1
Blemmer, T. 162–3, 166
Blunt, B.A. 261
Bode, R.H. 323

Bodenham, A.R. 258
Bom, A. 31–2
Bonsel, G.J. 101
Bontempo, F.A. 356–7
Booms, P. 472–4
Bose, R. 236–7, 316
Bouchard, A. 122
Bovill, J.G. 97
Boyd, O. 133–4, 334–5
Boyle, G. 36–7
Boysen, K. 162–3
Bradley, A.F. 106
Bradley, M. 31–2
Brain, A.I.J. 51–2, 414
Brandstater, B. 178
Brandstrup, B. 166
Brant, R.F. 143–4
Bray, R.J. 87
Brayley, N. 270–1
Brennan, M. 430
Brick, P. 176
Britt, B.A. 450–2, 458–60
Brunelli, A. 285
Brunner, E. 182, 184
Buch, N. 164–5
Bugge, L. 164–5
Bühling, F. 290
Bulut, M. 164–5
Bundgaard, L. 164–5
Burke, D.S. 332
Burm, A.G.L. 97
Butterworth, J.F. IV 206
Byrd, B.F. 122

C

Cahalan, M.K. 122
Caldera, D.L. 332
Caliebe, D. 232–3
Callesen, T. 162–3
Camboni, D. 299
Cameron, E. 428
Cameron, K. 31–2
Campbell, D.L. 323
Caplan, C.H. 332
Carabello, B. 332
Caramelli, B. 314
Carlisle, J. 159, 306–7
Carlsen, C.G. 164–5
Carlsson, P.S. 164–5
Carpenter, D. 472–4
Carpenter, M. 397–8
Cass, J.L. 323
Casson, F. 472–4
Chalkiadis, G.A. 438
Chan, M.T. 168, 242–4
Chassot, P.G. 230–1

Chayen, D. 204
Chayen, M. 204
Cheema, S. 210, 294
Cheng, S.C. 184
Chesnut, R.M. 261
Choi, P. 242–4
Chonette, D. 111
Chraemmer-Jørgensen, B. 124, 156
Christensen, A.M. 166
Christensen, L.J. 338–9
Chrolavicius, S. 242–4
Churasia, S. 420
Clark, D.L. 113
Clark, J.K. 31–2
Clark, L.C. Jr. 44–5
Clark, T. 157, 212
Clarke, M. 272–4
Coker, G.G. 14–15
Colam, B. 258
Collard, C.D. 240–1
Collins, V.J. 202
Conti, E. 176
Cook, D.R. 372
Cook, T.M. 215
Cooper, D.W. 397–8
Cooper, J.B. 117, 124, 156
Corall, I.M. 19–21
Coriat, P. 402
Cormack, R.S. 410
Cottingham, R. 270–1
Counsell, D. 215
Cravero, J. 436
Crestani, F. 190–1
Crofts, S. 428
Cromheecke, S. 228–9
Culnane, T.J. 438
Curley, G. 350–1

D

da Silva, R. 230–1
Davies, R.G. 297
Dawson, D. 149
De Bernoche, C. 314
De Blier, I.G. 228–9
De Hert, S.G. 228–9
Dehlie, B. 162–3
Dellagrammaticas, D. 258
Denborough, M.A. 448
Desai, S.P. 404
Desira, W.R. 397–8
Deufel, T. 461, 466–8, 469
Devereaux, P.J. 242–4
Devitt, H. 143–4
De Vries, A. 461
Dewar, J.H. 14–15

DeWolf, A.M. 372, 373
Diamond, G. 111
Dibb, W. 139
Dikranian, K. 426
Djernes, M. 124, 156
Dobsch, B.P. 373
Doig, C.J. 143–4
Donn, K.H. 93
Drake, C.G. 268–9
Drexler, B. 190–1
Dubois, M.C. 434
Du Chesne, I. 466–8
Duff, C. 458–60
Dullenkopf, A. 432
Durazzo, A.E.S. 314
Durward, Q.J. 268–9
Dwane, P. 145–6

E
Edmund, H. 36–7
Edwards, P. 270–1
Eger, E.I. II 70, 178
Ehrenwerth, J. 283
Eisenberg, H.M. 261
Ekberg, O. 28–30
El-Ganzouri, A.R. 406
Elkjaer, J. 162–3
el-Moalem, H. 145–6
Engbæk, J. 22–4, 25–7
Engbers, F.H.M. 97
Eriksson, L.I. 28–30
Errera, A. 443–4
Espersen, K. 124, 156

F
Fallon, M.B. 360–1
Farrell, B. 270–1
Faulkner, H.J. 194–5
Fawcett, J. 139, 149
Feilden, H. 31–2
Feist, Y. 466–8
Ferson, D.Z. 416
Finn, S.E. 188
Fischer, J.E. 432
Fleming, S.C. 147–8, 344–6
Forbes, A. 168
Forrester, J. 111
Fortunato, F.L. 358
Foss, N.B. 162–3, 347–9
Foulkes, M.A. 261
Franks, N.P. 176, 186, 192
Frantz, R.P. 362–4
Frascarolo, P. 230–1
Fraund, S. 232–3
Freeman, D.V. 323
Freeman, J. 358
Freiberger, D. 404
Frodis, W. 458–60
Fruergaard, K. 162–3
Fujii, J. 458–60
Futter, M. 157, 212

G
Gambus, P.L. 96
Gan, T.J. 145–6, 325

Ganz, W. 111
Garcia, C. 230–1
Gatt, S.P. 404
Gerber, A.C. 432
Gibbons, G.W. 323
Giovannelli, M. 160
Glass, P.S.A. 91, 93, 145–6
Glen, J.B. 76, 85
Gluud, C. 162–3
Gocht-Jensen, P. 164–5
Goldman, L. 332
Goldstein, R.M. 367–8
Golla, A. 461
Gonwa, T.A. 367–8
Goodale, D.B. 96
Goroll, A.H. 332
Gough, M. 258
Gough, M.J. 258
Gould, T.H. 340–1
Gouyet, L. 434
Grace, K. 340–1
Graham, J.M. 297
Gramkow, C.S. 166
Grände, P. 265–7
Granger, D. 44–5
Gration, P. 321
Graungaard, B. 166
Gravenstein, J.S. 124, 156
Gray, C. 109–10
Gray, T.C. 5–6, 11–13
Greenaway, C.L. 87
Greenblatt, E.P. 188
Greene, H.M. 38–9
Greenspan, L. 242–4
Greher, M. 440
Grimm, T. 466–8
Gross, G.J. 224–5
Grosse, C.M. 93
Grounds, R.M. 133–4, 149, 334–5
Gu, W. 234
Guggiari, M. 402
Gugino, L.D. 404
Guo, T.Z. 192
Guyatt, G. 242–4

H
Haas, M. 162–3
Hachenberg, T. 290
Haist, C. 450–2
Halpern, E.F. 323
Halsall, P.J. 472–4
Halton, J. 5–7
Hamer Hodges, R.J. 385–6
Hannallah, R.S. 430
Hansen, E.G. 164–5
Hanson, K.K. 188
Hanss, R. 232–3
Hardman, D. 93
Hardy, K.J. 336
Harris, R.A. 188
Harrison, G.G. 455–7
Harrison, N.L. 188
Harte, B.H. 420
Hartman, R.E. 426

Hartung, E.J. 466–8
Hartzenberg, M. 270–1
Hassink, E.A. 101
Hayllar, K.M. 365
He, J. 430
Heffernan, A. 350–1
Heltø, K. 164–5
Henneberg, S.W. 164–5
Hermens, Y. 160
Heslet, L. 124, 156
Hilden, J. 162–3
Hippeläinen, M. 141
Hirsch, N.P. 283
Hjortsø, E. 166
Hofmann, S. 299
Høgdall, C. 164–5
Hogg, M. 472–4
Holman, R. 272–4
Holte, K. 347–9
Hopkins, P.M. 472–4
Horbol, J.E. 342
Horrocks, M. 258
Hughes, M.A. 91
Hull, C.J. 19–21
Hull, R.D. 143–4
Hummer, K.A. 430
Hunt, R.W. 438
Hunter, J.M. 16–18
Hunter, S.C 85
Huraux, C. 402
Husberg, B.S. 367–8
Huth, C. 290

I
Ikeoka, D.T. 314
Iles, D. 461, 472–4
Ivankovich, A.D. 406
Iversen, L.H. 166
Izumi, Y. 426

J
Jacka, M. 143–4, 242–4
Jacobs, J.R. 91
Jacobsen, J. 162–3
James, S. 137–8
Jane, J.A. 261
Jenkins, A. 176, 186
Jenkins, C.S. 147–8, 344–6
Jennet, B. 249–51
Jennings, L.S. 367–8
Jensen, F.S. 164–5
Jensen, G. 162–3
Jensen, K.V. 164–5
Jensen, P.F. 124, 156, 162–3
Jeppesen, I.S. 166
Jevtovic-Todorovic, V. 426
Johannessen, N.W. 124, 156
Johansen, M.J. 416
Johansen, S.H. 124, 156
Johansson, G. 162–3, 164–5
Johnson, A.H. 263–4
Johnson, K.J. 461
Johnston, G. 428
Jones, J. 210, 294

Jones, R.M. 336
Jones, R.S. 16–18
Jørgensen, J. 162–3
Jørgensen, L. 162–3, 164–5
Julier, K. 230–1
Jurd, R. 190–1
Juul, A.B. 162–3

K
Kalkman, C.J. 101
Kalow, W. 450–2
Kamiyama, Y. 93
Kang, Y. 358, 371, 372, 373
Kapral, S. 217, 440
Kassel, N.F. 268–9
Katz, R.L. 107
Kawut, S.M. 360–1
Keating, J. 281–2
Keats, A.S. 120
Kehl, F. 234
Kehlet, H. 157, 212, 342, 347–9
Keller, C. 432
Kenny, G.N.C. 53, 94–5
Keramati, S. 408–9
Kerr, R.S.C. 272–4
Kersten, J.R. 224–5, 234,
    236–7, 316
Khamis, H. 270–1
Khanykin, B. 162–3
Kim, H.J. 292
Kim, J.A. 292
Kim, K. 292
Kim, M.J. 292
Kirby, A. 143–4
Kitz, R.J. 117
Klauber, M.R. 261
Klein, R. 418
Klintmalm, G.B. 367–8
Knight, R.F. 385–6
Knot, E.A.R 356–7
Knox, L. 143–4
Kofoed-Enevoldsen, A. 162–3
Koinig, H. 217
Kokri, M.S. 397–8
Koller, Carl 200–1
Koltchine, V.V. 188
Komolafe, E. 270–1
Korneluk, R.G. 458–60
Korshin, A. 164–5
Kozian, A. 290
Kram, H.B. 131–2
Krasowski, M.D. 188
Kretzschmar, M. 290
Krintel, J.J. 25–7
Krogstad, D. 332
Krolikowski, J.G. 234
Krowka, M.J. 360–1, 362–4
Kuylenstierna, R. 28–9

L
Laffey, J.G. 350–1, 420
Laloe, V. 270–1
Lam, A.M. 99
Lambert, S. 190–1

Landtwing, D. 287–9
Langeron, O. 402
Lanng, C. 166
Laporta, D.P. 143–4
Larrabee, M.G. 180
Layug, E.L. 309
Ledermann, B. 190–1
Lee, T.S. 131–2
Lee, V.-V. 240–1
Lehane, J. 410
Lehmann-Horn, F. 461, 466–8
Leslie, K. 168, 242–4
Levy, M. 367–8
Lewis, K.P. 323
Lewis, M. 408–9
Lewis, S.C 258
Liapis, C. 258
Lieb, W.R. 176, 186
Lim, T. 97
Linder, S. 170
Lindorff-Larsen, K. 166
Lindström, D. 170
Liu, L. 242–4
Liu, S.S. 218
Llewellyn, N. 441
LoGerfo, F.W. 323
Lomas, G. 270–1
Lossol, K. 342
Lovell, R.R.H. 448
Lu, J. 192
Lunardi, J. 463–5
Lund, C. 347–9
Lundbech, L.B. 164–5
Lundvall, L. 164–5
Lundy, J.S. 72
Lunn, T.H. 164–5
Lurz, F.W. 122

M
MacDonald, A.G. 55–6
Machado, F.S. 314
Macintosh, R.R. 40–1
MacKay, I.M. 46
MacLean, E.J. 31–2
MacLennan, D.H. 458–60, 461
MacMahon, S. 157, 212
Madsen, J.B. 162–3
Maharaj, C.H. 420
Mahmood, F. 236–7, 316
Málaga, G. 242–4
Malik, M.A. 420
Malinzak, E. 325
Mallampati, S.R. 404
Mandell, M.S. 360–1
Mangano, D.T. 309
Manzarbeitia, C. 360–1
Marcus, H. 111
Marhofer, P. 217, 440
Marmarou, A. 261
Maroof, M. 145–6
Marotta, P. 360–1
Marquez, J. 371
Marsh, B. 94–5
Marshall, L.F. 261

Martin, D. 371
Martinsen, K.R. 164–5
Marton, G. 93
Mascia, M.P. 188
Masso, E. 402
Matta, B. 99
Matyal, R. 236–7, 316
Mayberg, T.S. 99
Mazairac, G. 270–1
Maze, M. 192
McCarter, R. 430
McCarthy, R.J. 406
McCarthy, T. 469
McDonnell, J.G. 350–1
McFall, M.R. 147–8, 344–6
McGoon, M.D. 362–4
McKee, A. 157, 212
McManus, E. 139
McNally, C.M. 438
Mearns, A.J. 210, 294
Meindl, A. 461
Meitinger, T. 461
Mendelson, C.L. 380–1
Merkel, G. 70
Mertens, E. 228–9
Meyhoff, C.S. 164–5
Mihic, S.J. 188
Miles, W.F. 147–8, 344–6
Minto, C.F. 96
Mirakhur, R.K. 160
Miran, A. 162–3
Mitchell, J.D. 236–7, 316
Moen, J. 101
Moesgaard, F. 338–9
Moir, D.D. 389–90
Mølgaard, Y. 162–3
Møller, J.T. 124, 156
Mollerup, H. 164–5
Moloschavij, A. 238
Molyneux, A.J. 272–4
Monachini, M.C. 314
Monnier, N. 463–5
Montori, V.M. 242–4
Moppett, I. 160
Moretti, E. 145–6
Morgan, M. 208
Moriarty, A. 441
Morris, C. 139
Mortensen, C.R. 25–7
Mortensen, M.B. 162–3
Morton, N. 94–5, 428, 443–4
Morton, W.T.G. 60
Moulon, C.E. 336
Moult, M. 418
Mowbray, P. 397–8
Muir, A.W. 31–2
Müllenheim, J. 238
Müller, C.R. 466–8
Munksgaard, A. 162–3
Munoz-Sanchez, A. 270–1
Murat, I. 434
Murillo-Cabezas, F. 270–1
Murray, B. 332
Myles, P.S. 168, 397

Mynster, T. 338–9
Mythen, M.G. 135–6

N
Nakahiro, M. 182
Narahashi, T. 180
Nåsell, H. 170
Nathan, H. 204
Nayer, N 217
Neill, E.A.M. 19–21
Nelson, L.E. 192
New, W. Jr. 115
Newbower, R.S. 117
Newell, D.W. 99
Ngeow, J.E. 218
Nielsen, H.J. 338–9
Nielsen, L.L. 162–3
Nilsson, L. 28–30
Nisanevich, V. 348–9
Nolan, J. 332
Nordström, C.H. 265–7
Nørgaard, P. 162–3
Normandin, D. 287–9
Novack, V. 236–7, 316
Nussbaum, S.R. 332

O
Obal, D. 226
Øberg, B. 162–3
O'Donnell, B. 350–1
O'Grady, J.G. 365
Okholm, M. 166
Olldashi, F. 270–1
Olney, J.W. 426
Olsson, R. 28–9
O'Malley, T.A. 332
Ørding, H. 166
Osborn, I. 416
Østergaard, D. 22–4
Ovassapian, A. 416

P
Paech, M.J. 168
Pagel, P.S. 224–5, 234
Pais, P. 242–4
Palin, R. 31–2
Palmer, G.M. 438
Pan, W. 240–1
Pandit, J.J. 321
Panzica, P.J. 236–7, 316
Paracelsus 59
Pardo, M. Jr. 360–1
Parke, T.J. 87
Parsons, D.G. 418
Partidge, B.L. 281–2
Pasch, T. 230–1
Pascoe, E. 168
Pasquet, A. 255
Passerini, L. 143–4
Patel, K.M. 430
Pearse, R. 149
Pedersen, B.D. 124, 156
Pedersen, T. 124, 154–5, 156
Peerless, S.J. 268–9
Penfield, W. 255

Perdawid, S.K. 164–5
Perkins, E.J. 438
Perko, G. 162–3
Petersen, P.L. 162–3
Peyton, P. 168
Philipp, A. 299
Phillips, M. 458–60
Pierce, E.T. 323
Pineo, G.F. 143–4
Pinna, A. 373
Pinsky, M. 358, 371
Pintar, T. 240–1
Plotkin, J.S. 373
Poeling, J. 299
Pogue, J. 242–4
Pölönen, P. 141
Pomposelli, F. 236–7, 316, 323
Pongretz, D. 461
Ponzer, S. 170
Porte, R.J. 356–7
Posternak, J.M. 180
Pott, F. 162–3, 166
Poukinski, A. 164–5
Power, C. 350–1
Pöyhönen, M. 141
Preckel, B. 226, 238
Price, H.L. 74
Procaccio, V. 463–5
Puech-Leão, P. 314
Pulawska, T. 164–5

Q
Quill, T.J. 93
Quinnell, R.J. 472–4

R
Ramsay, M.A.E. 360–1
Rask, H. 164–5
Rasmussen, L.S. 124, 156, 164–5
Rasmussen, M.S. 166
Rasmussen, N.H. 124, 156
Ravlo, O. 124, 156
Rees, D.C. 31–2
Refai, M. 285
Reid, A.M. 8–9
Renner, J. 232–3
Reynolds, F. 395
Reza, J. 164–5
Rhodes, A. 149
Riber, C. 164–5
Rice, A.S. 87
Richardson, J. 210, 294
Riis, J. 166
Ringrose, C. 472–4
Riou, B. 402
Robbins, B.H. 64
Roberts, I. 270–1
Robertshaw, F.L 279–80
Robertson, K.M. 145–6
Robinson, R.L. 472–4
Rodgers, A. 157, 212
Rodrigus, I.E. 228–9
Rodt, S.A. 164–5
Roed, J. 25–7, 162–3

Roewer, N. 466–8
Roizen, M.F. 122
Rosenblatt, W.H. 416
Rosner, B.S. 113
Rosner, M.J. 263–4
Rosner, S.D. 263–4
Rothwell, P.M. 258
Rottensten, H.H. 166
Rovsing, M.L. 162–3
Rübsam, B. 466–8
Rudolph, U. 190–1
Ruokonen, E. 141
Ryall, D.M. 397–8

S
Sabanathan, S. 210, 294
Sabbatini, A. 285
Sadr Azodi, O. 170
Sage, D. 157, 212
Saidman, L.J. 178
Saint-Maurice, C. 434
Salas, N. 162–3
Salati, M. 285
Salvatierra, C. 281–2
Sandercock, P. 270–1, 272–4
Sandham, J.D. 143–4
Saper, C.B. 192
Sassano, J.J. 371
Satya-Krishna, R. 321
Saville, G. 157, 212
Schäfer, K.-L. 466–8
Schiller, N.B. 122
Schilling, T. 290
Schindelhauer, D. 461
Schlack, W. 226, 238
Schmeling, T.J. 224–5
Schmid, C. 299
Schmid, E.R. 230–1
Schnider, T.W. 96
Scholz, J. 232–3
Schrogendorfer, K. 217
Schug, S. 157, 212
Scott, V.L. 372, 373
Seldinger, S.I. 42–3
Sellick, B.A. 330, 412
Severinghaus, J.W. 68, 106
Shafer, S.L. 89, 96
Shah, R.D. 210, 294
Shakur, H. 270–1
Shapiro, W.A. 122
Shaw, B. Jr. 371
Shaw, M.A. 472–4
Shields, M. 160
Shimada, Y. 49
Shoemaker, W.C. 131–2
Shrimpton, J. 272–4
Siegwart, R. 190–1
Silbert, B.S. 168
Simonsen, I. 164–5
Sinclair, S. 137–8
Singer, M. 137–8
Sitzwohl, C. 440
Skovgaard, L.T. 25–7
Skovgaard, N. 164–5

Slater, E.E. 332
Slogoff, S. 120
Smith, G.B. 283
Smith, J.S. 122
Smith, K.R. 438
Smith, P.J. 87
Snow, J. 62–3
Soppitt, A. 145–6
Southwick, F.S. 332
Spahn, D.R. 230–1
Speers, L. 66
Stanley, G.D. 323
Starzl, T. 355, 369
Steele, D.S. 472–4
Stenlake, J.B. 14–15
Stevens, J.E. 87
Stevenson, C.A. 159
Stieglitz, P. 463–5
Stjernholm, P. 162–3
Stockman, B.A. 228–9
Stoffel, M.P. 360–1
Stratton, I. 272–4
Strebel, S. 99
Strichartz, G.R. 206
Subramaniam, B. 236–7, 316
Subramaniam, R. 420
Sudbrak, R. 466–8
Sun, D.A. 418
Sundar, E. 236–7, 316
Surgenor, S. 436
Svendsen, P.E. 164–5, 166
Svoboda, P. 270–1
Swan, H.J. 111
Swanson, K.L. 362–4
Swart, M. 306–8
Szur, A.J. 66

T
Takala, J. 141
Talmor, D.S. 236–7, 316
Tanaka, K. 49, 234
Tanck, E.N. 406
Tateo, I. 309
Taylor, Z. 44–5
Teasdale, G. 249–51
Teilum, D. 166
ten Broeke, P.W. 228–9
Terreau, M.E. 450–2
Terrell, R.C. 66
Thage, B. 166
Thämer, V. 226, 238
Thomas, M. 340–1
Thorne, G. 340–1
Todd, D.P. 78
Todo, S. 369
Tomlin, S.L. 186
Tønnesen, H. 166, 170
Torgerson, D. 258

Traub, R.D. 194–5
Treadwell, T.R. 66
Tuman, K.J. 406
Tunstall, M.E. 385–6, 391–2
Turina, M.I. 230–1
Tzakis, A. 369

U
Ucciardi, T.R. 66
Uemoto, S. 360–1
Umedaly, H.S. 418
Urwin, J. 14–15
Urwyler, A. 469
Utting, J.E. 11–12, 16–18, 109–10

V
Valentiner, L. 347–9
Valenzuela, C.F. 188
Van der Linden, P.J. 228–9
Van Egmond, J. 31–2
van Zundert, A. 157, 212
Varvel, J.R. 89
Vaughn, W.K. 240–1
Vedelsdal, R. 162–3
Verghese, C. 87
Verghese, S.T. 430
Viby-Mogensen, J. 22–4, 25–7
Villar, J.C. 242–4
Viner, S. 143–4
Virji, M.A. 371, 372
Visser, K. 101
Vletter, A.A. 97
Vogt, K.E. 190–1
von Segesser, L.K. 230–1
Vuyk, J. 97

W
Waigh, R.D. 14–15
Wakeling, H.G. 147–8, 344–6
Waldmann, C.S. 87
Walker, L.R. 164–5
Walker, N. 157, 212
Wallace, A. 309
Walli, A. 164–5
Wallin, L. 166
Wang, L.P. 162–3
Waraksa, B. 404
Ward, S. 19–21
Warlow, C.P. 258
Warltier, D.C. 224–5, 234
Warren, J.C. 60
Warriner, C.B. 418
Warty, V.S. 371
Wasserberg, J. 270–1
Waterman, P. 371
Waxman, K. 131–2
Weatherley, B.C. 19–21
Webb, A.R. 135–6

Weinstabl, C. 217
Weiss, M. 432
Welte, T. 290
West, S. 469
Wetterslev, J. 162–3, 164–5
Whalen, K. 436
Whall, R. 139
White, M. 53, 94–5
Whittington, M.A. 194–5
Wiberg-Jørgensen, F. 124, 156
Wick, M.J. 188
Wiebe, K. 299
Wiesner, R.H. 362–4
Wildsmith, J.A.W. 200, 215
Williams, R. 365
Wilson, J. 139
Winkel, P. 162–3
Winnie, A.P. 202
Winter, P.M. 371
Witt, H. 28–30
Wladis, A. 170
Wolf, R. 44–5
Woods, I. 139
Woods, W.G. 147–8, 344–6
Worton, R.G. 458–60
Wourali 5
Wozniak, D.F. 426

X
Xavier, D. 242–4
Xiumé, F. 285
Xu, S. 242–4

Y
Yadav, Y. 270–1
YaDeau, J.T. 218
Yang, H. 242–4
Yang, M. 292
Yarvitz, J.L. 430
Yates, D. 270–1
Ye, Q. 188
Yeh, J.Z. 182
Yelderman, M. 115
Yi, C.A. 292
Yndgaard, S. 162–3
Yoshiya, I. 49
Youngs, E.J. 96
Yusuf, S. 242–4
Yutthakasemsunt, S. 270–1

Z
Zaric, D. 162–3
Zaugg, M. 190–1, 230–1
Zeldin, R.A. 287–9
Zhang, M.Q. 31–2
Zollinger, A. 230–1
Zorumski, C.F. 426
Zorzato, F. 458–60

Subject Index

Note: page numbers in *italics* refer to figures and tables.

3-in-1 blocks, ultrasound guidance 217

A
abdominal aortic aneurysm repair
  endovascular (EVAR) 304–5
  postoperative survival prediction 306–8
abdominal surgery 329
  transversus abdominis plane block 350–1
  see also colonic surgery; colorectal cancer surgery;
      liver resection; liver transplantation
acceleromyography 13
acetaminophen *see* paracetamol
adrenaline, preoperative oxygen delivery
    optimization 139–40
age, influence on propofol pharmacodynamics 96
airway assessment
  difficult mask ventilation, prediction 402–3
  Mallampati classification 404–5
  multivariate risk index 406–7
  optimal assessment of oropharyngeal class and
    mandibular space length 408–9
airway management 401
  cricoid pressure 330–1, 412–13
  difficult intubation in obstetrics 410
  GlideScope® Video Laryngoscope 418–19
  intubation in patients with cervical spine
    immobilization 420–1
  laryngeal mask airway 414–17
Airwayscope®, intubation in patients with cervical
    spine immobilization 420–1
alfentanil, pharmacokinetics and pharmacodynamics 89
  interaction with propofol 97–8
alpha 1-subunit of DHPR 463–5
alphaxalone 190
althesin 83
Anaesthesia, 25 most highly cited papers 476–7
anaesthetic equipment 35
  Boyle's machine 36–7
  failures 117–19
  Fluotec vaporizer 46–8, *47*
  laryngeal mask airway 51–2
  Macintosh blade laryngoscope 40–1
  polarography 44–5
  propofol infusion system 53–4
  pulse oximeter 49–50
  safety 56
  Seldinger technique 42–3
  spinal needles 38–9
  Tec vaporizers 48
anaesthetic postconditioning, halothane 226–7
anaesthetic preconditioning
  attenuation by hyperglycaemia 234–5
  sevoflurane 230–3
anaesthetic–protein interactions 175
  firefly luciferase inhibition 176–7

Anesthesia and Analgesia, 25 most highly cited
    papers 478–9
Anesthesiology, 25 most highly cited papers 480–1
aneurysms, intracranial, ISAT 272–4
angiography, Seldinger technique 42–3
anticholinesterases 3–4, 7
antiemetics, prophylactic use 159
arterial catheterization, Seldinger technique 42–3
arteriovenous fistula construction, regional
    anaesthesia 325–6
aspiration prevention, cricoid
    pressure 330–1, 412–13
aspiration risk
  obstetric anaesthesia 380–1
  relationship to TOFR 28–30
atenolol, effect on postoperative mortality and
    morbidity 309–10
atorvastatin, effect on cardiovascular events 314–15
atracurium 3
  conception and inception 14–15
  elimination models 19–*20*
  fixed dosing 21
  pharmacokinetics 19–21, *20*
  side effects 15
  storage 15
  use in renal failure 16–18
awake craniotomy 255–7
awareness, obstetric anaesthesia 386, 390

B
'balanced anaesthesia' concept 73
benzodiazepines, and gamma oscillations 194–5
beta-blockers, perioperative use 223, 242–4, 309–10
  in diabetic patients 162–3
  POISE trial 311–13
blood gas machines 106
blood loss
  in liver resection, relationship to CVP 336–7
  in liver transplantation 356–7
blood oxygen tension measurement,
    polarography 44–5
blood transfusion, risk of postoperative
    complications 338–9
bowel surgery *see* colonic surgery; colorectal cancer
    surgery
brachial plexus anaesthesia
  in children, US guidance 440
  subclavian perivascular technique 202–3
brain death 247
  diagnosis 252–4
brain development, effects of neonatal anaesthetic
    exposure 426–7
brain injury, secondary 261–2
British Journal of Anaesthesia, 25 most highly cited
    papers 482–3

bromoform, inhibition of firefly luciferase 176–7
bupivacaine
  post-thoracotomy analgesia 210–11, 294–6
  toxicity 393–4

C

Caesarean section
  spinal anaesthesia, effects of phenylephrine and
    ephedrine 397–8
  see also obstetric anaesthesia
calcium levels, depletion during liver transplantation 371
capnography monitoring, avoidance of adverse
  outcomes 117–19
cardiac catheterization, Swan–Ganz catheter 111–12
cardiac output, relationship to mortality
  risk 131–2, 334–5
cardiac risk assessment 332–3
cardiac surgery
  goal-directed haemodynamic therapy 141–2
  perioperative plasma volume expansion 135–6
cardioprotection 223
  comparison of volatile and intravenous
    anaesthetics 228–9
  continuous insulin infusion 236–7
  halothane, effect on reperfusion injury 226–7
  isoflurane 224–5
  metoprolol (POISE trial) 242–4
  sevoflurane 230–3
  statins 240–1
  xenon 238–9
  see also anaesthetic postconditioning; anaesthetic
    preconditioning
cardiopulmonary exercise testing, prediction of
  survival after AAA repair 306–8
cardiovascular morbidity
  effect of continuous perioperative insulin
    infusion 316–17
  effect of perioperative atenolol 309–10
  effect of perioperative atorvastatin 314–15
  effect of perioperative metoprolol 311–13
carotid endarterectomy
  comparison of superficial, intermediate, and deep
    cervical plexus block 321–2
  general versus local anaesthesia
    (GALA trial) 258–60, 318–20, 319
catheter exchange method, Seldinger technique 42–3
caudal anaesthesia see central neuraxial blockade
central neuraxial blockade
  effects on postoperative mortality and
    morbidity 212–14
  major complications 215–16
  post-thoracotomy analgesia 210–11
  use of opioids 208–9
central venous pressure (CVP), relationship to blood
  loss during liver resection 336–7
cerebral autoregulation, effects of isoflurane,
  desflurane, and propofol 99–100
cerebral perfusion pressure (CPP) management 263–4
cervical plexus block, comparison of superficial,
  intermediate, and deep block 321–2
cervical spine immobilization, intubation 420–1
Child–Turcotte–Pugh score, and portopulmonary
  hypertension 363–4
chloroform anaesthesia

Snow's account 62–3
vaporizers 48
citrate toxicity, during liver transplantation 371–2
Clark electrode 44, 45
coagulation disorders, in liver transplantation 356–7
cocaine, early use 200–1
colonic blood flow, effect of thoracic epidural
  anaesthesia 340–1
colonic surgery
  Doppler-guided fluid therapy 147–8, 344–6
  fast-track multimodal rehabilitation 342–3
  liberal versus restrictive fluid regimens 166–7, 347–9
  transversus abdominis plane block 350–1
colorectal cancer surgery, prognostic factors 338–9
complication rates
  effect of high perioperative oxygen fraction 164–5
  effects of intravenous fluid restriction 166–7
  effect of nitrous oxide avoidance 168–9
  effect of perioperative smoking cessation 170–1
complications of anaesthesia 153
  impact of neuraxial blockade 157–8
  impact of pulse oximetry 156
  risk factors 154–5
  see also postoperative nausea and vomiting (PONV)
confidential enquiries into maternal deaths 382–4, 410
conscious level, Glasgow Coma Scale 247, 249–51
context-sensitive half time 75, 91–2
conus medullaris, damage during spinal
  anaesthesia 395–6
Copper Kettle, chloroform administration 48
coronary artery bypass surgery
  preoperative statins 240–1
  sevoflurane preconditioning 230–3
coronary artery disease, liver transplant patients 373
corticosteroids, intravenous, in head injury
  (CRASH trial) 270–1
craniotomy, combined regional and general
  anaesthesia 255–7
CRASH trial 270–1
Cremophor 76, 77, 83
  adverse effects 85, 86
cricoid pressure 330–1, 412–13
critical incident analysis 117–19
critical incidents, distribution by type 118
cuffed endotracheal tubes, use in small children 432–3
'curare deaths' 78, 79
cyclodextrins (CDs) 31–2

D

dantrolene sodium, in malignant hyperthermia 455–7
death from anaesthesia 78–9
decrement time 83, 90
  context-sensitive half time 91–2
depth of anaesthesia monitoring 6
  EEG changes 113–14
desflurane 67
  cardioprotection 228–9
  effect on cerebral autoregulation 99–100
  Tec mark 6 48
dexmedetomidine, in awake craniotomy 256
DHPR, alpha 1-subunit mutation 463–5
diabetes, cardioprotection 225
  impairment of anaesthetic preconditioning 234–5
  perioperative beta blockade 162–3

diazepam, and gamma oscillations 194–5
difficult airway, definition 401
difficult intubation 401
  GlideScope® Video Laryngoscope 418–19
  in obstetrics 410–11
  patients with cervical spine immobilization 420–1
  prediction 404–9
  use of LMA-Fastrach™ 416–17
difficult mask ventilation (DMV) 401
  prediction 402–3
dopexamine hydrochloride infusion 133–4, 139–40,
  334–5
Doppler-guided fluid therapy 135–6, 137–8, 145–6
  major bowel surgery 147–8, 344–6
double burst stimulation (DBS) 22–4
double-lumen endobronchial tubes 279–80
  margin of safety 281–2
  positioning 283–4

E
electroencephalogram (EEG) 113–14
emergence agitation, children 436–7
emergency surgery, optimization study 137–8
encapsulation technique, reversal of neuromuscular
  blockade 31–2
endovascular coiling, intracranial aneurysms 272–4
enflurane 67
  GABA receptor modulation 182
ephedrine, fetal and maternal effects 397–8
epidural anaesthesia
  bupivacaine and etidocaine toxicity 393–4
  effects on postoperative mortality and
    morbidity 212–14
  paediatric 441–2
  post-thoracotomy 210–11, 294–8
  relationship to POPC risk 27
  safety benefits 157–8
  thoracic, effect on colonic blood flow 340–1
  see also central neuraxial blockade
epidural opioids 208–9
equipotency studies, halothane and halopropane 70–1
errors 117–19
  distribution by type 118
ether
  first recorded use 60
  obstetric anaesthesia 385–6
etidocaine toxicity 393–4
etomidate 83
  optical isomers 186–7
European Malignant Hyperpyrexia Group 453–4
  guidelines for molecular detection of MH 469–71
EVAR (endovascular aneurysm repair) trial 304–5
explosions 55–6
eye opening, Glasgow Coma Scale 249

F
failed intubation drill, obstetric anaesthesia 391–2
  fast-track rehabilitation, colonic surgery 342–3
femoral to distal artery bypass, effect of anaesthesia
  type 323–4
fentanyl, pharmacokinetics and pharmacodynamics 89
fetal acidosis, spinal anaesthesia, effects of
  phenylephrine and ephedrine 497–8
fingertip oxygen saturation measurement 49–50
firefly luciferase, inhibition by bromoform 176–7

fires 55–6
fluid management
  children 434–5
  Doppler-guidance 135–8, 147–8, 344–6
  goal-directed 145–6
  pneumonectomy patients 289
fluid restriction 347–9
  effect on postoperative complications 166–7
fluorinated hydrocarbons, study of anaesthetic
  properties 64–5
Fluotec vaporizer 46–8, 47
Fluothane see halothane
fulminant hepatic failure, prognostic indicators 365–6

G
gaboxadol see THIP
GALA trial 247, 258–60, 318–20, 319
gamma-aminobutyric acid (GABA) receptors 175
  action of THIP (gaboxadol) 184–5
  β3 subunit mutations 190–1
  effect of etomidate 186–7
  effect of general anaesthetics 182–3
  role in sedative response to general anaesthetics 192–3
  sites of anaesthetic action 188–9
  gamma oscillations, effect of anaesthetic agents 194–5
Glasgow Coma Scale 247, 249–51
GlideScope® Video Laryngoscope 418–19
glyburide, effect on myocardial preconditioning 224, 225
glycaemic control 223
  continuous insulin infusion 236–7, 316–17
glycine receptors, sites of anaesthetic action 188–9
goal-directed haemodynamic therapy 141–2
goal-directed intraoperative fluid administration 145–6
  during major bowel surgery 147–8
goal-directed postoperative therapy 149–50
'golden compromise' solution, paediatric fluid
  therapy 434
graft patency, lower limb arterial bypass, effect of
  anaesthesia type 323–4
gut mucosal perfusion, effect of perioperative plasma
  volume expansion 135–6

H
haemodialysis patients, use of atracurium 16–18
haemodynamic therapy, goal-directed 141–2
haemostasis, in liver transplantation 356–7
halogenated methyl ethyl ethers, study of anaesthetic
  properties 66–7
halopropane, comparison with halothane 70–1
halothane (Fluothane)
  for Caesarean section 389–90
  comparison with halopropane 70–1
  development 65
  effect on reperfusion injury 226–7
  GABA receptor modulation 182
  introduction 46, 48
  minimum alveolar concentration 178–9
headache, post lumbar puncture, prevention 38–9
head injury 247–8
  brain oedema management 265–7
  cerebral perfusion pressure management 263–4
  effect of IV corticosteroids (CRASH trial) 270–1
  outcome, role of secondary brain injury 261–2
hepatic resection, CVP, relationship to blood
  loss 336–7

hepato-pulmonary syndrome (HPS), outcome after
  liver transplantation 360–1
hepato-renal syndrome, liver transplantation 367–8
hip surgery, ultrasound-guided regional anaesthesia 217
Hofmann elimination 14
humidification, safety 56
hyperglycaemia, attenuation of isoflurane
  preconditioning 234–5
hypertension, relationship to myocardial
  ischaemia 120–1, *121*
hypotension
  epidural-related 340–1
  post-reperfusion syndrome 358–9
  relationship to myocardial ischaemia 120–1, *121*
  role in head injury outcome 261–2
hypovolaemia, intraoperative 344
hypoxia, role in head injury outcome 261–2

I

ICI 35 868 *see* propofol
ignition, necessary criteria 55
inferior vena cava occlusion, pregnancy 387–8
inhaled anaesthetics
  chloroform, Snow's account 62–3
  ether, first documented use 60–1
  fluorinated hydrocarbons 64–5
  GABA receptor modulation 182–3
  halogenated methyl ethyl ethers 66–7
  MAC, comparison of halothane and halopropane 70–1
  nitrous oxide, rate of uptake 68–9
  see also halothane (Fluothane); isoflurane; nitrous
    oxide; sevoflurane
ionic hypocalcaemia, during liver transplantation 371
ionized hypomagnesaemia, during liver
  transplantation 372
insulin, continuous perioperative infusion,
  cardioprotection 236–7, 316–17
interventional lung assist iLA 299–300
'Intocostrin' 5
intracranial aneurysms, ISAT 272–4
Intralipid 83
intrathecal opioids 208–9
intravenous anaesthesia
  cardioprotection 228–9
  propofol (ICI 35 868), development 76–7
  thiobarbiturates 72–3
  thiopentone, distribution 74–5
  see also propofol; thiopentone; total intravenous
    anaesthesia
intubating laryngeal mask airway 416–17
intubation
  cuffed endotracheal tubes, use in small children 432–3
  difficult *see* difficult intubation
  failed intubation drill, obstetric anaesthesia 391–2
intubation techniques 401
in vitro muscle contracture testing
  discordance with genetic analyses 466–8
  malignant hyperthermia 450–4
ISAT (International Subarachnoid
  Aneurysm Trial) 248, 272–4
isoflurane 67
  effect on cerebral autoregulation 99–100
  GABA receptor modulation 182
  optical isometry 187
isoflurane–nitrous oxide anaesthesia, PONV risk 101–2

isoflurane preconditioning 224–5
  attentuation by hyperglycaemia 234–5

K

K_{ATP} channels, role in preconditioning 224–5
ketamine, gamma oscillation disruption 194–5
'King's College Criteria', liver transplantation 366

L

lactate concentration, goal-directed haemodynamic
  therapy 141–2
laryngeal mask airway 51–2, 401, 414–15
  in awake craniotomy 257
  LMA CTrach®, intubation in patients with cervical
    spine immobilization 420–1
  LMA-Fastrach™ 416–17
laryngoscopy
  Macintosh blade *40*–1
  McCoy blade 41
  see also difficult intubation; intubation
laudanosine 14, 15
liberal fluid administration, colonic surgery 347–9
lidocaine, mechanism of action 207
lignocaine, reduction of propofol injection pain 428–9
liver failure, acute, prognostic indicators 365–6
'Liverpool technique' 7
liver resection, CVP, relationship to blood loss 336–7
liver transplantation 355
  citrate toxicity 371–2
  coexisting coronary artery disease 373
  haemostasis 356–7
  patient selection 365–6
  piggyback method 369–70
  post-reperfusion syndrome 358–9
  preoperative hepato-pulmonary syndrome 360–1
  preoperative portopulmonary hypertension 360–4
  survival, effect of pre-transplant renal function 367–8
LMA CTrach®, intubation in patients with cervical
  spine immobilization 420–1
LMA-Fastrach™ airway 416–17
local anaesthesia 199
  brachial plexus, subclavian perivascular
    technique 202–3
  cocaine, early use 200–1
  complications of central neuraxial block 215–16
  intrathecal and epidural opioids 208–9
  molecular mechanisms 206–7
  postoperative central neuraxial blockade, effects on
    outcome 212–14
  post-thoracotomy analgesia 210–11
  psoas compartment block 204–5
  ultrasonic guidance 217, 218–19
lower limb arterial bypass, effects of anaesthesia
  type 323–4
lumbar plexus, psoas compartment block 204–5
lumbar puncture, prevention of postpuncture
  headache 38–9
lung resection
  predicted versus observed postoperative lung
    function 285–6
  protective ventilation strategy 292–3

M

magnesium levels, depletion during liver
  transplantation 372

malignant hyperthermia 447
  alpha 1-subunit of skeletal muscle DHPR
    mutation 463–5
  dantrolene sodium 455–7
  discordance between IVCT results and genetic
    analyses 466–8
  European Malignant Hyperpyrexia Group 453–4
  first description 448–9
  genetic heterogeneity of susceptibility 461–2
  genetic variation in *RYR1* and MH phenotypes
    472–4, *473*
  ryanodine receptor gene 458–60
  susceptibility testing 469–71, *470*
  in vitro muscle contracture testing 450–4
Mallinckrodt right-sided double lumen tube, margin
  of safety 281
Mallampati classification 404–5
mandibular space length, optimal assessment 408–9
Marsh pharmacokinetic model for propofol 83, 94, 95
mask ventilation, difficult *see* difficult mask
  ventilation (DMV)
maternal deaths, confidential enquiries 382–4, 410
McCoy blade laryngoscope 41
mechanical ventilation
  protective ventilation strategy 292–3
  pulmonary immune effects 290–1
mechanisms of anaesthesia 175, 192–3
  action on synapses and axons 180–1
  etomidate, optical isomers 186–7
  firefly luciferase inhibition 176–7
  GABA analogue (THIP/gaboxadol) 184–5
  GABA$_A$ receptor 188–9, 190–1, 192–3
  GABA receptor modulation 182–3
  gamma oscillation disruption 194–5
  glycine receptor 188–9
  local anaesthesia 206–7
  sedative component 192–3
mechanomyography 13
MELD (model for end-stage liver disease) scores 368
  and portopulmonary hypertension 362–4
methylprednisolone, in traumatic brain injury
  (CRASH trial) 270–1
metoprolol, perioperative use
  in diabetic patients 162–3
  POISE trial 242–4, 311–13
Meyer–Overton correlations 175
Microcuff PET tube 432–3
minimum alveolar (end-tidal) concentration
  (MAC) 71, 178–9
  comparison of halothane and halopropane 70
mivacurium 3
monitoring 105
  avoidance of adverse outcomes 117–18
  blood gases 106
  EEG changes 113–*14*
  neuromuscular blockade 107–10
  pulse oximetry 115–16, 124–5
  Swan–Ganz catheter 111–12
  transoesophageal echocardiography 122–3
morphine, gamma oscillation disruption 194–5
morphine infusions, paediatric use 443–4
Morris, Lucien, Copper Kettle 48
mortality risk from anaesthesia 78–9, 154–5
  confidential enquiries into maternal deaths 382–4

  impact of neuraxial blockade 157–8
  perioperative metoprolol, use in diabetic
    patients 162–3
motor response, Glasgow Coma Scale *249*, 250
muscle relaxants *see* neuromuscular
  blockade
myocardial ischaemia, perioperative 223
  detection 122–3
  halothane, effect on reperfusion injury 226–7
  relationship to postoperative myocardial
    infarction 120–1
  see also cardioprotection
myocardial preconditioning 224–5

N
N265M mutation, GABA$_A$ receptor β3 subunit 190–1
Na$^+$ channels, effect of local anaesthetic
  agents 206–7
NA97 *see* pancuronium bromide
nasal remifentanil 430–1
National Audit Project 215–16
nausea and vomiting *see* postoperative nausea and
  vomiting (PONV)
Nellcor N-100 pulse oximeter *116*
neonates
  anaesthetic exposure, effects on brain
    development 426–7
  paracetamol pharmacokinetics 438–9
  see also paediatric anaesthetics
neostigmine 4
  timing of administration 18
neuraxial blockade, safety benefits 157–8
  see also central neuraxial blockade
neuroanaesthesia 247–8
  awake craniotomy 255–7
  cerebral autoregulation, effects of anaesthetic
    agents 99–100
  GALA trial 258–60
neuromuscular blockade 3–4
  associated deaths 78, 79
  atracurium 14–21
  depth monitoring 6
  d-tubocurarine 5–7
  pancuronium bromide 8–10
  pharyngeal function 28–30
  reversal by encapsulation 31–2
  urinary excretion of agents 16
  use of artificial ventilation 5
  see also residual neuromuscular block
neuromuscular blockade monitoring techniques
  double burst stimulation 22–4
  peripheral nerve stimulation 107–*8*
  single twitch and tetanic responses 8–9
  train-of-four ratio 11–13
  train-of-four ratio (TOFR) 109–10
neuromuscular blockade reversal,
  sugammadex 4, 31–2, 160–1
nitrous oxide
  avoidance, effect on complication rates 168–9
  effects on cerebral blood flow 99
  rate of uptake 68–9
noble gases, cardioprotection 238–9
non-invasive ventilation, in awake craniotomy 257
Novalung iLA 299–300

O

obstetric anaesthesia 377
  aspiration risk 380–1
  awareness 386, 390
  bupivacaine and etidocaine toxicity 393–4
  Caesarean section, use of halothane 389–90
  confidential enquiries into maternal deaths 382–4
  difficult intubation 410–11
  effects of phenylephrine and ephedrine 397–8
  failed intubation drill 391–2
  general anaesthesia 385–6
  inferior vena cava occlusion 387–8
  spinal anaesthesia, conus medullaris damage 495–6
oesophageal Doppler-guided fluid therapy 135–8,
  147–8, 344–6
oesophageal sphincter tone, investigation during
  neuromuscular blockade 28–30
one-lung ventilation (OLV)
  inflammatory response 290–1
  protective ventilation strategy 292–3
opioids
  alfentanil, pharmacodynamic interaction with
    propofol 97–8
  intrathecal and epidural use 208–9
  paediatric use 443–4
  remifentanil, pharmacokinetics and
    pharmacodynamics 93
opioid selection, application of pharmacokinetics and
  pharmacodynamics 89–90
optical isometry
  etomidate 186–7
  isoflurane 187
optimization studies 129
  cardiac output and oxygen delivery 131–2
  dopexamine hydrochloride infusion 133–4
  Doppler-guided fluid therapy 145–6, 147–8, 344–6
  fluid restriction 166–7
  goal-directed haemodynamic therapy 141–2
  oxygen delivery 334–5
  perioperative plasma volume expansion 135–6
  postoperative goal-directed therapy 149–50
  preoperative oxygen delivery 139–40
  proximal femoral fracture repair, intraoperative
    fluid management 137–8
  pulmonary artery catheterization 143–4
Org 25969 (sugammadex) 31–2
oropharyngeal class
  Mallampati classification 404–5
  optimal assessment 408–9
oximetry, avoidance of adverse outcomes 117–19
oxygen, 80%, impact on complications rates 164–5
oxygen delivery
  perioperative optimization 139–40, 334–5
  relationship to mortality risk 131–2, 133–4
oxygen saturation
  polarography 44–5
  pulse oximetry 49–50

P

paediatric anaesthesia 425
  cuffed endotracheal tubes 432–3
  emergence agitation, comparison of sevoflurane and
    halothane 436–7
  epidural infusion analgesia 441–2

  infraclavicular brachial plexus block, US guidance 440
  nasal remifentanil 430–1
  neonatal anaesthetic exposure, possible detrimental
    effects 426–7
  opioid infusions 443–4
  paracetamol pharmacokinetics 438–9
  perioperative fluid therapy 434–5
  propofol infusion 87–8, 94–5
  propofol injection pain reduction 428–9
pancuronium bromide 3
  first use 8–10
  risk of postoperative pulmonary complications 25–7
paracetamol, pharmacokinetics in neonates 438–9
paracetamol-induced liver failure, prognostic
  indicators 365–6
paravertebral block, post-thoracotomy
  analgesia 210–11, 294–8
pCO$_2$ monitoring 106
Pentax AWS®, intubation in patients with cervical
  spine immobilization 420–1
percutaneous catheterization, Seldinger
  technique 42–3
perioperative deaths 153
petaline, Hofmann elimination 14
pharmacodynamics
  interaction between propofol and alfentanil 97–8
  opioids 89–90
  propofol, changes with age 96
pharmacokinetics
  atracurium 19–21
  context-sensitive half time 91–2
  Marsh model for propofol 83, 94, 95
  opioids 89–90
  remifentanil 93
  Schnider model 84
  thiopentone 74–5
pharyngeal function, investigation during
  neuromuscular blockade 28–30
phenylephrine, fetal and maternal effects 397–8
piggyback orthotopic liver transplantation 369–70
plasma volume expansion, preservation of gut mucosal
  perfusion 135–6
pneumonectomy
  postoperative pulmonary oedema 287–9
  predicted versus observed postoperative lung
    function 285–6
pO$_2$ monitoring 106
POISE (PeriOperative ISchemic Evaluation)
  trial 242–4, 311–13
polarography 44–5
portopulmonary hypertension (POPH)
  outcome after liver transplantation 360–1
  screening prior to liver transplantation 362–4
postconditioning, halothane 226–7
postdural puncture headache, prevention 38–9
postoperative analgesia, thoracotomy 210–11
postoperative goal-directed therapy 149–50
postoperative infections
  blood transfusion as risk factor 338–9
  effect on prognosis after colorectal cancer
    surgery 338–9
postoperative mortality and morbidity
  effect of perioperative atenolol 309–10
  effect of perioperative atorvastatin 314–15

effect of perioperative metoprolol 311–13
effects of central neuraxial blockade 212–14
postoperative myocardial infarction, relationship to
     perioperative myocardial ischaemia 120–1
postoperative nausea and vomiting (PONV)
  comparison of propofol with isoflurane–nitrous
       oxide 101–2
  effect of nitrous oxide avoidance 168
  prophylactic antiemetics 159
postoperative survival prediction, abdominal aortic
     aneurysm repair 306–8
postpneumonectomy pulmonary oedema 287–9
post-reperfusion syndrome, liver transplantation 358–9
post-thoracotomy analgesia 294–8
potency of anaesthetic agents
  MAC 70–1
  minimum alveolar (end-tidal) concentration
       (MAC) 178–9
preconditioning
  attenuation by hyperglycaemia 234–5
  isoflurane 224–5
  sevoflurane 230–3
pregnancy
  inferior vena cava occlusion 387–8
  see also obstetric anaesthesia
propofol 83–4
  in awake craniotomy 256
  cardioprotection 228–9
  development 76–7
  effect on cerebral autoregulation 99–100
  injection pain reduction in children 428–9
  lipid formulation 85–6
  paediatric infusion model 94–5
  pharmacodynamic interaction with alfentanil 97–8
  pharmacodynamics, changes with age 96
  PONV risk 101–2
  use in neurosurgery 106
propofol infusion syndrome 99, 100
propofol infusion system 53–4
protective ventilation strategy 292–3
proximal femoral fracture repair, intraoperative fluid
     management 137–8
PROXI trial 164–5
psoas compartment block 204–5
pulmonary artery catheterization 131–2, 134
  trial of use 143–4
pulmonary complications
  effect of high perioperative oxygen fraction 164–5
  risk factors 25, 26, 27
  risk from residual neuromuscular blockade 25–7
pulmonary oedema, postpneumonectomy 287–9
pulse oximetry 49–50
  evaluation 115–16, 124–5, 156
  Nellcor N-100 pulse oximeter 116
pumpless interventional lung support 299–300

Q
quaternary ammonium compounds, Hofmann
     elimination 14

R
raised intracranial pressure, management of brain
     oedema 265–7
rehabilitation, accelerated, colonic surgery 342–3

remifentanil
  in awake craniotomy 256
  nasal administration in children 430–1
  pharmacokinetics 93
renal dysfunction, effect on liver transplantation
     outcome 367–8
renal failure
  and atracurium 16–18
  and sugammadex 32
reperfusion injury, effect of halothane 226–7
residual neuromuscular block, risk of postoperative
     pulmonary complications 25–7
restrictive fluid administration, colonic surgery 347–9
right heart catheterization, diagnosis of
     portopulmonary hypertension 362–4
rocuronium 3
  reversal by encapsulation 31–2
Rusch right-sided double lumen tube, margin of
     safety 281
ryanodine receptor gene (RYR)
  genetic variation, relationship to MH
       phenotype 472–4, 473
  role in malignant hyperthermia 458–61

S
safety 56
  mortality risk from anaesthesia 78–9
sarcoplasmic reticulum calcium release channel 458
Schnider model for propofol 83, 96
secondary brain injury 248
  role in head injury outcome 261–2
sedation
  mechanism of action of general anaesthetics 192–3
  propofol infusion system 87–8
segmental wall motion anomalies (SWMAs) 122–3
sevoflurane 67
  emergence agitation 436–7
sevoflurane preconditioning 228–9
  coronary artery bypass surgery 230–3
  interrupted administration 232–3
simulation-based training, difficult intubation in
     obstetrics 410–11
site-directed mutagenesis, GABA$_A$ receptor 188–9
smoking cessation, perioperative, effect on
     complication rates 170–1
sodium channels, effect of local anaesthetic agents 206–7
solubility of agents, relationship to rate of uptake 68–9
spinal anaesthesia
  Bier's development 378–9
  conus medullaris damage 395–6
  development 39
  effects on postoperative mortality and
       morbidity 212–14
  obstetric, effects of phenylephrine and
       ephedrine 397–8
  safety benefits 157–8
  see also central neuraxial blockade
spinal needles 38–9
spinal opioids 208–9
splanchnic blood flow, effect of thoracic epidural
     anaesthesia 340–1
Starling equation 287
static electricity, safety precautions 56
statins, perioperative use 223, 240–1, 314–15

stroke volume output fluid algorithm *345*

subarachnoid haemorrhage
  induced hypertension and hypervolaemia 268–9
  ISAT 272–4
  triple-H therapy 247

subclavian perivascular technique 202–3

sufentanil, pharmacokinetics and pharmacodynamics 89

sugammadex (Org25969) 4, 31–2, 160–1

supine hypotension, pregnancy 387–8

surgical site infection rates, effect of high perioperative
  oxygen fraction 164–5

SvO$_2$ (mixed venous oxygen saturation), goal-directed
  haemodynamic therapy 141–2

swallowing, investigation during neuromuscular
  blockade 28–30

Swan–Ganz catheter 111–12

synaptic effects of anaesthetics 180–1

T

tachycardia, relationship to myocardial ischaemia 120–*1*

target controlled infusion systems 53–4

TECOTA (Temperature Compensated
  Trichloroethylene Air) vaporizer 48

Tec vaporizers 48

tetanic responses, neuromuscular monitoring 8–9

thiobarbiturates 72–3

thiopentone
  distribution in the body 74–5
  gamma oscillation disruption 194–5
  introduction 72, 73
  obstetric anaesthesia 385–6

THIP (4,5,6,7-tetrahydroisoxazolo
  [5,4-c]pyridin-3-ol) 184–5

thoracic anaesthesia 277–8
  double-lumen endobronchial tubes *279*–84
  interventional lung assist 299–300
  mechanical ventilation, pulmonary immune
    effects 290–1
  postoperative analgesia 210–11, 294–8
  postpneumonectomy pulmonary oedema 287–9
  predicted versus observed postoperative lung
    function 285–6
  protective ventilation strategy 292–3

thoracic epidural anaesthesia, effect on colonic blood
  flow 340–1

total intravenous anaesthesia (TIVA) 83–4
  delivery devices 53–4
  PONV risk 101–2

train-of-four (TOF) twitch technique 3
  alphabetic labelling *12*

train-of-four ratio (TOFR) 3, 11–13, 109–10
  limitations 22
  relationship to DBS ratio 23–4

relationship to pharyngeal function 28–30
relationship to POPC risk *26*

transoesophageal echocardiography (TOE), detection
  of SWMAs 122–3

transversus abdominis plane (TAP) block 350–1

traumatic brain injury (TBI)
  brain oedema management 265–7
  cerebral perfusion pressure management 263–4
  effect of IV corticosteroids (CRASH trial) 270–1
  secondary brain injury 261–2

Traumatic Coma Data Bank 247, 261

trephination 247

tuberomammillary nucleus (TMN), role in sedative
  response to general anaesthetics 192–3

d-tubocurarine 3
  contraindications 6
  first use 5–7

Tuffier's line 395

U

ultrasound-guided regional anaesthesia
  3-in-1 blocks 217
  brachial plexus block, children 440
  systemic review 218–19

uptake rate, nitrous oxide 68–9

V

vaporizers 48
  see also Fluotec vaporizer

vascular access surgery, regional anaesthesia 325–6

vascular surgery 303
  atorvastatin, effect on cardiovascular events 314–15
  continuous insulin infusion 316–17
  EVAR trial 304–5
  lower limb arterial bypass, effect of anaesthesia
    type 323–4

vasospasm, in subarachnoid haemorrhage 268–9

vecuronium 3
  partial paralysis, investigation of pharyngeal
    function 28–30
  sugammadex reversal 32

ventrolateral preoptic nucleus, role in sedative
  response to general anaesthetics 192–3

verbal response, Glasgow Coma Scale *249*, 250

volatile anaesthetics
  cardioprotection 228–9
  see also desflurane; halothane (Fluothane);
    sevoflurane

vomiting *see* postoperative nausea and vomiting
  (PONV)

X

xenon, cardioprotection 238–9